ANNALS OF
THE NEW YORK ACADEMY
OF SCIENCES

Volume 572

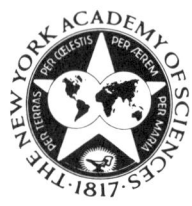

EDITORIAL STAFF

Executive Editor
BILL BOLAND

Managing Editor
JUSTINE CULLINAN

Associate Editor
ANGELA C. FINK

The New York Academy of Sciences
2 East 63rd Street
New York, New York 10021

THE NEW YORK ACADEMY OF SCIENCES
(Founded in 1817)

BOARD OF GOVERNORS, 1989

WILLIAM T. GOLDEN, *Chairman of the Board*
LEWIS THOMAS, *President*
CHARLES A. SANDERS, *President-Elect*

Honorary Life Governors

| SERGE A. KORFF | H. CHRISTINE REILLY | IRVING J. SELIKOFF |

Vice-Presidents

| MARVIN L. GOLDBERGER | DAVID A. HAMBURG | CYRIL M. HARRIS |
| DENNIS D. KELLY | | PETER D. LAX |

HENRY A. LICHSTEIN, *Secretary-Treasurer*

Elected Governors-at-Large

| GERALD D. LAUBACH | JOHN D. MACOMBER | NEAL E. MILLER |
| LLOYD N. MORRISETT | GERARD PIEL | JOSEPH F. TRAUB |

FLEUR L. STRAND, *Honorary Past Chair*   HELENE L. KAPLAN, *General Counsel*

OAKES AMES, *Executive Director*

OCCUPATIONAL HEALTH IN THE 1990s
DEVELOPING A PLATFORM FOR DISEASE PREVENTION

ANNALS OF THE NEW YORK ACADEMY OF SCIENCES
Volume 572

OCCUPATIONAL HEALTH IN THE 1990s
DEVELOPING A PLATFORM FOR DISEASE PREVENTION

Edited by Philip J. Landrigan and Irving J. Selikoff

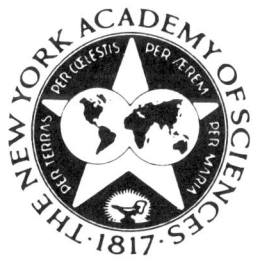

The New York Academy of Sciences
New York, New York
1989

Copyright © 1989 by the New York Academy of Sciences. All rights reserved. Under the provisions of the United States Copyright Act of 1976, individual readers of the Annals *are permitted to make fair use of the material in them for teaching and research. Permission is granted to quote from the* Annals *provided that the customary acknowledgment is made of the source. Material in the* Annals *may be republished only by permission of the Academy. Address inquiries to the Executive Editor at the New York Academy of Sciences.*

Copying Fees: For each copy of an article made beyond the free copying permitted under Section 107 or 108 of the 1976 Copyright Act, a fee should be paid through the Copyright Clearance Center, Inc., 21 Congress St., Salem, MA 01970. For articles of more than 3 pages the copying fee is $1.75.

⊚ *The paper used in this publication meets the minimum requirements of American National Standard for Information Sciences—Permanence of Paper for Printed Library Materials, ANSI Z39.48-1984.*

Library of Congress Cataloging-in-Publication Data

Occupational health in the 1990s.

  (Annals of the New York Academy of Sciences, ISSN 0077-8923 ; v. 572)
  Result of a workshop held by the New York Academy of Sciences on Jan. 21–23, 1988 in Washington, D.C.
  Includes bibliographical references.
  1. Industrial hygiene—United States—Congresses.
2. Occupational diseases—United States—Prevention—Congresses.   I. Landrigan, Philip J.   II. Selikoff, Irving J.   III. New York Academy of Sciences.
IV. Series.   [DNLM: 1. Occupational Diseases—prevention & control—congresses.   W1 AN626Y1 v. 572 / WA 440 01485 1988]
  Q11.N5 vol. 572   [RC963.7.U6]   500s   89-13548
                                    [613.6'2'0973]
  ISBN 0-89766-523-6 (alk. paper)
  ISBN 0-89766-524-4 (pbk. : alk. paper)

BiC/PCP
Printed in the United States of America
ISBN 0-89766-523-6 (cloth)
ISBN 0-89766-524-4 (paper
ISSN 0077-8923

ANNALS OF THE NEW YORK ACADEMY OF SCIENCES

Volume 572
December 29, 1989

OCCUPATIONAL HEALTH IN THE 1990s
DEVELOPING A PLATFORM FOR DISEASE PREVENTION[a]

Editors and Workshop Organizers
PHILIP J. LANDRIGAN AND IRVING J. SELIKOFF

CONTENTS

Address of Welcome. *By* PHILIP J. LANDRIGAN	1
Part I. Occupational Disease: Nature and Extent	
Keynote Address. *By* IRVING J. SELIKOFF	4
Epidemiologic and Toxicologic Evidence of Occupational Cancer in Metalworking and Transportation Equipment Industries: Undercounting Occupational Disease. *By* FRANKLIN E. MIRER, ROBERT M. PARK, AND MICHAEL A. SILVERSTEIN	10
Legal vs. Medical Criteria for Determining Causation in Occupational Disease Claims. *By* LESLIE CHEEK, III	17
Medical and Legal Causation. *By* DAVID OZONOFF	23
Current Magnitude of Occupational Disease in the United States: Estimates from New York State. *By* PHILIP J. LANDRIGAN AND STEVEN MARKOWITZ	27
Occupational Diseases: New Workforces, New Workplaces. *By* BRUCE A. FOWLER AND ELLEN K. SILBERGELD	46
Discussion: Part I	55
Part II. Workplace Regulation and Disease Prevention	
Workplace Regulation Gone Wrong. *By* EULA BINGHAM	61
Public Funding for Worker Education in Occupational Health and Safety. *By* BARBARA BERNEY AND DEBORAH NAGIN	67
Discussion: Part II	72
Round Table 1: Risk Assessment and Regulation	
Opening Statement. *By* WILLIAM J. NICHOLSON	74

[a] This volume is the result of a workshop entitled Occupational Health in the 1990s: Developing a Platform for Disease Prevention, held by the New York Academy of Sciences on January 21–23, 1988 in Washington, D.C.

Outcome versus Process in Decision Making. *By* NICHOLAS A. ASHFORD 76

Risk Assessment and Occupational Health: Conceptual Problems. *By* FRANK N. LAIRD 79

Round Table 1: Discussion 84

Round Table 2: Generic Standards–Prospects and Pitfalls

Opening Statement. *By* BERTRAM ROBERT COTTINE 89

Generic Standards: Prospects and Pitfalls. *By* R. HAYS BELL 90

An Industrial Hygienist's Perspective on Generic Standards. *By* JEFFREY S. LEE 93

Occupational Safety and Health Standards. *By* RICHARD A. LEMEN, LAWRENCE F. MAZZUCKELLI, RICHARD W. NIEMEIER, AND HEINZ W. AHLERS 100

Round Table 2: Discussion 107

Special Address. *By* SCOTT LILLY.................................... 110

Part III. Right to Know and Disease Prevention

The Right to Know in the Workplace: The Moral Dimension. *By* J. DONALD MILLAR 113

Round Table 3: High-Risk Worker Notification and the Prevention of Occupational Disease

High-Risk Worker Notification: A Necessary Public Health Program. *By* JAMES M. MELIUS 124

The Politics of the Worker-Notification Bill. *By* MARTIN F. CONNOR 126

The High-Risk Disease Notification and Prevention Program: Role of Personal Physicians. *By* ALAN L. ENGELBERG 130

The Case for Worker Notification. *By* KNUT RINGEN................... 133

Round Table 3: Discussion 142

Worker-Notification Activities at the National Institute for Occupational Safety and Health: Past and Present. *By* EDWARD L. BAKER, PAUL A. SCHULTE, AND JEAN G. FRENCH 144

Round Table 4: The Consequences of High-Risk Worker Notification

The High-Risk Occupational Disease Notification and Prevention Act: From Primary to Secondary Prevention—From Paternalism to Autonomy. *By* PAUL W. BRANDT-RAUF AND SHERRY I. BRANDT-RAUF 151

The Worker's Place in Enforcing OSHA. *By* ANTHONY MAZZOCCHI 155

Notification of Workers at High Risk: Design and Implementation of a Program to Address Their Needs. *By* DAVID K. PARKINSON......... 157

Predicting the Consequences of the High-Risk Occupational Disease Notification and Prevention Act. *By* MARK A. ROTHSTEIN 160

Round Table 4: Discussion 163

Depoliticizing Occupational Health: Can It Be Done? Should It Be Done? *By* ANDREW MAGUIRE 166

Part IV. Worksite Inspection and Disease Prevention

The Insurrection of Vestigial Failures against OSHA. *By* SHELDON W. SAMUELS 172

Round Table 5: Worksite Inspection and the Control of Occupational Disease

Worksite Inspection and the Control of Occupational Disease: The OSHA Experience. *By* JOHN R. FROINES 177

The Role of the Worksite Inspection under the Occupational Safety and Health Act: Reflections of 17 Years of OSHA Experience. *By* MORTON CORN 184

Is Regulation Effective? A Case Study of Underground Coal Mining *By* JAMES L. WEEKS 189

Occupational Disease Prevention in Canada: A Change of Direction? *By* GORDON ATHERLEY 200

Occupational Health Sciences and Practice in the 1990s: International Perspectives. *By* M. A. EL BATAWI 207

Lessons from the UK. *By* MORRIS GREENBERG 212

Worker Safety: A Role for the Court? *By* T. ALEXANDER HICKMAN...... 216

Round Table 5: Discussion 221

Round Table 6: A Blueprint for Effective Workplace Inspection in the United States

The Future is Now: Developing Effective Workplace Inspection in the United States. *By* DAVID H. WEGMAN 224

Unlocking OSHA's Potential: An Inspection Strategy for the 1990s. *By* LESLIE I. BODEN 228

An Invitation to Act. *By* MARGARET SEMINARIO 235

Round Table 6: Discussion 237

Part V. Workers' Compensation, Litigation, and the Prevention of Occupational Disease

Workers' Health, Safety, and Compensation in Historical and Cross-National Perspective. *By* RAY H. ELLING 240

New Developments in Workers' Compensation Law. *By* T. FORREST FISHER 256

Tort Litigation: A Goal, a Source of Polarization, and a Possible Tool for
  Prevention. *By* RONALD SIMON 261

*Round Table 7: Restructuring Workers' Compensation to Prevent
Occupational Disease*

Workers' Compensation and the Prevention of Occupational Disease. *By*
  DAVID L. MALLINO... 271

Workers' Compensation and the Prevention of Occupational Disease. *By*
  PETER S. BARTH 278

Restructuring Workers' Compensation to Prevent Occupational Disease.
  By EDWARD J. BURGER, JR. 282

Making the Law Responsive. *By* ROBERT STEINGUT................... 284

Restructuring Workers' Compensation to Prevent Occupational Disease.
  By DOMINICK J. TUMINARO...................................... 286

Round Table 7: Discussion 291

Closing Remarks. *By* PHILIP J. LANDRIGAN 295

Index of Contributors 296

Financial assistance was received from:
- AFL-CIO/INDUSTRIAL UNION DEPARTMENT/WORKPLACE HEALTH FUND
- AMERICAN PUBLIC HEALTH ASSOCIATION/OCCUPATIONAL SAFETY AND HEALTH SECTION
- ASSOCIATION OF SCHOOLS OF PUBLIC HEALTH
- ENVIRONMENTAL PROTECTION AGENCY (U.S.)
- NATIONAL INSTITUTE FOR OCCUPATIONAL SAFETY AND HEALTH
- NATIONAL INSTITUTE OF ENVIRONMENTAL HEALTH SCIENCES
- NEW YORK STATE DEPARTMENT OF HEALTH
- SOCIETY FOR OCCUPATIONAL AND ENVIRONMENTAL HEALTH
- STATE OF NEW JERSEY DEPARTMENT OF HEALTH

The New York Academy of Sciences believes it has a responsibility to provide an open forum for discussion of scientific questions. The positions taken by the participants in the reported conferences are their own and not necessarily those of the Academy. The Academy has no intent to influence legislation by providing such forums.

Address of Welcome

PHILIP J. LANDRIGAN

*Division of Environmental and Occupational Medicine
Department of Community Medicine
Mount Sinai School of Medicine
New York, New York 10029*

Our task is to discuss the current status of occupational disease in the United States. How much occupational disease is there? Where is it? Which workers are suffering from it? What factors account for its perpetuation in 1988? And, most importantly, what can be done to prevent and ameliorate occupational disease in the decade ahead?

The timing of this Workshop is fortuitous. We are at the beginning of an election year. We are at the start of a new session of Congress. We are at a point in history where the status of occupational disease and occupational disease legislation are under intensive scrutiny.

Substantial progress has been made in the prevention of occupational disease in the United States in the 18 years that have elapsed since passage of the Occupational Safety and Health Act in 1970. Some of the worst abuses have been curbed; standards have replaced guidelines; requirements have replaced recommendations; secrecy is less prevalent; and an ineradicably high level of expectation now exists in occupational health.

Nevertheless, success in eliminating work-related disease has remained elusive. Cancer mortality is increasing, and occupational exposures appear to account for at least part of this trend.[1] Death rates in underground mining have increased.[2] Asbestos, although used less frequently than in the past, remains widely dispersed; approximately 10,000 asbestos-related deaths are expected to occur in the United States each year for the remainder of the century.[3] Silicosis is still common among miners and foundry workers[4]; a recent review indicated that levels of silica exposure in 43% of American ferrous foundries remain above legally mandated standards.[5] Finally, there is substantial uncertainty about the hazards of the future workplace and the possible health risks of new technologies.

Why, when they are so eminently preventable, do occupational diseases continue to exist in the United States? A series of factors account for this persistence.[6]

1. Despite two decades of increased public, regulatory, and scientific awareness and effort, *relatively little is known about the potential health effects of most synthetic chemicals*. Most attention and research have focused on relatively few well-known hazards, such as asbestos, lead, and vinyl chloride and their associated diseases. A recent study by the National Research Council found no information available on the toxicity of approximately 80% of the 50,000 chemical substances in commercial use.[7] Even for groups of substances that are most closely regulated—drugs and foods—reasonably complete information on possible untoward effects is available for only a minority of agents. Premarket evaluation of new chemical products is notably inadequate.

2. *Physicians are not trained to suspect work as a cause of disease.* Most physicians do not routinely obtain histories of occupational exposure for their patients that would allow them to identify the occupational origin of disease.

Recent surveys indicate that adequate occupational histories are recorded on fewer than 10% of hospital charts.[8] In consequence, many diseases of occupational origin are mistakenly assigned to other causes, such as old age or cigarette smoking, and opportunities for early prevention and treatment are lost.

3. *Physicians do not receive adequate training in occupational medicine.*[9] Very little time is devoted in American medical schools to teaching physicians to recognize the symptoms of occupational toxins or to recall the known associations between exposures such as asbestos or mercury and their outcomes, impaired lung function and neurologic disorders. The average American medical student receives only 4 hours of training in occupational medicine during the 4 years of medical school.[9]

4. *Workers are often exposed to more than one hazardous substance and are often not informed that they have been exposed at all.* The symptoms of many work-related conditions develop only many years after onset of exposure. During this 15- to 25-year latency (incubation) period, workers may switch jobs often; they may forget materials with which that have not worked for many years, and because they have not been provided with adequate information, they may be unable to give their physicians a complete history of past exposures.

5. The Occupational Safety and Health Administration (OSHA) and the National Institute for Occupational Safety and Health (NIOSH) are authorized to investigate hazardous working conditions in specific worksites. *Resource limitations*, however, have reduced their ability to do so. The budget of NIOSH has been decreased more than 50% since 1980. Workplace inspections now are largely restricted to a few high risk industries and to sporadic investigations of complaints.

6. *Fragmented, unreliable, and outdated surveillance programs* produce significant underestimates of the actual number of cases of occupational illness. These programs have tended to focus more on occupational injuries than on diseases and to collect data primarily on acute illnesses. As a result, the picture they produce does not convey an appropriate sense of urgency about reducing the burden of occupational disease.

In summary, a profound lack of information on chemical toxicity, insufficient and inappropriate education of physicians and workers, and incomplete surveillance of workplaces impede all attempts to reduce the impact of occupational disease in the United States. A coherent plan to improve the surveillance, prevention, diagnosis, and treatment of occupational disease is sorely needed.

The changing character of our nation's economic and industrial base underscores the importance and the timeliness of developing a sound plan to address the problem of occupational disease. Changing technology, whether applied in "high technology" industries or used to reinvigorate traditional manufacturing industries, entails continued exposure to hazardous substances and processes. The service industry presents a unique set of occupational hazards, including ergonomic problems and stress. Responsible management increasingly recognizes the impact of occupational hazards on productivity and costs, and it seeks the expertise and resources to provide an efficient and cost-effective approach to preventing occupational disease. Our national commitment to economic development must be matched by a commitment to keeping our workers healthy and productive and to providing industry with a rational system to control occupational diseases and their costs.

Those are the issues that we intend to discuss. Specific topics that we shall cover include the medical and legal definitions of occupational illness; the current magnitude of the occupational disease problem; regulation and enforcement as tools for the prevention of occupational disease; the role of risk assessment in disease prevention; the current status of legislative proposals for right-to-know and high-risk worker notification; the role of worksite inspection; and last but not least, the role of workers' compensation and tort litigation in the prevention of occupational illness.

We anticipate that the discussions that will take place during this Workshop will be a prelude to discussions of these same issues that will occur throughout the presidential and congressional campaigns. Workplace health issues are an important parameter of social policy. Candidates who desire to be responsive to the social needs of working men and women must seriously address issues of occupational health and safety. We hope that the discussions that will be presented here will help to guide the shaping of appropriate platform planks.

In conclusion, I am pleased on behalf of the Mount Sinai School of Medicine and the Division of Environmental and Occupational Medicine to welcome you to this Workshop. I should like publicly to acknowledge the great debt of gratitude we owe to the New York Academy of Sciences for having chosen to sponsor this Workshop and to the many organizations that have provided support. I wish all of us the very best success in our deliberations.

REFERENCES

1. BAILAR, J. C. III & E. M. SMITH. 1986. Progress against cancer? N. Engl. J. Med. **314:** 1226–1232.
2. WEEKS, J. L. & M. FOX. 1983. Fatality rates and regulatory policies in bituminous coal mining, United States, 1959–1981. Am. J. Public Health **73:** 1278–1280.
3. NICHOLSON, W. J. 1985. Cancer from occupational asbestos exposure: Projections 1965–2020. *In* Disability Compensation for Asbestos-Associated Disease in the United States. I. J. Selikoff, Ed. Environmental Science Laboratory. Mt. Sinai School of Medicine. New York.
4. LANDRIGAN, P. J. *et al.* 1986. Silicosis in a grey iron foundry: The persistence of an ancient disease. Scand. J. Work Environ. Health **12:** 32–39.
5. OUDIZ, J. *et al.* 1983. A report on silica exposure levels in United States foundries. Am. Ind. Hyg. Assoc. J. **44:** 374–376.
6. ROSENSTOCK, L. & P. J. LANDRIGAN. 1986. Occupational health: The intersection between clinical medicine and public health. Ann. Rev. Public Health **7:** 337–356.
7. NATIONAL RESEARCH COUNCIL. 1984. Toxicity testing—strategies to determine needs and priorities. National Academy Press. Washington, DC.
8. ROSENSTOCK, L. 1981. Occupational medicine: Too long neglected. Ann. Intern. Med. **95:** 774–776.
9. LEVY, B. S. 1985 The teaching of occupational health in United States medical schools: Five-year follow-up of an initial survey. Am. J. Public Health **75:** 79–80.

PART I. OCCUPATIONAL DISEASE: NATURE AND EXTENT

Keynote Address

IRVING J. SELIKOFF

*Department of Community Medicine
Mount Sinai School of Medicine
New York, New York 10029-6574*

The major question before us today is: Why do we still have occupational disease?

The goal of this meeting is to seek answers to that question and to gather insights that will enable us to prevent occupational disease in the 1990s, so that the constraints, the problems, the defeats, and the omissions that impeded us in the past will not block us in the future. I am optimistic. When I think of how much has been accomplished, despite the meager resources we have had and the difficulties we have encountered, I believe that we shall make progress against occupational disease in the next decade.

MOST OCCUPATIONAL DISEASES ARE OF RELATIVELY RECENT ORIGIN

Although we can go back in history to Agricola and to Ramazzini and find traces of occupational diseases such as lead poisoning and silicosis in centuries past, most of our problems are of very recent origin. The first man-made chemical was created only in 1856, when Perkins, who had been a student of Von Hoffman in Germany, produced an aniline dye, mauvine. In the 1860s and early 1870s, factories to manufacture this dye developed in Germany and Switzerland. In 1895, Rehn, a German surgeon, found the first three cases of bladder cancer in exposed workers. That discovery is almost within the lifetime of persons here today. When World War I broke out and we could no longer import these dyes from Germany and Switzerland, DuPont built the great Chambers Works in southern New Jersey in 1916 to supply the need. Fifteen years later, in 1931, certainly within our lifetimes, the first cases of bladder cancer were seen in workers employed in that plant. And though in the next decade controls were instituted, and although eventually the plant was razed and buried, we are still seeing cases of cancer from the Chambers Works, part of the so-called "cancer alley" of New Jersey. The problem of occupational cancer, like so many problems in occupational medicine, is recent.

The chemical industry, of course, has vastly expanded. The American Chemical Society announced several years ago that they were registering new chemicals at the rate of 70 per hour. The U.S. Environmental Protection Agency has, under the provisions of the Toxic Substances Control Act, registered more than 60,000 unique chemical substances and more than 4 million mixtures, formulations, and blends. While most never enter commerce (there are only about 500 new products per year), the problem has become almost overwhelming. And it is compounded by the fact that most of these chemicals have never been tested for their toxicity.

THE CASE OF ASBESTOS: DOSE-RESPONSE AND LATENCY

To further answer the question of why occupational diseases are still with us, it is useful to review the case of asbestos, to learn what happened in the past so that we can prevent repetition in the future.

Once more, we are dealing with a recent event. In 1899, Dr. Montague Murray in England examined a man who had worked in one of the new asbestos factories, had become very short of breath and soon died. When Dr. Murray was asked about this case by a Departmental Committee of the British Parliament in 1906, and whether lung scarring from asbestos should be compensable, he said no, there would be no reason for such compensation. "Now that we know that asbestos can kill people, it will not happen any more." His optimistic advice was taken and asbestosis was not included in the list of compensable diseases in Great Britain.

In 1924, Dr. W. E. Cooke examined the postmortem findings of a young woman who had worked in an asbestos textile factory in Rochdale, England and who died of scarring of the lungs. This case was reported in the *British Medical Journal*. Additional cases in this plant were studied by the Factory Medical Department under the leadership of Dr. E. R. A. Merewether, and much disease was found. By 1930, asbestosis was recognized as a problem; a vast literature rapidly developed, primarily in Britain, but also with an occasional case reported in the United States in the early 1930s.

Two enormously important factors became evident in the early studies on asbestos. The first is dose-response. While we can argue about how many fibers cause how much disease, the principle to be used in judgment is dose-response: the more asbestos, the more disease. Data on the incidence of asbestos disease in one factory, where people worked in 1941–1945 and were traced to 1987, show clearly that the longer people worked, the greater the number of cases of asbestosis developed. The same principle holds true for lung cancer. The data demonstrated that less than one month of employment was enough to cause doubling of lung cancer rates, but that if people worked longer, proportionally more disease ensued. The same holds when dose is expressed in terms of fibers per cubic millimeter; even 6 fiber-years of exposure to asbestos were enough to double the incidence of lung cancer. The findings are consistent with a linear dose-response.

The second major principle, evident in early studies and still important today, is latency. Deaths due to asbestosis, when examined by time from first exposure, are rare during the first 10 or 15 years. The same is true for mesothelioma, which is rare during the first 20 years. After that, there is an extraordinary burgeoning of the problem. The concept of latency has affected all of us in this field: industry, scientists, government agencies. Dr. Wilhelm Hueper of the U.S. Public Health Service wrote in the 1950s that latency is a very difficult thing to appreciate, particularly for people in industry. Even today, it is not fully understood, although it is becoming better known to everyone, including lawyers. Oliver Wendell Holmes once wrote that even a dog knows the difference between being stumbled over and being kicked. That may be so, if there are only seconds between cause and effect, but when there are 30 or 40 years between cause and effect, the distinction is not all that simple.

An example of a misstep may be instructive. Philip Drinker, an excellent scientist and head of the industrial hygiene department at Harvard, was asked by the Navy to investigate hazards of insulation work in U.S. Navy shipyards in 1945. He reported that there was no significant problem. It was not appreciated that, of more than a thousand people examined, almost all had begun work less than three years previously. Only a handful had worked for even 10 years. The assurance that was given influenced many people not to give this problem the attention it deserved. In clinical terms, the results have been serious. Our files overflow with examples: an insulation worker who began work in 1945 and who presented in 1975 with mesothelioma—a 30-year latency; a plasterer, a healthy man when he went to work in 1950, who assumed that everything was under control, yet in 1982, after a 32-year period of latency, died of lung cancer; another insulation worker who went to work for a company as a manager developed disabling asbestosis 35 years later; a construction worker who went to work after World World II in the construction industry 35 years later developed a peritoneal mesothelioma for which we have no cure. We have no treatment for this disease; it is invariably fatal. These fatalities are the result not only of exposure to asbestos, but also of our failure to adequately grasp the concept of latency which prevented us from properly handling a problem that we knew existed in 1924.

ETHICAL BARRIERS TO THE RECOGNITION OF OCCUPATIONAL DISEASE

Why did we fail so long to recognize diseases caused by asbestos? One sometimes hears that industrialists are rogues who sat in board rooms and conspired to keep relevant information from public health officials, from scientists, from society in general, from workers, and from unions. Could this be the fact? I don't believe it. Of course, there may have been conspiracies in regard to asbestos and some chemicals, but conspiracy alone could not have withstood the explosion of information on asbestosis which began in 1930.

How did we go astray more recently with asbestos cement, for example? We had been reassured that it was "tightly bound in." Yet when Dr. Murray Finkelstein at the Ontario Workers' Compensation Board examined workers from an asbestos cement plant in Canada, he found exactly the same pattern of lung disease and cancer that had been seen in those working with insulation. Very shortly, Dr. Raffn and her colleagues in Denmark will publish results of their study of deaths in the one asbestos cement plant in Alborg.[a] They found the same thing: lung cancer, mesothelioma, and asbestosis. We had been misled. But was industry also misled? Conspiracy could not have been the whole story. Were physicians not allowed to publish? The philosopher Giordano Bruno, who sacrificed his own life, said that "Science has many saints but few martyrs." Does this apply to physicians?

Another aspect was recorded by Paul Brodeur. It involved an episode at a meeting at which the physician for an asbestos company in Tyler, Texas was present. "I'm sorry I can't speak to you, because it's a question of patients' rights." "Patients' rights? Do you mean Pittsburgh Corning?" "Why yes. If they don't want me to talk to you, there's nothing I can do." This raised the question of who is the patient. That's a fair question because in American society the understanding is that company physicians have a special responsibility to the company.

---

[a] RAFFN, E., E. LYNGE, K. JUEL & B. KORSGAARD. 1989. Incidence of cancer and mortality among employees in the asbestos cement industry in Denmark. Br. J. Ind. Med. **46** (2): 90–96.

Yet a question is now being posed by many company physicians: exactly what is their ethical position? Perceptions are changing in many places.

SCIENTIFIC BARRIERS TO THE RECOGNITION OF OCCUPATIONAL DISEASE

Why have science and scientists had difficulty in recognizing occupational disease? One reason may be that epidemiologic techniques are quite recent and have been applied to the study of occupational disease only in the past three decades. It was only in 1954 that the first cohort study of an occupational group was reported: Case's rubber workers' study.

Another problem has been that it has taken pathologists time to learn about the occupational diseases. One of the greatest cancer pathologists, Rupert Willis, author of *The Spread of Tumors in The Human Body*, questioned the existence of mesothelioma. Dr. Willis was reflecting on his experiences and publications in 1925, 1935, and 1945. There were very few cases of mesothelioma at the time. Not appreciated was that there were very few asbestos workers who had begun work in 1920 or 1930. The pathologists, too, failed to appreciate the importance of latency.

When Cochrane and Webster in South Africa studied 107 consecutive cases of mesothelioma (and themselves spoke to the patients), they learned that 106 had had asbestos exposure. But virtually no cases of mesothelioma had appeared in the 1920s, '30s, and 40s. Willis could not have seen them. Mesothelioma is a relatively new phenomenon.

Similarly, we have recently had the advantage of an analysis of all cases in the Danish Cancer Registry from its beginning in 1945. Very few cases of mesothelioma were recorded in the early years; they have appeared more recently. Again, mesothelioma is a new phenomenon.

Especially illustrative is the case of coal workers' pneumoconiosis. In this country there were probably around 700,000 coal miners in the early 1900s. Nobody knows what happened to them. Early studies were done by the U.S. Public Health Service in the 1930s, but then, quiet: quiet with regard to research in all of the pneumoconioses. Nobody really knows why. Funds were not available. The first $100,000 for coal workers' research in the United States was provided only in 1963. Could it be, then, that the absence of scientific work explains our failure to recognize these diseases for so many years?

The British were far ahead of us. In 1963, Europe was spending 9 million dollars (which, of course, was also far too little).

It has been said that occupational disasters do not occur from miscalculation, they result from very careful calculations, many of which are wrong. Examples of the *hubris* of scientists: Dr. Pedley and Dr. Cunningham wrote in the *Canadian Journal of Public Health* in 1930 that there was no problem with asbestos in Canada. Anthony Lanza, reporting his study for the asbestos industry, said, "Yes there is now disease, but it's not going to occur anymore." And Dr. Merewether, after his brilliant studies in 1929 and 1930, said something like "Well it's all over now. We know. We have good regulations now; there's not going to be any more disease." And Dr. Dreessen's study in the United States for the Public Health Service in 1934 and in 1935 again announced "There are not going to be more problems." These statements were considered, thought about, and utilized by many. And the latest, of course, has been the 1984 report of the Ontario Royal Commission that asbestosis will become a disease of the past.

GOVERNMENTAL BARRIERS TO PREVENTION OF OCCUPATIONAL DISEASE

To summarize, then, I don't think industry conspiracies fully explain what happened. I don't think that absence of science is the whole explanation. Could the culprit be the U.S. Public Health Service? Here I would immediately except NIOSH; NIOSH has always done its best. But apart from NIOSH, could it have been the failure of the various agencies in the Deparment of Labor and elsewhere? What happened from 1935 to 1965? Nobody has looked into this gap. We don't know. Vicki Trasko of the Public Health Service was in charge of pneumoconiosis statistics for our country, and she complained in 1961 that we had no national statistics. Ten years ago, Congress asked NIOSH to study and report on statistics in occupational health. They found that there was no national overall information.

How can this phenomenon be characterized? Perhaps by analogy to Plato's Ring of Gyges, alleged to make men invisible. When the wearer turned it the proper way, he became invisible and could do anything he wanted. He could take anything, do anything, kill people, because he couldn't be seen. And that's what may happen in many agencies; faceless people who can make decisions, without personal responsibility.

Is it that, for a variety of reasons, the agencies don't enforce the regulations they establish and that Congress legislates? It's possible. Some may not appreciate the intense disappointment that labor has in many instances with OSHA. They fought extraordinarily hard in 1970 to put OSHA in place. Congress did a superb job in fashioning the agency that we now have. Yet, when labor looked at the first results in 1972, they found that the Department of Labor had given OSHA 41 cents per worker per year for its work. There were 9,000 inspections at 14 million workplaces; 80% had violations. George Taylor, who used to be in charge of occupational health for the AFL/CIO, noted that the hopes that they had in 1970 had been distorted by legal legerdemain.

With regard to asbestos, 10 years ago, it was written in *Lancet* that the 1931 regulations, in which Dr. Merewether had such confidence, were wonderful regulations. The only trouble was that they were not used and that from the outset, the requirements had been no more than "pious aspirations." Is the cause of our failure then that we don't use what we have? A recent headline in the *New York Times* (January 10, 1988) read "Whose job is the safety of the American workplace?" Imagine that question being asked in 1988 when the OSHAct was passed in 1970!

One can easily sympathize with the people in the agencies. They elected to work in these agencies that try to do a good job. They don't take their jobs in order to hurt people.

THE FAILURE OF WORKERS' COMPENSATION TO PREVENT OCCUPATIONAL DISEASE

Dr. Cooke's case in 1924 gave the disease its name, pulmonary asbestosis. The patient was Nellie Kershaw, who deserves to be commemorated. She had to stop working because she was short of breath. Her physician, Dr. Walter Scott Joss, diagnosed "asbestos poisoning." She sought what we would now call social security, and was refused because she had an industrial disease and should seek workers' compensation. She wrote to the company that had employed her, saying that she had had no money for 9 weeks and needed nourishment. They refused to help and fought successfully to prevent asbestos poisoning's being labeled a compensable disease. How important could workers' compensation have been? Could it have alerted workers, management, and the public that asbestos exposure could cause death? Would control efforts have been expedited?

In this country, reformers fought successfully soon after the turn of the century to have workers' compensation laws passed in Massachusetts, New Jersey and New York. These were rapidly brought to the Supreme Court. The principal case, *New York Central Railroad* v. *White*, was heard in 1917. The issue was that in workers' compensation, workers were asked to give up an essential right. The Supreme Court said: "Yes, that's true. It will take from them what had been sought for 400 years, legal redress. But for giving up that right, workers would be assured of a certain and speedy remedy, they would not have to prove liability, and they would get adequate compensation." Thus, the Supreme Court held that workers' compensation was legal and that a large group of people—workers— would be different from all others in our country and no longer have their right to a day in court, if injured; but, in return, they would have adequate, certain, and speedy renumeration. Workers' compensation, however, has failed. We don't have adequate compensation, we don't have certainty, and we often do not have speed—some cases can remain in litigation for 5 to 7 years. One remembers the dial painters who used to lick brushes and paint radium compounds onto the faces of watches. When they developed cancer of the mouth, jaw and other bones, they were like Nellie Kershaw. Little or no workers' compensation was given. Dr. Harrison Martland of Newark wrote in 1929 that "The only advantage [in] this terrible mess has been, as usual, to the legal profession."

In 1961, when Ms. Trasko wrote to all state health departments, she found that altogether they were aware of 72 persons who were receiving compensation for pneumoconiosis. At that same time, however, the Social Security Administration was providing funds to 15,000 people for pneumoconioses disability.

CONCLUSION

As we go into the 1990s we might well ask, how did this happen? How did we fail to recognize and prevent occupational disease? Probably no one factor can be blamed, but rather an interaction of multiple factors. What Sir William Osler said about tuberculosis—that it was a social disease with medical aspects—may now be true also for occupational disease.

Epidemiologic and Toxicologic Evidence of Occupational Cancer in Metalworking and Transportation Equipment Industries

Undercounting Occupational Disease

FRANKLIN E. MIRER, ROBERT M. PARK, AND
MICHAEL A. SILVERSTEIN

*Health and Safety Department
United Auto Workers
Detroit, Michigan 48214*

A wave of one-hundred-thousand or million-dollar OSHA citations for falsifying injury reports has exposed the massive undercounting of occupational injuries and illnesses in the United States. These citations began when Union Carbide was caught covering up instances of workers affected by chemical leaks, and they spread through the list of major corporations, including the auto industry. On the basis of revised information now available, the recorded traumatic injury rate will probably soon be four times that currently reported by the Bureau of Labor Statistics (BLS). The injury cover-up has had harmful effects on the effort to make workplaces safe and healthy. For example, major attacks on safety and health protections, such as the Schweiker bill in 1980, have been based on small shifts in the BLS injury rate that we now know to be completely unreliable.

The same reasons for not counting injuries are also used to avoid counting cases of occupational disease, and the same people do the counting. The undercounting has supported similar attacks on health and safety protections. Occupational diseases have been underreported in these ways: first, simply omitting obvious cases; second, discounting illnesses that may also be found in the general population; and third, attributing illnesses that may have multiple causes exclusively to nonoccupational causes.

In short, each case is scrutinized with a "workers' compensation mentality," in which any hint of nonoccupational origin is grounds for exclusion. This mentality is given a scientific gloss in the treatment of epidemiologic evidence of occupational origins of disease, some of which require that extremely high-risk ratios or precise exposure-response relations be demonstrated before a causal association will be accepted.

The principal focus of this report is a review of recent epidemiologic and toxicologic findings regarding occupational cancer in the metalworking and transportation equipment industries. This review supports the OSHA disclosures about underreporting. Findings of excess cases of cancer among workers and the carcinogenicity of common industrial materials in laboratory studies indicate that the threat to public health from exposure to chemicals is probably greater in chemical-using occupations than in the chemical manufacturing industry. Recent attempts to minimize the fraction of cancer due to occupational exposure generally fail to recognize the large populations with exposures to mixed chemicals for which excess cases of cancer have been detected and also the growing number of widely used materials found to be carcinogenic in laboratory studies.

However, big as it is, occupational cancer is really old business and is probably a minor fraction of the occupational disease burden borne by American workers. Expanding the view of occupational health beyond counting the bodies of victims of cancer and fibrotic lung disease will create major new opportunities for improving the lives of workers and, incidentally, the efficiency of business and industry.

Addressing the evident occupational cancer problem through coordinated public health interventions, such as new standards to limit exposure, improved control technology including substitution, worker training, medical surveillance, and continuing research, is a major and immediate part of the unfinished business in occupational health. This can be accomplished in the 1990s.

Probably the greatest opportunity to prevent work-related disability lies in the area of repeated trauma disorders. Illnesses like carpal tunnel syndrome, caused by the physical stresses of repetitive jobs designed without people in mind, also cost workers and employers millions of dollars in lost work time and medical care. The redesign of jobs through worker participation programs promises to improve the quality of life of workers as well as the efficiency of production and the quality of the product. Yet the failure of mainstream occupational medicine to accept complaints of symptoms by workers as real, the constant effort to explain any diagnosed case by nonoccupational factors, and the lack of effective epidemiologic treatment of data are enormous obstacles to identifying and eliminating the job factors that cause the illness. A similar picture can be painted for occupational asthma, dermatitis, neurologic effects of solvents and metals, and other endpoints. Until our occupational medical system is transformed so that physicians are willing and able to identify such effects in living workers through routine medical contacts and to accept occupational causation, our progress will be limited.

These views find quantitative expression in the experience of the United Auto Workers representing 1,000,000 American workers, principally in the metalworking and transportation equipment industries. This report focuses on occupational cancer, because quantitative data from mortality studies are available and because an adequate scientific basis exists to connect laboratory results to present workplace conditions. Recent findings regarding the processes and chemical exposures in these industries illustrate the extent to which 10- and 20-year-old ideas about the extent and locus of chemical hazards must be revised. During this period, studies in our industry have identified excess cases of cancer likely due to occupation in a wide variety of plants. These findings have considerably broader significance because the chemical agents and processes studied resemble those in other manufacturing industries, other economic sectors including the construction and service sectors, as well as home and community exposures.

The types of operations of current concern include machining, foundry, plating and die cast, model and pattern shops, vehicle assembly, electronics, and maintenance welding.

The occupational cancer problem in machining is often considered to be confined to skin cancer, a relic of Victorian England and poorly refined petroleum lubricants. [1-3] However, recent data demonstrate an association of stomach cancer and perhaps cancer of other parts of the digestive tract with exposure to the more modern water-based cutting and grinding fluids. There are estimated to be 1.3 million workers in machining plants and an additional 10 million exposed to oils, abrasives, and grinding dust in the United States. [4-8]

Excess mortality from lung cancer and nonmalignant respiratory disease is found among workers in modern, high-production foundries. [9-13] The cancer mortality may be attributed in part to combustion products and perhaps agents like formaldehyde, but our work showed elevated cases of lung cancer among cleaning room workers whose principal exposure was silica-containing dust.[14]

Excess lung cancer found among workers in an automotive parts plant, in which the principal processes were chrome, nickel, and copper plating and zinc die cast, was shown by a case-control investigation to be likely associated with exposure to reputedly noncarcinogenic chromic acid mist.[15]

Even workers in the highest skilled jobs in the industry, the pattern and model shops of the design staffs of the auto companies, have been shown to have excess mortality and morbidity from colon cancer. Exposures included wood dust, a variety of adhesive systems and resins, machining, and solvents, all at low levels compared to existing OSHA Permissible Exposure Limits.[16-18]

The largest group of workers in the auto industry, those in assembly plants, were shown to have an excess of lung and lymph cancer in a large, industry-sponsored proportional mortality study. This group was the control population for an investigation of the experience of spray painters possibly exposed to chromate pigments. Exposures in assembly plants are diverse, and no clear associations between exposure and cancer mortality have since emerged.[19]

In addition to epidemiologic studies, a new body of laboratory studies has identified a number of common materials, many used in megaton amounts, to be carcinogenic in animals by conventional criteria.

Methylene chloride has long been thought to be the least toxic chlorinated hydrocarbon solvent, with toxicity in oral dosing studies discounted. However, it has now been shown to cause lung and liver cancer in mice, breast cancer in rats, as well as liver toxicity, at inhalation exposure levels not greatly above the current OSHA standard.[20,21]

Silica is another agent long considered to pose no carcinogenic risk despite considerable epidemiologic evidence. Studies now show that it causes lung cancer in rats by inhalation alone and in hamsters when instilled in conjunction with polynuclear aromatic hydrocarbons.[22-25]

Probably the greatest public health concern comes from recent inhalation studies of petroleum distillates including gasoline, showing kidney cancer and toxicity in rats and liver cancer in mice at relatively low exposure levels.[26,27]

The epidemiologic and laboratory findings taken together constitute a warning of a possibly massive problem that is not being adequately addressed by regulation or other public health interventions to reduce exposure.

The relationship between relative and absolute risk in correlating laboratory and epidemiologic studies must be considered in order to appreciate the difficulty of seeking "confirmation" of animal studies through human experience. The following simplified illustration will demonstrate the often ignored implications of quantitative risk extrapolations.

In a standard cancer bioassay, the animals must experience an incidence of 1 in 10 for the observation to achieve statistical significance. Elevated risk less than this level can be directly observed only in specialized studies involving very large numbers of animals or for certain rare tumors, but risk assessments commonly extrapolate well below this level. Sensitivity to detecting the carcinogenicity of specific chemicals is achieved by the ability to expose animals to large doses.

Different *assumed* (or hypothetical) exposure-response relationships will give widely varying doses estimated to cause attributed lifetime risks in the 1 in 1,000 range and below or different estimated risks at any given dose. Risks in the 1 in 1,000 range are considered very large by public health agencies, and extrapolations to 1 in 1,000,000 are routinely made. The relation of the observable range to the extrapolated range is shown schematically in FIGURE 1.

By contrast, epidemiology typically looks at relative risks rather than attributed risks. Imagine a group of workers exposed at a particular level to a chemical suspected of causing lung cancer. Imagine that the actual risk of lung cancer attributed to exposure at that level is 1 in 100. This risk must be compared to a background level of a lifetime risk of lung cancer among American males of about 6 in 100. (This background must be attributed to all the other lung carcinogens to which workers are exposed, which includes but is not limited to cigarette smoking.) Consider the following "thought" epidemiologic study comparing the observed mortality and that expected from the general population.

The observed risk will be the background plus that attributed to exposure. In this case it would be 1 in 100 attributed plus 6 in 100 background for a total of 7 in

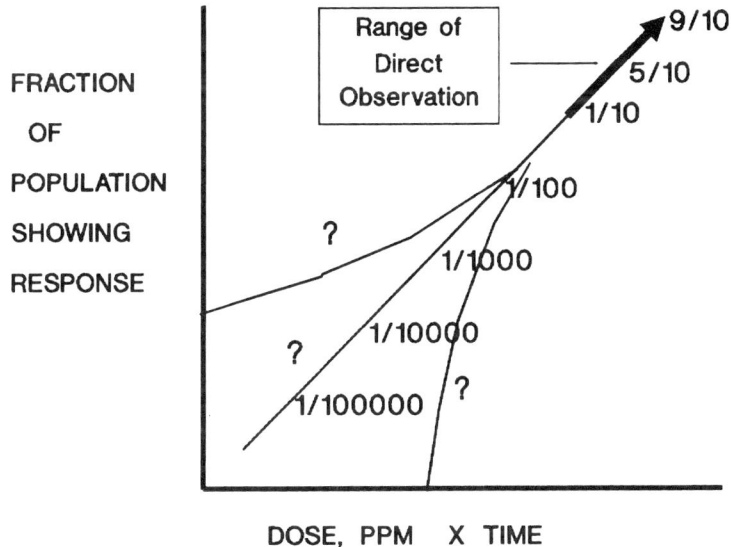

FIGURE 1. Dose-response relationship.

100. Compared to expected risk, the ratio is 1.17, a 17% excess. Even if statistically significant, in a very large population, this number is a very difficult one to get epidemiologists to credit. This relationship is shown schematically in FIGURE 2.

Therefore, if a chemical agent causes a common tumor in people, such as a lung, colon, or breast tumor, it will be detectable in an epidemiologic study only if there are large absolute risks. Many chemical industry studies should be viewed in this light. Furthermore, when an association is found for a common site tumor, even at high human exposure levels, then absolute risks will be important (although probably not directly observable) at most lower measurable exposure levels. For many chemical agents, occupational cancer risks are unlikely to be directly observed through epidemiologic studies showing both high relative risks and exposure-response relations at prevailing exposure levels.

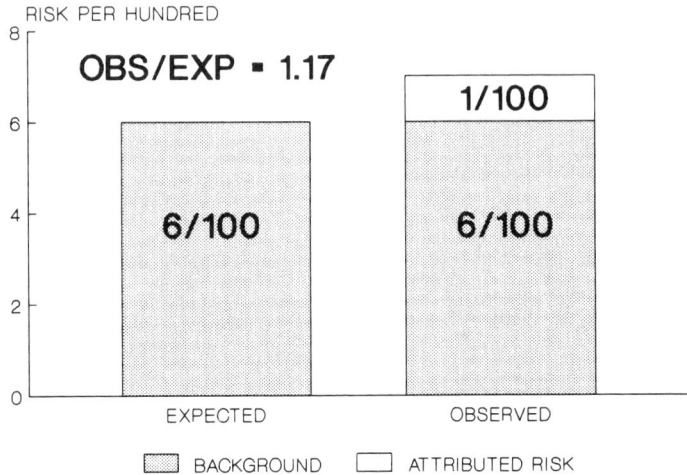

FIGURE 2. "Thought" epidemiology. Observed = background + attributed risk.

CONCLUSIONS

1. Many workers are employed in the chemical-using industries for which observations of excess cancer mortality have been reviewed or reported in this paper. These workers are not generally thought to be exposed to chemicals at levels that pose a carcinogenic risk, yet there is considerable evidence that such a risk exists.

2. Estimates of the fraction of cancer due to occupational exposures that depend on extrapolation of risk from the number of workers exposed to known single carcinogenic agents may understate the risk.

3. Mortality studies in industrial populations outside the chemical industry should be expanded. Repeated studies of processes that employ large numbers of workers may be productive because exposure histories and employment patterns may differ widely from plant to plant; large facilities should be emphasized for statistical power.

4. Documentary evidence needed to determine quantitative exposure to chemicals in studied cohorts is not generally available. Field and laboratory industrial hygiene studies to model and reconstruct these exposures are needed. Such studies would also provide a basis for a control strategy.

5. Laboratory toxicology should be driven by these epidemiologic findings. Lacking are animal studies of the effects of chronic exposure to basic materials in industry to which large numbers of workers are exposed. More priority should be given to mixed chemical exposures that are shown to pose a hazard by epidemiologic findings. Important candidates identified by the studies reported herein are wood dust, solvents, foundry particulates, die release agents, coatings, and cutting fluids.

REFERENCES

1. MASTROMATTEO, E. 1955. Cutting oils and squamous-cell carcinoma. Part I: Incidence in a plant with a report of six cases. Br. J. Ind. Med. **12:** 240–243.
2. WATERHOUSE J. A. H. 1971. Cutting oils and cancer. Ann. Occup. Hyg. **14:** 171–180.
3. IARC. 1984. Mineral oils (lubricant base oils and derived products). IARC Monographs **33:** 87–151.
4. DECOUFLÉ, P. 1978. Further analysis of cancer mortality patterns among workers exposed to cutting oil mists. J. Natl. Cancer Inst. **61:** 1025–1030.
5. JARVHOLM, B., L. LILIENBERG, G. SALLSTEN, G. THIRINGER & O. AXELSON. 1981. Cancer morbidity among men exposed to oil mist in the metal industry. J. Occup. Med. **23:** 333–337.
6. VENA, J. E., H. A. SULTZ, R. C. FIEDLER & R. E. BARNES. 1985. Mortality of workers in an automobile engine and parts manufacturing complex. Br. J. Ind. Med. **42:** 85–93.
7. PARK, R. M., D. H. WEGMAN, M. A. SILVERSTEIN, N. A. MAIZLISH & F. E. MIRER. 1988. Causes of death among workers in a bearing plant. Am. J. Ind. Med. **13:** 569–580.
8. SILVERSTEIN, M., R. PARK, M. MARMOR, N. MAIZLISH & F. MIRER. 1988. Mortality among bearing plant workers exposed to metalworking fluids and abrasives. J. Occup. Med. **30:** 706–714.
9. EGAN-BAUM, E., B. A. MILLER & R. J. WAXWEILER. 1981. Lung cancer and other mortality patterns among foundrymen. Scand. J. Work Environ. Health **7:** (Suppl. 4): 147–155.
10. PALMER, W. & W. SCOTT. 1981. Lung cancer in ferrous foundry workers: A review. Am. Ind. Hyg. Assoc. J. **42:** 329–340.
11. FLETCHER, A. C. & A. ADES. 1984. Lung cancer mortality in a cohort of English foundry workers. Scand. J. Work Environ. Health **10:** 7–16.
12. GIBSON, E. S., R. H. MARTIN & T. N. LOCKINGTON. 1977. Lung cancer in a steel foundry. J. Ocup. Med. **19:** 807–812.
13. TOLA, S., R. S. KOSKELA & S. HERNBERG. 1979. Lung cancer mortality among iron foundry workers. J. Occup. Med. **21:** 753–760.
14. SILVERSTEIN, M., N. MAIZLISH, R. PARK, B. SILVERSTEIN, L. BRODSKY & F. MIRER. 1986. Mortality among ferrous foundry workers. Am. J. Ind. Med. **10:** 27–43.
15. SILVERSTEIN, M., F. E. MIRER, D. KOTELCHUCK, B. SILVERSTEIN & M. BENNETT. 1981. Mortality among workers in a die casting and electroplating plant. Scand. J. Work Environ. Health **7** (Suppl. 4): 156–165.
16. ROBINSON, C., R. J. WAXWEILER & C. MCCANNON. 1980. Pattern and modelmakers: proportionate mortality 1972–1978. Am. J. Ind. Med. **1:** 159–165.
17. SWANSON, G. & S. BELLE. 1982. Cancer morbidity among woodworkers in the U.S. automotive industry. J. Occup. Med. **24:** 315–319.
18. SWANSON, G. M., S. H. BELLE & R. W. BURROWS. 1985. Colon cancer incidence among modelmakers in the automobile manufacturing industry. J. Occup. Med. **27:** 567–569.
19. CHIAZZE, L., L. D. FERENCE & P. H. WOLF. 1984. Mortality among automobile assembly workers. II. White males. J. Occup. Med. **26:** 215–221.
20. NATIONAL TOXICOLOGY PROGRAM. 1986. Toxicology and Carcinogenesis Studies of Dichloromethane (Methylene Chloride) in F344/N Rats and BCG3F1 Mice (inhalation studies) NTP TR-306, NIH Publication 86–2562.
21. BUREK, J., K. NITSCHKE, T. BELL, D. WACKERLE, R. CHILDS, J. BEYER, D. DITTENBER, L. RAMPY & M. MCKENNA. 1984. Methylene chloride: A two-year inhalation toxicity and oncogenicity study in rats and hamsters. Fund. Appl. Toxicol. **4:** 30–37.
22. GOLDSMITH, D. F., D. M. WINN & C. M. SHY, EDS. 1986. Silica, Silicosis and Cancer. Prager. Basel, Switzerland.
23. DAGLE, G. E., A. P. WEHNER, M. L. CLARK & R. L. BUCHSBON. 1986. Chronic inhalation exposure of rats to quartz. *In* Goldsmith *et al.*[22] :255–266. Prager. Basel, Switzerland.

24. HOLLAND, L. M., J. J. WILSON, M. I. TILLERY & D. M. SMITH. 1986. Lung cancer in rats exposed to fibrogenic dusts. *In* Goldsmith *et al.*[22] :267–279. Prager. Basel, Switzerland.
25. NEIMEIER, R. W., L. T. MULLIGAN & J. ROWLAND. 1986. Cocarcinogenicity of foundry silica sand in hamsters. *In* Goldsmith *et al.*[22] :215–228. Prager. Basel, Switzerland.
26. MEHLMAN, M. A., G. P. HEMSTREET, J. J. THORPE & N. K. WEAVER. 1984. Renal Effects of Petroleum Hydrocarbons. Princeton Scientific Publishers. Princeton, NJ.
27. MACFARLAND, H. N., C. E. ULRICH, C. E. HOLDSWORTH, D. N. KITCHEN, W. H. HALLIWELL & S. C. BLUM. 1984. A chronic inhalation study with unleaded gasoline vapor. J. Am. Coll. Toxicol. **3:** 231–248.

Legal vs. Medical Criteria for Determining Causation in Occupational Disease Claims

LESLIE CHEEK, III[a]

Crum & Forster Insurance Companies
Washington, D.C. 20036

Both of the Nation's legal mechanisms for compensating the victims of workplace exposure to hazardous substances are close to foundering on the same rocks—the difficulties of proving workplace causation of harm in occupational disease claims.

These difficulties have rendered the nonfault workers' compensation system as litigation-bound and transaction cost-intensive as the fault-based common law of torts. They have also spawned new bases for compensation plainly aimed at finessing causation issues by permitting recovery in the absence of demonstrable harm. Twenty-seven states' workers' compensation laws now recognize claims for disabling mental stress unaccompanied by physical injury, and, in a handful of states, tort damages may be sought for such ephemera as "cancerphobia," statistically increased risk of disease, medical surveillance, and loss of the quality of life.

My thesis is that the integrity of both workers' compensation and the common law of torts is being severely compromised by the absence of empirical *medical* and *scientific* data essential to the fulfillment of the traditional *legal* requirement of proof of causation to a reasonable certainty by a preponderance of the relevant evidence.

Unless we can fashion a workable surrogate for the missing medical and scientific data needed to make rational compensation decisions, we risk surrendering our entire legal system to the crackpots and charlatans who are already making a mockery of both science and law in their zeal to find "causation" where no empirical basis for it exists.[1]

Put another way, we must find some means of fashioning *legal certainty* of just compensation in an environment of *medical* and *scientific uncertainty*. If we do not, we risk crippling the capacity of workers' compensation to deal with occupational disease claims and making our tort system so speculative and unpredictable that it becomes uninsurable at any price.

A leading scholar in the occupational health field, Dr. Leslie I. Boden, has rightly observed that many occupational diseases:

> ... may be caused by both occupational and nonoccupational factors. It is often difficult or impossible to determine which of these factors caused the disease in a specific case, or even to determine their relative contribution.... Even when epidemiological studies are able to determine very accurately excess risks of disease in *populations*, they are not able to determine which *individuals* in those populations would not have developed the disease without occupational exposure. In many cases, this uncertainty cannot be resolved.[2]

---

[a] Address for correspondence: Federal Affairs Department, Crum & Forster Insurance Co., Suite 414, 1025 Connecticut Avenue, N.W., Washington, D.C. 20036.

Boden argues that disease causation presumptions and medical panels will not solve the problem of proving causation in occupational disease claims. He urges instead, "strengthening the evidentiary status of epidemiological and toxicological studies,"[3] on the grounds that "[t]he use of experts in clinical medicine to offer opinions about whether a particular person's lung cancer was caused by workplace exposure is a form of dishonesty required by inappropriate evidentiary requirements."[4] Boden suggests that:

> . . .[a] way of further strengthening the position of claimants is to design presumptions that shift the burden of persuasion based on reasonable inferences from scientific and statistical studies, without the development of the more specific types of evidence normally required to demonstrate individual cause. . . . Here, as with specific disease presumptions and medical panels, the problem is one of design and implementation, not a conceptual one. Clearly, both the quality of studies entered as evidence and the levels of excess risk that are implied by such studies should be important determinants of the weight given to them.[5]

Although some have argued, and in absolute terms may be correct, that statistical evidence of disease incidence among an exposed population is "of little use in judging the condition of a specific worker,"[6] epidemiologic studies, properly conducted and properly used, can provide meaningful guidance as to the *probability* that a particular worker's disease was caused by chemical exposure.

The crucial phase in this formulation is "properly conducted and properly used," for, as an abstract matter, in many chronic diseases, including most cancers, it is impossible to be absolutely sure that *any* individual's disease was caused by chemical exposure:

> . . . At least three factors make certainty unlikely: (1) no symptom of the disease will be peculiar to the exposure (the exceptions including diseases such as asbestosis whose peculiar symptoms label them as asbestos-caused); (2) factors other than exposure to the chemical from any manufacturer's [or employer's] activities, including genetics, other than exposures such as diet, and even exposures to the same chemical from natural background sources, may have caused disease; and (3) it will be the cumulative exposure to the chemical of interest, and not any particular day's [or employer's] dose, that is likely to be related to disease.[7]

Thus, given the uncertainty surrounding the harmful potential of the 50,000 or so chemicals in industrial use, the issue in many occupational disease and toxic tort claims is not only the traditional one of whether the *claimant's* injury was the result of a chemical exposure, but also the more fundamental one of whether exposure to the suspect chemical *can* cause the injury of which the claimant complains.

This problem has often been characterized as the "Can, Does, Did Triad"[8]: *Can* substance X cause disease Y? *Does* the claimant have disease Y? *Did* substance X cause the claimant's disease Y? Assuming proper diagnosis, the "Does" question can almost always be answered. But except in a handful of known cause-and-effect relationships, the "Did" question, as we have seen, can almost never be answered with certainty. What about the "Can" question? What can be learned about it that could help answer the "Did" question?

Here is where epidemiology, properly conducted and properly used, can play an important role. Generally speaking, results of epidemiologic studies can be expressed in terms of the *relative risk* of disease associated with exposure. If exposure is not associated with disease, the relative risk is 1. That is, the exposed person is no more likely to have the disease than is a nonexposed person. But if the relative risk is, for example, 2, an exposed person is approximately twice as likely to become diseased.[9]

It is a basic characteristic of statistics that relative certainty is directly related to sample size. In a properly designed epidemiologic study, the chance factor in small samples can be quantified through the calculation of levels of significance designed to eliminate the random or stochastic nature of cancer.[10]

It is also important in using epidemiology on disease causation issues that the relative risk demonstrated by a particular study show a strong association between the suspect chemical and the disease at issue. For example, if epidemiologic studies indicate that the relative risk of developing cancer X from exposure to 100 units of chemical Y is 4, and worker A had 100 units of exposure to chemical Y, there will be a three out of four (or 75 %) chance that worker A's cancer X is due to chemical Y. However, if the relative risk from 100 units of chemical Y is only 1.1, then there will be only a 1 out of 11 (or 9%) chance that the cancer is due to the chemical exposure.

Yet even properly performed population and epidemiologic studies cannot by themselves serve as the basis of a biologic inference that a causal relationship exists: "[T]he epidemiologist must integrate additional scientific information. The derivation of such an inference requires rigorous consideration of laboratory, experimental, demographic and epidemiologic data,"[11] widely shorthanded as the Henle-Koch-Evans Postulates.[12]

How can these *scientific* principles be integrated with traditional *legal* principles of causation, which essentially require a claimant plaintiff to prove, by a preponderance of the evidence, that it is more likely than not that the defendant's conduct caused his harm?

The essentially *qualitative* legal test can be, and has been, expressed in *quantitative* terms. An extensive 1950's study proposing how courts should decide cases concerning radiation-induced leukemias concluded:

> . . . If as little as 2.5 rems exposure of a fetus and from 25 to 50 rems exposure of an adult doubles the incidence of leukemia, then a person so exposed could claim . . . that if he should develop leukemia . . . the chances are better than fifty-fifty that his leukemia resulted from the radiation exposure, rather than from all other causes together. Therefore "more probably than not" his leukemia was caused by the radiation to which he was exposed.[13]

But a purely *quantitative* scientific analysis, even one based on rigorous adherence to the Henle-Koch-Evans Postulates, cannot serve by itself as a surrogate for the *qualitative* legal standard of "more likely than not" on disease causation issues:

> The Henle-Koch-Evans Postulates do not, by themselves, provide a complete legal standard because the determination of legal causation requires consideration of the degree of certainty required to meet the plaintiff's burden of proof. This deficiency can be remedied, however, by requiring in addition that the attributable risk for the factor at issue be greater than .50. . . . If, in an exposed population, more than half the cases of a disease can be attributed to the exposure, and if the postulates are satisfied, then absent other information about a diseased individual, it is more likely than not that his or her illness was caused by the exposure.[14]

A correct *qualitative legal* standard thus would be one in which both the *quantitative*, scientifically determined *increased* risk and *attributable* risk exceeded the 51% or "more likely than not" test. And in cases in which exposure in sufficient amounts and durations is certain, "any relative risk greater than 2 would lead to an attributable risk of more than .50."[15]

If it is thus possible to scientifically quantify the qualitative legal test of "more likely than not" through rigorous adherence to the Henle-Koch-Evans Postulates and attributable risk analysis, what weight should be given to what even the advocates of statistical evidence concede is nothing more than a biologic inference that a causal relation exists between a particular chemical exposure and a particular disease?

Certainly, such evidence, even if impeccably prepared, cannot serve as the foundation for a presumption, conclusive or otherwise, that a worker's or a tort plaintiff's exposure to chemical X caused his or her disease Y. Presumptions, either medically or legally speaking, exist to reflect reality, not create it.

If responsibly conducted epidemiologic studies, however, can demonstrate that there is a greater than twofold higher risk of contracting a particular disease as a member of a workplace or other population exposed to a particular chemical in specified concentrations and durations, than as a member of a general population shouldn't that demonstration have some "added value" in the adjudicative process?

My answer is "Yes," quickly followed by the question, "How much added value?" Returning to the "Can, Does, Did Triad," it seems to me that if responsibly conducted epidemiologic studies can establish that there is a greater than twofold increased risk (over that of the general population) of contracting a particular disease as a result of being a member of a particular population exposed in requisite duration to a particular concentration of a particular chemical, then a member of that exposed population who can present such evidence should be deemed to have met the burden of proving the first element of the "Can, Does, Did Triad": Chemical X, in sufficient concentrations and durations, can cause disease Y.

It would then be up to the claimant to establish the two other elements of the triad—that he in fact does have disease Y, and that given the duration and concentration of his exposure to chemical X, it is more likely than not that X did cause his particular Y.

The employer or defendant in this formulation could contest the bases on which the increased risk and attributable risk analyses were made.[16] In addition, the employer or defendant would be free, as they now are, to argue that notwithstanding the increased or attributable risk occasioned by the exposure, factors other than the exposure were predominant in the disease etiology.

Moreover, as in other fields of expertise, there is "room for responsible epidemiologists to differ significantly on many of the key choices and assumptions to be made in analyzing [a] causal relationship,"[17] and expert witnesses would be needed to explore the complexities of detailed application of the Henle-Koch-Evans Postulates.[18]

Thus, even an epidemiologically derived standard for establishing inferences of causation would not eliminate the contentiousness in occupational disease or toxic tort claims. But among members of a similarly exposed group, it would go a long way toward eliminating the individual expense of having to establish, on a case-by-case basis, that exposure to chemical X can cause disease Y.

It would also avoid the adoption of other surrogates that would do greater damage to both science and law, such as presumptions of causation based on exposure in excess of regulatory limits or presumptions based on animal or tissue culture studies.

Strengthening the evidentiary status of epidemiologic evidence in the adjudicatory process will mean little to claimants or plaintiffs, however, unless epidemiologic evidence exists. What can be done to assure the availability of the needed studies?

In my judgment, H.R. 162 and S. 79 of the current Congress, the proposed High Risk Occupational Disease Notification and Prevention Act, should be promptly enacted. The enactment of these bills would encourage insurers and self-insured employers to undertake clinical and epidemiologic studies of exposed worker populations to determine what is and, equally important, what is not dangerous to workers' health.

If these studies show that particular concentrations or durations of exposure, or both, do not create increased risks of work-related disease, then it follows that they can be used not only to forestall unnecessary notifications under the Act, but also to controvert spurious occupational disease and toxic tort claims.

By the same token, if these studies show that there are increased risks in such exposures, then they can be used not only for insurance underwriting, rating, and loss prevention purposes, but also as compensability guidelines by workers' compensation tribunals and courts.

The proposed Act offers the business community as a whole—and insurers in particular—the opportunity to help the proposed Risk Assessment Board do for the prevention of occupational disease and the rationalization of occupational disease compensation what Underwriters Laboratories, ANSI, ASTM, and, most recently, OSHA have done for the prevention of traumatic injury by countless products and materials both inside and outside the workplace.

The reason is that the medicoscientific and procedural framework within which the Risk Assessment Board would operate would enable the Board, over time, to establish a rational basis not only for preventing occupational disease, but also for determining, for compensation purposes, what conditions do or do not increase the risk of occupational disease.

The Act, in my judgment, would eventually assure the availability, to employer and employee representatives alike, of a centralized source of the very best medical and scientific information on how to prevent, treat, and compensate for occupational diseases. The bill's scientific and procedural provisions would give all affected interests a tremendous opportunity to advance their collective knowledge of chronic and latent workplace disease.

Society is likely to find *cures* for most long-latency diseases before it fully understands their *causes*. But until these cures are found, sufferers of diseases caused by exposure to chemicals in the workplace and elsewhere must be compensated on a fair and rational basis.

If those of us with a stake in the survival of the workers' compensation and tort systems fail to devise that fair and rational basis, the courts, administrative tribunals, and legislatures will find other means, perhaps unfair and irrational, of achieving compensation objectives.

Although properly conducted and properly used epidemiologic data cannot provide all the answers, they can nonetheless provide some useful guidance. Every step should be taken to assure its proper integration into the adjudicative process.

Similarly, Congress should encourage the needed clinical and epidemiologic studies by enacting the proposed High Risk Occupational Disease Notification and Prevention Act.

NOTES AND REFERENCES

1. See, for example, *Gicas* v. *United States*, 50 F. Suppl. 217 (E.D. Wis. 1981).
2. "Compensating Victims of Pollution: The Workers' Compensation Experience," statement of Leslie I. Boden, Assistant Professor of Economics, Occupational Health Program and Department of Health Policy and Management, Harvard School

of Public Health, before the Subcommittee on Commerce, Transportation and Tourism of the Committee on Energy and Commerce, U.S. House of Representatives, November 22, 1983, at 6 [emphasis in original].)
3. *Idem* at 12.
4. *Idem* at 12–13.
5. *Idem* at 13.
6. Note, "Compensating Victims of Occupational Disease," 93 Harv. L. Rev. 916, 931, n. 108 (1980).
7. HARDY, T. S. 1982. Determination of Causation in Compensation of Persons Chronically Injured by Toxic Substances Exposures. Unpublished manuscript, at 13 (January 7).
8. See, generally, GOTS, R. E. 1983. Medical/Scientific Decision-Making in Occupational Disease Compensation. Appendix I. Role of the State Workers' Compensation System in Compensating Occupational Disease Victims, Crum and Foster (June).
9. HARDY, op. cit. *supra* n. 7, at 12.
10. See HAVENDER, W. R. 1982. Assessing and controlling risks. *In* Social Regulation, Bardach and Kagan, Eds. . . . "[A]mong a group of similarly exposed persons, only some of them—seemingly at random—will actually develop cancer. Not every smoker of high-tar cigarettes contracts lung cancer (in fact, only one in five does), and not every worker who worked with asbestos comes down with mesothelioma." *Idem* at 24–25.
11. BLACK & LILIENFELD. 1985. Epidemiologic proof in toxic tort litigation. 52 Fordham L. Rev. 732, 762.
12. *Idem* at 763.
13. STASON, E. B. *et al.* 1959. Atoms and the law, at 498. See also, note, Tort Action for Cancer: Deterrence, Compensation, and Environmental Carcinogenesis. 1981. 90 Yale L.J. 840, 861.
14. BLACK & LILIENFELD. op. cit. *supra* n. 11 at 767 [footnotes omitted].
15. *Idem* at 768 [footnote omitted].
16. "In using the Henle-Koch-Evans Postulates as constrained by attributable risk, great care must be taken in defining the exposure and the exposed population. In some instances, the focus should be on the total exposure above a certain level; in other cases the extent of exposure at any given time may be more important. The population of interest should be limited to individuals exposed at or beyond the level or extent at issue." *Idem* at 767, n. 143.
17. *O'Gara* v. *United States*, 560 F. Suppl. 786 (E.D. Pa. 1983).
18. "[T]he witnesses through whom the evidence is introduced must be suitably qualified. . . . Precedent . . . supports a rule requiring that a medical expert be qualified as an epidemiologist before testimony on causation is admitted. . . ." Black and Lilienfeld, op. cit. *supra* n. 11 at 769 [footnotes omitted].

Medical and Legal Causation

DAVID OZONOFF

Environmental Health Section
Boston University School of Public Health
Boston, Massachusetts 02118

It is an interesting and revealing circumstance that one of the first sessions in a workshop entitled "Occupational Health in the 1990s" should concern the problem of medical versus legal causation. This, no doubt, is some measure of the importance that litigation has already assumed as a driving force for much that is both good and bad in medicine in general and occupational health in particular. The directions that disease prevention takes in the 1990s may well be determined in large part by how the question of medical causation evolves. I will attempt to justify this rather rash statement at the end of my brief discussion of the causation problem.

Although differences between medical and legal causation are apparent in several contexts, including regulation, my remarks deal primarily with tort actions, which require plantiffs to demonstrate that a defendant was the "legal" cause of an occupational illness. In contrast to the usual case of occupational injury, which calls for evidence that a specific, concrete event or condition gave rise to the plantiff's harm, in many cases of suspected occupational disease there may be considerable uncertainty about the relation between exposure to a toxic agent and the plaintiff's disease. When this uncertainty exists or is claimed to exist by defendants, scientific evidence about causation becomes an essential part of the case.

I do not have space here to examine the differences between legal and medical causation in detail.[1] Indeed, part of what I would like to claim is that most attempts to set out such differences must shoot at a moving target. Causation is a much abused, but little understood concept, considerably more complex and sophisticated a notion than we generally give it credit for. I do not believe that we can give a good accounting of it yet, the volume of writing on the subject notwithstanding. There are, however, some things we can say about the misunderstandings of causation.

First, causation is a characteristic of a relationship, not an empirical characteristic. Calling a relationship "causal" is a judgment, one based on both theory and empirical evidence. Since much, if not all, empirical evidence is itself theory-laden, causality is ultimately tied intimately to a base in theory. There is no way that causation can be "discovered" without the essential participation of theory. This holds for all kinds of causation, in the laboratory, in the real world, or wherever. The oft-heard pronouncement that epidemiology can reveal only associations, not causation, is fundamentally wrongheaded and mistaken. It is, in some trivial sense, true, but this is a property it shares with every other empirical science as well. Hill's well-known guidelines on causation[2] are just that, guidelines to help make a judgment about causality, not postulates that must be fulfilled for causality to hold.

The confusion over the nature of causation is compounded when two cultures meet, as in the courtroom. That causation means something different in law and in science is well known and will not be belabored here. The point I wish to emphasize is that not only are the notions different but also there is no fixed meaning in either discipline. In both cases, the notion of causality is both created and modified as the consequences of earlier decisions become evident and are tested in new situations, in the one case by additional experiments or observations of the real world and in the other by testing its appropriateness in new legal cases and situations.

Hence there are many reasons why the topic of this panel, medical and legal causation, is ambiguous and ill-defined. Because causation is a judgment call, we must ask whose judgment will prevail and for what purposes. The judge's judgment is incorporated into his or her decisions on the admissibility of testimony and evidence, and the instructions to the jury, which in turn are based on a body of rules, law, and precedent concerning the nature and requirements for legal causation. The jury's judgment is constrained by the previous decisions of the judge, but it involves in addition a complex web of tacit presumptions and analogies from everyday experience. Rather than discuss the interesting question of legal judgments, however, let us look at scientific judgments.

First, let me address the issue of scientific consensus with respect to causation. When a rough consensus exists in the scientific community, arrived at by whatever method, controversy about legal causation will be lessened, but not necessarily eliminated (e.g., cancer trauma cases.)[3] On many issues such consensus does exist, but on many more there is substantial controversy. One feature that tends to set off those subjects for which there is controversy from those for which there is little or none is the existence of substantial consequences, that is, controversy tends to exist whenever the stakes are high, independent of the degree of "scientific certainty" involved. Stakes can be high because of scientific importance, perhaps because a result calls into question conventional views, or because of practical consequences, for example, it will affect regulation or result in large liability.

The causation issue in an occupational disease suit can be approached in two ways: one from the general or universal point of view, the second from the particular or clinical point of view. In the first approach, an attempt is made to prove that exposures similar to the plaintiff's would cause the observed health effects in the general case, that is, at other worksites, under different conditions, in different populations, via other routes of exposure, and so forth. The plaintiff then becomes merely a special case. This is the type of causation of which Hill speaks in giving us his criteria for causal associations, one of which is consistency with other results in other populations, settings, and the like. The second approach is particularistic: Did exposure cause harm to this worker at this time? This kind of causal judgment is the norm, not the exception. This is the usual clinical situation in which a physician diagnoses the individual person. Clearly the two approaches are related, but they are not identical.

The difference is not as stark in the case of a single worker as it is when groups of workers are involved. Consider, for example, a large group of workers exposed to an organic solvent. These workers complain of a wide variety of problems, from heart disease to depression to frequent respiratory problems. One way to establish causation is to perform an epidemiologic study to demonstrate that this group of workers, taken together, had an illness experience different from that of a suitable comparison group. Although this is possible, and in fact forms the bread and butter of the occupational epidemiologist, the constraints and difficulties of this approach are well known. Success even in the face of a real and substantial effect is often meager, and the result is still difficult to apply because it pertains to the group, not necessarily to all individuals within the group. However, we could also imagine putting each worker through a battery of tests, from neuropsychologic tests to complete cardiovascular workups to immune panels. The results of this battery in each case would be examined to determine if they were consistent with exposure to the solvent in question.

I can already hear the objections to this way of proceeding. It will be called anecdotal, unscientific, too uncertain, and unrigorous a judgment on which to rest weighty matters of dollars and sense. But let me emphasize again that it differs little from the usual instance of clinical diagnosis that occurs thousands of times daily. Drugs are prescribed or withdrawn, tests are ordered, and surgery is performed, each time on the basis of the same kind of causal judgment but with far less evidence than is present in these cases. Moreover, this happens even when we know that there are parties that stand to gain or lose in the process, and that there are significant practical consequences to these decisions for the patient. We recognize that we cannot wait indefinitely for some unstated threshold of proof to be crossed before a patient is treated, and furthermore that professional judgment is itself a powerful intellectual tool that can divine connections in particular instances without a standard algorithm that can be routinely applied to every case. This situation is no less true in court than in a doctor's office. And because of the adversary process, there is always a "second opinion." Ultimately the jury, like the patient, must decide.

I make these remarks in defense of clinical causation, not to disparage the attempt to establish universal or general propositions, but only to suggest that this is not the only practically significant standard of causation that we use. Most of my professional life is taken up with trying to establish such general propositions about the effects of chemical exposure on populations, and hopefully the results will be useful to those who must apply them clinically to individuals as well as to the public health community. But to use the criteria for this purpose for causal decisions about individuals places a heavy burden on a clinician or a community.

The population approach, however, must show that the particular case represents a general phenomenon. This is an appropriate objective for science, but a heavy burden for a community, plaintiff group, or single patient to bear. In some cases, such a demonstration may be beyond the limits of our tools. A rare disease or idiosyncratic reaction following a rare exposure, such as aplastic anemia after chlordane exposure, may be obvious from case reports but may not be demonstrable by epidemiologic study.

To return briefly to the significance of this element to occupational disease prevention in the 1990s, I believe that conceiving the causation problem from the clinical rather than the epidemiologic point of view will allow many more plaintiffs to obtain some compensation for harm. Whether this is good or bad depends, I suppose, on whose ox is being gored. More importantly, however, it will also result in the same kind of defensive behavior on the part of employers that is now so typical of medical practitioners faced with the specter of a malpractice claim. Conversely, requiring an epidemiologic standard of proof in these cases will essentially foreclose on the ability of many truly injured workers to recover any damages. The result will be to remove what apparently is one of the more potent driving forces behind workplace preventive measures.

The fear of liability is certainly not the only lever that can move the heavy weight of prevention. But it is an important ingredient in employer decision-making, and factors that affect it may in turn advance or retard the introduction of preventive measures in the workplace. The appearance of this panel's subject matter in this workshop was a recognition of these complex connections.

NOTES AND REFERENCES

1. There is a large literature on this subject. For a guide to some of this research and a recent statement about it, cf. BODEN, L. I., R. MIYARES & D. OZONOFF. 1988. Science and persuasion: Environmental disease in US Courts. Soc. Sci. Med. **27:** 1019–1029.
2. HILL, A. B. 1971. Principles of Medical Statistics, 9th ed. Oxford University Press. New York.
3. TILEVITZ, O. E. 1977. Judicial attitudes towards legal and scientific proof of cancer causation. Columbia J. Environ. Law. **3:** 353.

Current Magnitude of Occupational Disease in the United States

Estimates from New York State

PHILIP J. LANDRIGAN[a] AND STEVEN MARKOWITZ

Division of Environmental and Occupational Medicine
Department of Community Medicine
Mount Sinai School of Medicine
New York, New York 10029

Occupational diseases encompass a broad range of human illness. They include lung cancer and mesothelioma in asbestos workers, cancer of the bladder in dye workers, leukemia in workers exposed to benzene, chronic bronchitis in workers exposed to dust, disorders of the nervous system in workers exposed to solvents, chronic kidney disease in workers exposed to lead, heart disease in workers exposed to carbon monoxide, impairment of reproductive function in men and women exposed to lead and pesticides, and chronic disease of the musculoskeletal system in workers who suffer repetitive trauma.

Occupational exposures have been estimated to cause 100,000 deaths and 400,000 cases of illness each year in the United States.[1] However, no empirical data exist on the current incidence or prevalence of occupational disease in the United States. Currently available surveillance systems for occupational illness have been described as "fragmented, unreliable and 70 years behind the times."[2]

Effective prevention of occupational disease requires accurate data on incidence, prevalence, and time trends. Long experience with the communicable diseases has demonstrated the value of effective, sensitive disease surveillance systems. Data from such systems have been essential for the global eradication of smallpox[3] and for the control of measles in the United States.[4] If occupational diseases are to be similarly controlled, similar data will be required.

In an initial effort to obtain more accurate data on the incidence and prevalence of occupational disease in one large state—New York—our group from the Mount Sinai School of Medicine, with support from the New York State Departments of Health and Labor and the New York State Legislature, has undertaken a statewide survey of occupational disease. This study made use of data from the New York State Workers' Compensation Board, the U.S. Occupational Safety and Health Administration (OSHA), disease registries maintained by the New York State Department of Health, and physicians' reports.

This report presents the results of our evaluation[b] and suggests approaches for extrapolating these data to derive improved national estimates of the incidence and prevalence of occupational disease in the United States.

---

[a] Address for correspondence: Philip J. Landrigan, M.D., Mount Sinai School of Medicine, Division of Environmental and Occupational Medicine, 1 Gustave L. Levy Place, Box 1058, New York, N.Y. 10029.

[b] The full presentation of these data is included in a report entitled "Occupational Disease in New York State: Proposal for a Statewide Network of Occupational Disease Diagnosis and Prevention Centers," Mount Sinai School of Medicine, New York City, 1987. This report is available from the authors at no cost.

MORTALITY

Accurate data on mortality from occupational disease are largely lacking. In the absence of such data, we used a proportionate attributable risk approach to estimate occupational disease mortality in New York State.

Estimated percentages of each disease attributable to occupation were applied to disease-specific mortality totals to obtain estimates of total numbers of deaths due to occupational exposures; 10% of all cancer, 100% of all pneumoconioses, and 1-3% of all chronic respiratory, cardiovascular, neurologic, and renal disease deaths were ascribed to occupational causes[5-14] (TABLE 1). Application of these percentages leads to the conclusion that between 4,686 and 6,592 deaths each year in New York State are the result of occupational exposures.

TABLE 1. Annual Estimates of Occupational Disease Mortality, New York State

Cause of Death	Average Total Annual Mortality, NYS 1979–1982	Estimated Proportion and Number of Deaths Associated with Occupation		Average Annual Occupational Disease Deaths Reported by Workers' Compensation
		%	n	
Cancer	37,081	10	3,708	3
Pneumoconioses	25	100	25	34
Chronic respiratory disease	4,104[a]	1–3	41–123	3[b]
Cardiovascular disease, renal disease, and neurologic disorders	91,213	1-3	912–2,736	176
Other conditions	34,631	—	—	17
Total	167,054	—	4,686–6,592	233

SOURCES: Vital Statistics of New York State, 1979–1982; Compensated Cases Closed, State of New York Workers' Compensation Board Division of Research and Statistics, Bulletins Nos. 40–43, 1979–1982.

[a]Includes emphysema, asthma, bronchitis, bronchiectasis, and allergic alveolitis (ICD 490–496).

[b]Includes all nontoxic respiratory system conditions.

This range is probably a low estimate of total occupational disease mortality in New York State. A low estimate is generated, because proportional risks were applied to deaths from only six conditions: cancer, pneumoconioses, cardiovascular disease, chronic respiratory disease, neurologic illness, and renal disease. Furthermore, in each instance, conservative proportional risk estimates were selected from the range of figures available.

It is important to consider these results in the context of overall mortality data. There are 167,000 deaths in New York State each year. The estimated 5,000–7,000 deaths attributable to work-related exposures therefore constitute 3–4% of total deaths. Every year, twice as many people die from work-associated diseases as die from homicide and suicide combined, 1.5 times as from accidents, and more than twice as many have died of occupational diseases in New York State each year as have died from AIDS since that disease was first identified in 1981.

TABLE 1 also provides data on the average number of occupational disease deaths reported annually by the New York State Workers' Compensation Board between 1979 and 1982. Although the worker's compensation system provides an intuitively appealing and widely employed resource for occupational disease surveillance, its records are not accurate; they produce a significant underestimate of the number of persons affected by occupational disease, as well as misleading information on the pattern of occupational illness. Of the 233[c] occupational disease deaths reported on average each year by the Workers' Compensation Board, only 3 were cancer deaths. By contrast, data from other sources indicate that in 1979, nearly 80 deaths in New York State resulted from mesothelioma, a single relatively rare type of cancer that is nearly always caused by occupational exposure to asbestos.[15] Hospital discharge data, to be discussed herein, also indicate that Workers' Compensation data are incomplete.

MORBIDITY

Estimates of the incidence of nonfatal occupational illness are inherently less precise than are those of mortality. Estimates of the occurrence of work-related illness in New York State, however, are facilitated by the existence of several data sources in New York, in other states, and nationally. These data allow crude estimates of disease incidence and prevalence despite their weaknesses. TABLES 2 through 7 present the results of several approaches to the estimation of occupational disease morbidity in New York State, based on Workers' Compensation data, hospital discharge records, state disease registries, employers' OSHA reports, and California physicians' reports.

New York State-Specific Data

TABLE 2 shows the distribution of disease and the average number of new cases of nonfatal occupational illness reported annually by the New York State Workers' Compensation Board. These figures represent only closed cases of occupational disease—cases in which benefits have been awarded by the Workers' Compensation Board—not all claims submitted to the Board. These estimates are almost certainly too low.

Easily recognized, acute conditions, such as skin disease and musculoskeletal conditions, are relatively overrepresented; chronic disease is underreported. Only six cases of work-related cancer were compensated annually. The total of 3,765 new cases reported by Workers' Compensation is the lowest of the three illness estimates developed in the study.

Data from the New York State Department of Health's Heavy Metals Registry is useful for assessing the completeness of the workers' compensation data. Physicians, medical laboratories, and health care facilities are required to report excessive urine and blood levels of lead, cadmium, mercury, and arsenic to the Heavy Metals Registry. As shown in TABLE 3, in 1985, the registry reported 575 cases with elevated blood lead levels alone in 1985 and a total of 1,061 cases of excessive absorption of all four metals requiring reporting to the registry in that

---

[c] All nontraumatic accidental conditions have been incorporated into the disease category (e.g., heart attacks and infectious diseases are included under "diseases").

TABLE 2. Occupational Disease Morbidity Reported by the New York State Workers' Compensation Board, 1979–1982 Annual Averages

Condition	Average Annual Workers' Compensation Awards, NYS 1979–1982
Infectious and parasitic diseases	156
Cancer	6
Mental disorders	67
Nervous system and sensory organ conditions	
Hearing loss	627
Eye disease	20
Other	168
Circulatory system diseases	
Heart attacks	446
Stroke and other	34
Respiratory system diseases	
Pneumoconioses	
Asbestosis	14
Silicosis	28
Other	10
Other respiratory conditions	93
Musculoskeletal system conditions	968
Accidental poisonings	447
Skin diseases	639
Other	42
Total	3,765

SOURCES: Compensated Cases Closed, State of New York Workers' Compensation Board, Division of Research and Statistics Bulletins Nos. 40–43, 1979–1982.

year. The Workers' Compensation Board, however, recorded an average of 446 cases of all "systemic poisonings," including other causes besides heavy metal exposure, during the years 1979–1982.

Hospital discharge data, compiled by the Statewide Planning and Research Cooperative System (SPARCS) of the State Department of Health, provide an-

TABLE 3. Comparative Frequency of Occupational Heavy Metals Poisonings Reported by the Workers' Compensation Board and the NYS Heavy Metals Registry

Metal	NYS Heavy Metals Registry Reports 1985	Average Annual Workers' Compensation Awards for Systemic Poisonings, 1979–1982
Lead	575	—
Mercury	454	—
Arsenic	30	—
Cadmium	2	—
Total	1,061	446

SOURCES: New York State Heavy Metals Registry 1985; Compensated Cases Closed, State of New York Workers' Compensation Board, Division of Research and Statistics Bulletins Nos. 40–43, 1979–1982.

other means of judging the completeness of the information collected by the Workers' Compensation Board. According to the SPARCS data base, 599 hospital discharges for pneumoconioses were reported in New York State (TABLE 4). By contrast, workers' compensation benefits were initiated for an average of 52 individuals with pneumoconioses each year between 1979 and 1982. Clearly, the number of hospital discharges is not equivalent to the number of individuals with pneumoconioses. However, the likelihood that hospital discharges may overestimate the numbers of workers with pneumoconioses is counterbalanced by the fact that only the more severe cases of pneumoconioses require hospitalization, and thus represent only a small proportion of all cases of the disease. Hence, it is likely that workers' compensation data significantly underestimate the burden of pneumoconiosis in the State of New York.

TABLE 4. Pneumoconioses Cases Reported by the Statewide Planning and Research Cooperatiave System and the NYS Workers' Compensation Board

Pneumoconiosis	Average Annual Hospital Discharges 1980–1985	Average Annual Workers' Compensation Awards, 1979–1982
Asbestosis	210	14
Silicosis	298	28
Other	91	10
Total	599	52

SOURCES: Statewide and Research Cooperative System data; Compensated Cases Closed, State of New York Workers' Compensation Board, Division of Research and Statistics, Bulletins Nos. 40–43, 1979–1982.

National Data Extrapolated to New York

TABLE 5 provides an estimate of the occupational disease burden in New York State based on reports made by nongovernmental employers to the U.S. Department of Labor, Bureau of Labor Statistics (BLS) in 1984. The estimate of 11,687 new occupational illnesses in New York State was obtained by multiplying the U.S. incidence rate for each industry by the number of workers employed in that industry in New York State in 1984.

TABLE 6 illustrates the distribution of new cases of occupational disease in New York State by health condition. The two conditions reported most frequently by employers were skin diseases and musculoskeletal conditions. The Bureau of Labor Statistics data on which this estimate is based are limited almost entirely to easily recognizable, acute conditions and include virtually no cases of cancer or of other chronic or long latency occupational diseases.

California Physicians' Reports Extrapolated to New York State

California is unusual among the states in requiring physicians to report all cases of occupational disease treated and in publishing the resulting information. The "Doctors' First Report of Injury or Illness," from which the California

TABLE 5. Estimates of Occupational Disease Incidence by Industry Based on 1984 Bureau of Labor Statistics Data

Industry	U.S. Rate of New Cases Per 10,000 Workers 1984	New York State Employees, 1984	Estimated Number of New Cases of Occupational Disease in NYS, 1984
Agriculture, forestry, and fishing	43.8	95,000	416
Manufacturing			
Durable goods	38.6	736,400	2,843
Nondurable goods	38.4	589,900	2,265
Construction	16.3	255,200	416
Services	14.1	1,966,100	2,772
Mining	13.0	6,800	9
Transportation and public utilities	11.8	418,500	494
Government	9.0[a]	1,318,200	1,186
Wholesale and retail trade	6.5	1,576,900	1,025
Finance, insurance, and real estate	3.7	704,400	261
Total	15.2	7,667,400	11,687

SOURCE: Occupational Injuries and Illnesses in the United States by Industry, 1984. U.S. Dept. of Labor, Bureau of Labor Statistics, Bulletin 2259, May 1986.

[a]BLS data exclude government employees. This rate is the average of the rates for employees in the following industries: transportation and public utilities; wholesale and retail trade; finance, insurance, and real estate; and services.

incidence rates were calculated, encompasses first treatments given for all work-related conditions.[16] TABLE 7 uses data from California physicians' reports to estimate the frequency of occurrence of occupational illness in New York State.

Using this approach, it is estimated that 27,985 new cases of occupational disease occur each year in New York State. To develop this estimate, disease-specific California incidence rates were multiplied by the total number of workers

TABLE 6. Estimates of Occupational Disease Incidence by Illness Category Based on 1984 Bureau of Labor Statistics Data

Condition	Estimated Number of New Cases in New York State, 1984
Skin disease or disorders	4,056
Disorders associated with repeated trauma	2,675
Respiratory conditions due to toxic agents	1,052
Disorders due to physical agents	832
Poisoning	465
Dust diseases of the lung	139
All other occupational illnesses	2,468
Total	11,687

SOURCE: Occupational Injuries and Illnesses in the United States by Industry, 1984. U.S. Department of Labor, Bureau of Labor Statistics, Bulletin 2259, May 1986.

in New York State. The distribution of new cases of disease reported by physicians (TABLE 7) is similar to that of diseases reported by employers (TABLE 6). The almost 28,000 illnesses estimated on the basis of physicians' reports include primarily acute conditions, especially skin diseases, and almost no cases of cancer.

The morbidity estimates presented in TABLES 2 to 7 range from a low of 3,765 cases to a high of 27,985 cases. Because all of these estimates exclude occupational cancer, the range should more properly extend from 10,345-34,565 new cases of work-related disease each year, assuming that 10% of all new cases of cancer are due to occupational factors. The resulting figure of 34,565 cases annually is probably the most accurate estimate currently available on the incidence of work-related illness in New York State. Nevertheless, because the occupational origin of work-related illness is so often overlooked by both physicians and other medical providers, even this figure may represent a conservative estimate.

TABLE 7. Occupational Disease Incidence Estimates Based on California "Doctors' First Report" Data, 1983

Condition	New Disease Rate per 10,000 California Workers[a]	Estimated Number of New Cases, New York State, 1984[b]
Skin conditions	12.2	9,354
Eye conditions	11.2	8,587
Systemic poisonings	3.0	2,300
Respiratory conditions	3.0	2,300
Chemical burns	2.4	1,840
Exposure to toxic materials	0.7	537
Ear conditions	0.6	460
Circulatory system conditions	0.6	460
Other	2.8	2,147
Total		27,985

[a]Occupational Disease in California, 1983. State of California Department of Industrial Relations, Division of Labor Statistics and Research, San Francisco, California, September 1985.

[b]There were 7,667,300 workers in New York State in 1984 (NYS Department of Labor).

In New York State, as elsewhere, there is little or no coordination among data sources on occupational disease, and the information they provide is fragmentary and unreliable. The occurrence of occupational disease is underreported for a variety of reasons, including workers' fears of losing their jobs, employers' fears of legal and financial liability, lack of recognition by physicians of the occupational origin of a patient's condition, the fact that workers are often unaware of or unable to recall their exposure to dangerous materials, and the frequently long latency period that elapses between exposure and the development of recognizable symptoms of disease.

Although the available data on occupational disease are limited, they are sufficient to demonstrate that occupational disease is a serious problem in New York State.

HAZARDOUS WORKPLACE EXPOSURES IN NEW YORK STATE

The identification and characterization of hazardous workplace exposures are necessary for understanding patterns of occupational disease in New York State and for formulating prevention strategies. Hazard surveillance complements occupational disease surveillance. Indeed, given the general underdiagnosis of occupational disease, systematic examination of work-related hazards in industries and occupations across the state can provide an important guide as to the location and nature of possible work-related illness.

In 1985, approximately 7.9 million people were employed in New York State—8% of the total United States workforce. Of these 7.9 million people, 1.3 million (16%) were employed in the manufacturing sector and another 285,000 (4%) in construction. Many fewer people were employed in other economic sectors important in terms of occupational health: 99,000 in agriculture and 6,700 in mining. The most populous economic sectors in New York in 1985 were the service industry, with 2.0 million workers, and wholesale and retail trade, with 1.6 million workers.

A total of 158,804 New Yorkers were employed in the 50 most hazardous industries (identified by 4-digit Standard Industrial Classification code) in 1985 according to the Inspection-Based Exposure Rating (IBER) system.[17] The limitation of the list to 50 industries is arbitrary and is not meant to imply that other industries do not present hazards. Over 75% of the workers in these industries are concentrated in 14 of New York State's 62 counties. In descending order, the counties with the highest employment in hazardous industries are: New York City (includes five counties), 32,900 workers; Erie, 23,700 workers; Niagara, 10,200 workers; Suffolk, 9,100 workers; and Onondaga, 9,100 workers.

A second hazard ranking scheme was proposed in 1983 by Pederson, Young, and Sundin of the National Institute for Occupational Safety and Health (NIOSH). This was the Industry Risk Index (IRI).[19] In contrast to the IBER approach, the IRI is based on the National Occupational Hazard Survey. Conducted by NIOSH between 1972 and 1974, the National Occupational Hazard Survey (NOHS) was a walk-through survey of a national sample of over 4,600 workplaces. Trained surveyors visited each of these 4,600 employment sites and described the chemical, physical, and biological hazards present in each workplace.[20] Over 8,000 potentially hazardous chemical agents and 86,000 trade-name products were observed to be in use in the workplaces visited. Because no actual measurements of exposures were performed as part of the survey, the extent of worker exposure to the inventoried hazards was not determined. Hence, the NOHS considered only "potential exposure." The term "potential exposure" indicates that a worker is situated in proximity to a hazardous material for a minimum number of hours per week. Despite this limitation, NOHS represented a landmark achievement in the creation of a national data base describing the magnitude and distribution of hazardous agents in the workplace. The survey was repeated during 1981 to 1983 as the National Occupational Exposure Survey, but those results are not expected to be available before 1990.

The IRI combines the industry-specific exposure profile provided by NOHS with a judgment on the toxicity of specific chemical agents as well as with information about the number of potentially exposed workers to create a ranking of industries according to the degree of hazard. The level of toxicity of a given agent was determined by its ability to cause cancer, mutations, birth defects, and acute harm as recorded in the Registry of Toxic Effects of Chemical Substances.[21] Distribution of workers by industry was obtained from County Business Patterns data. One of the main strengths of the IRI is its attempt to incorporate comprehensive toxicologic information on a vast array of agents into a hazard-ranking scheme.

A total of 746,806 workers in New York State were employed in the 50 most hazardous specific industries according to a modified IRI. Selected industries were deleted from the original IRI list, because they were judged to involve relatively minor actual hazards and distorted the overall employment figures because of large numbers of employees in these industries in New York State. The deleted industries include accounting and auditing, real estate, and legal services, which employed over 150,000 workers in 1985.

Hospitals and health care facilities (Standard Industrial Classification codes 8062 and 8099) employed the largest numbers of workers on the IRI list with a combined total of 405,000 workers, or 54% of all workers on the list. Other common hazardous industries are building maintenance, car repair, and pharmaceutical manufacture. Counties with the largest numbers of workers in hazardous industries include New York City, Suffolk, Nassau, and Erie. Nearly half of all workers employed in the IRI's 50 most hazardous industries reside in these counties.

There is a lack of overlap between the two lists of most hazardous industries, a difference that reflects the different methods used to create the two indexes. Each method has different strengths and weaknesses; they can be used in complementary fashion to gain a broad view of the relative hazards present in different industries. Both indexes demonstrate that a significant number of workers in New York State are employed in hazardous trades. Furthermore, the distribution of workers in hazardous industries throughout the state is similar, regardless of the index used. Use of either index would lead to similar conclusions about the need for and optimal location of occupational health services across the state.

COSTS OF OCCUPATIONAL DISEASE IN NEW YORK STATE

Estimates of the costs of illness and death associated with certain occupationally related conditions were made using the human capital approach to the calculation of the costs of illness.[22–28]

The human capital method divides costs into two categories: direct and indirect. *Direct costs* are the value of resources that could be allocated to other uses in the absence of disease. They include expenditures for hospitalization, physicians' services, nursing home care, drugs, medical appliances, and related expenses. *Indirect costs* are the value of the lost output of workers and retirees suffering premature death or disability, measured in terms of the wages they would have earned if they had not contracted occupational diseases. In addition to earnings loss, indirect costs include the lost value of household production services caused by disability and death from occupational disease, measured according to the market wages that would be paid to outsiders for those services.

The human capital approach can be used to estimate the costs of illness and death associated with occupationally related cancer and, to a more limited extent, stroke, heart disease, pneumoconioses, chronic respiratory disease, and renal failure.

Cancer

The estimates of occupational cancer discussed earlier were used to obtain an estimate of the annual direct costs of occupational cancer in New York State. Cost estimates were averaged over specific cancer diagnostic categories to obtain average direct costs by age and sex. National medical care cost data in 1975 dollars[29] were adjusted to account for the higher costs of medical care in New York State. These adjusted cost estimates were then applied to the New York incidence estimates and adjusted to 1985 dollars, using the medical care price index specific to the New York region.[30] Future costs were discounted at 6%. As shown in TABLE 8, the average direct cost per case of occupational cancer was $31,255 in New York State in 1985.

Additional costs of occupational cancer—foregone earnings—were ascertained by measuring lost productivity owing to cancer morbidity over the patient's expected life span, and comparing this to expected productivity and life expectancy of a matched cancer-free population.[29] These estimates were adjusted to take into account the 12.3% difference in average annual pay between New York State and U.S. workers. Future lost earnings were discounted at 6%. Total annual foregone earnings were $44,272 per cancer victim, as shown in TABLE 8.

Adding together direct costs and foregone earnings for all workers diagnosed with occupationally related cancer during a 12-month period, the total annual cost of occupational cancer in New York State was approximately $497 million in the early 1980s (TABLE 9).

Coronary Heart Disease and Stroke

Because incidence rates for coronary heart disease (CHD) and stroke were not available by age and sex in New York State, it was impossible to conduct as comprehensive an analysis for these diseases as for occupational cancer. Nevertheless, mean per-capita direct and indirect cost estimates,[29] averaged over age and sex categories, can be adjusted to New York 1985 dollars; it is therefore possible to obtain an approximate lower-bound indication of the costs of occupational deaths in New York State attributable to the major diagnostic categories that constitute cardiovascular disease. These cost estimates were applied to the work-related CHD and stroke mortality estimates discussed earlier. The resultant

TABLE 8. Direct and Indirect Costs per Person of Various Occupational Disease Diagnostic Categories in 1985

Diagnosis	Indirect Cost[a]	Direct Cost	Total Cost
Cancer[b]	$44,272	$31,255	$75,527
Coronary heart disease[c]	36,062	11,219	47,281
Stroke[c]	34,105	24,413	58,518
End-stage renal disease[c]	—	33,000	33,000[d]
Chronic respiratory disease[c]	—	8,058	8,058[d]
Pneumoconiosis	—	6,009[e]	6,009[d]

[a]Present value of future costs, discounted at 6%.
[b]Cases.
[c]Deaths.
[d]Direct costs only.
[e]Cost per hospital admission only.

TABLE 9. Cost of Occupational Diseases in New York State by Diagnostic Category

Diagnosis	Number of Cases/Deaths	Costs per Case	Total Costs
Cancer[a]	6580	75,527[b]	$496,960,000
Coronary heart disease[c]	600–1800	47,281[b]	28,368,600–85,105,800
Stroke[c]	102–306	58,518[b]	5,968,836–17,906,508
End-stage renal disease[c]	18–56	33,000[d]	594,000–1,848,000
Chronic respiratory disease[c]	120–400	8,058[e]	966,960–3,23,200
Pneumoconiosis	599[f]	6,009[g]	3,599,384
Total			$536,457,780–$605,043,508

[a]All cases.
[b]Indirect and direct costs.
[c]Deaths only.
[d]Direct costs only; indirect cost estimates are not available.
[e]Hospitalization cost only.
[f]Number of hospital admissions for pneumoconioses.
[g]Average cost per hospital admission.

summary cost figures do not fully account for costs of these illnesses, however, because more people suffer from these diseases than actually die from them.

Total economic costs of work-related CHD were obtained by combining and averaging the direct and indirect costs for the three major categories of CHD for which economic data are available: myocardial infarction, coronary insufficiency, and uncomplicated angina pectoris. The total cost per patient in New York State was estimated to be $47,281 in 1985 dollars, adjusted for differentials in New York State wages, hospital costs, physician fees, and other medical prices (TABLE 8). Approximately 25% of these costs, or $11,281, were direct costs, with the remaining 75%, or $36,062, due to earnings foregone as a result of heart disease, using a discount rate of 6% for lost future earnings. The total lower-bound estimate of the costs of occupational CHD in New York thus ranges from $28,368,600 to $85,105,800 (TABLE 9).

Average total per capita costs for completed strokes (including hemorrhagic and infarctive events, but excluding transient ischemic attacks) were estimated to be approximately $58,518 (1985 dollars) in New York State, using an adjustment methodology similar to that detailed earlier. This per capita cost included $24,413 in direct costs and $34,105 in indirect costs (TABLE 8). The lower bound range of costs due to occupationally related stroke deaths in New York in 1985 is thus conservatively estimated to be between $6 million and $18 million.

In summary, the total annual economic costs of occupational heart disease and stroke in New York State are estimated to be between $34 million and $103 million.

End-Stage Renal Disease

The annual cost of medical care for end-stage renal disease (ESRD) was estimated in 1982 to be approximately $26,000 per patient.[31] Adjusting this figure to 1985 dollars and using the medical care component of the Consumer Price Index for the New York region, the average estimated cost of direct medical care for patients with ESRD was approximately $33,000 per year. Accurate data on the etiology of ESRD are available for fewer than 50% of cases.[14] Epidemiologic estimates in an earlier section of this presentation, however, attribute 18 to 56 deaths caused by kidney disease per year in New York State to occupational causes. Thus, estimates of the medical cost of ESRD due to occupational exposures range between $594,000 and $1,848,000. Indirect costs cannot be calculated.

Pneumoconioses and Other Chronic Respiratory Diseases

Between 1980 and 1985 in New York State, the average annual number of hospital discharges for the pneumoconioses (ICD codes 500–505) was 599 (TABLE 4), accounting for approximately 7,724 annual inpatient days. At a cost of $466 per day, hospitalizations for pneumoconioses cost $3,599,384 in 1985.

Between 120 and 400 deaths per year in New York State are attributable to occupationally related chronic respiratory disease. In a recent study of the cost of care for patients with chronic lung disease, investigators found that the average patient used a total of $6,979 in health care resources during a 12-month period.[32] There were an average of 10.1 hospital days per patient year, which accounted for approximately one half the health care costs. Adjusting these data to New York State prices, the estimate of direct medical care expenses for deaths from occupationally related chronic lung disease in New York State was between $996,000 and $3,223,000.

In summary, the total estimated cost of occupational disease in New York State is between 540 and 604 million dollars per year.

SUPPLY OF OCCUPATIONAL HEALTH SERVICES AND PERSONNEL IN NEW YORK STATE

Trained Personnel

Clinical occupational health services concentrating on the detection and prevention of occupational disease are in short supply in New York State. In 1985, only 73 of the more than 52,000 licensed physicians in New York State were board certified in occupational medicine.[33,34] Thus, there is one occupational medicine physician for every 108,000 workers in the state.

The distribution of occupational medicine physicians throughout the state further accentuates their inaccessibility. Nearly two thirds, or 46, of the board-certified occupational medicine physicians in New York State are located in three counties: 23 in New York County, 16 in Monroe County, and 7 in Westchester County. Furthermore, at least two thirds of occupational medicine physicians are not involved in direct patient care. Most of these physicians work in administrative, research, or teaching positions. Important industrial counties such as Nassau, Onondaga, and Steuben have no occupational medicine specialists who provide direct patient care.

A larger number of physicians identify occupational medicine as their primary specialty than are board certified in the field. In New York State, 121 physicians involved in direct patient care list their primary speciality as occupational medicine.[35] The majority are not board certified in occupational medicine. Regardless of whether they are qualified to diagnose occupational disease, many self-designated occupational medicine physicians spend most of their time performing preemployment physical examinations or periodic evaluations, treating acute occu-

pational injuries, or delivering general medical care in an occupational setting or to identified occupational groups. Although these activities are necessary, they provide only limited sources for the diagnosis and treatment of chronic occupational diseases. Hence, it is unlikely that this larger group of occupational medicine physicians significantly increases the availability of services established specifically for the diagnosis and treatment of occupational disease.

Industrial hygienists are more common than are occupational physicians in New York State. The American Industrial Hygiene Association (AIHA), the major professional organization of industrial hygienists, lists 292 active industrial hygienists as members in New York State, including 91 who are certified.[36] Since 85% to 90% of all industrial hygienists are members of AIHA,[37] the estimated number of industrial hygienists in New York is 325 to 345.

Despite their greater numbers, however, industrial hygienists are not much more accessible than are occupational medicine physicians. TABLE 10 shows the type of employer or professional activity of industrial hygienists in New York. Two thirds, or 176, of the industrial hygienists in New York State are employed by corporations, mostly large companies such as IBM, which employs 22 industrial hygienists, Kodak, which employs 19, and General Electric, which employs 7. Various levels of government employ another 15% of the industrial hygienists

TABLE 10. Type of Employer or Professional Activity of Industrial Hygienists in New York State, 1985–1986

Affiliation	Number	Percent
Private corporation	176	63
Government	42	15
Private consultant	35	13
University	35	9
Total	278	100

SOURCE: American Industrial Hygiene Association Membership Directory, 1985–1986; excludes 14 industrial hygienists who did not indicate professional activity.

in New York State; universities employ 9%, especially New York University, which employs 10, the University of Rochester, which employs 7, and Columbia University, which employs 5. Only 35 industrial hygienists are primarily consultants.

Hence, large institutions employ the majority of industrial hygienists in New York State. Few industrial hygienists are available to the vast majority of employers, unions, occupational health programs, and community groups, who have an intermittent need for industrial hygiene services.

Institutional Resources

New York State has only one fully functioning hospital-based center specializing in the diagnosis and treatment of occupational disease. This facility is located at Mt. Sinai Medical Center in New York City. Specialty clinics at other medical centers in Rochester, Buffalo, and Long Island are being initiated, but currently they offer only limited services.

The extent to which company-based health services are currently available in New York State is unknown. However, a nationwide study conducted by NIOSH in 1981–1983 indicated that 24% of all industries sampled had inplant health services, an increase of 10% since the early 1970s. For small (1–99 employees) and medium-size (100–499 employees) industries, rates of established health facilities were approximately 5% and 35%, respectively.[38] Although access to some type of health services within the plant has improved overall, most workers are still employed in plants without on-site health services. It is unlikely that industries in New York State have established inplant health facilities significantly more frequently than have industries in the remainder of the country.

The growing interest in occupational disease and the increasing need to screen groups of workers with known hazardous exposures, such as exposure to asbestos, have led to the rise of for-profit health care corporations that specialize in periodic medical examinations. Their previous emphasis on providing general preventive evaluations for occupational groups such as executives and selected blue collar workers is being broadened to include a focus on occupational diseases. The quality of such services may, however, be limited.[39,40]

Various unions have developed health care centers for their membership that provide general services as well as selected specialty care. Unions in New York State with such facilities include the International Ladies' Garment Workers Union, the International Brotherhood of Teamsters, and the Service Employees International Union. Although these facilities do care for large numbers of workers with hazardous occupational exposures, they have not obtained expertise in occupational medicine and do not focus on the possible occupational diseases for which their members are at risk.

Local and county health departments throughout New York State do not offer diagnostic services in occupational medicine.

Training of Occupational Health Professionals

Given the present inadequate supply and lack of availability of occupational medicine physicians and industrial hygienists in New York, what are the prospects for the future? Only two occupational medicine residency programs exist in New York State, both in New York City. Columbia University School of Public Health graduates an average of 1.5 occupational medicine physicians per year. The Mount Sinai School of Medicine program averages 3 new occupational medicine physicians annually. Thus, 4.5 new occupational medicine physicians enter the workforce each year. Although this number is small, it represents approximately 10% of all new occupational medicine physicians trained each year in the United States.[41] Clearly, occupational medicine is an underserved specialty.

DISCUSSION AND RECOMMENDATIONS

The major finding of this study is that occupational disease is a major problem in New York State despite the fact that 18 years have now elapsed since passage of the Occupational Safety and Health Act in 1970. We estimate that each year in New York State occupational exposures are responsible for 5,000 to 7,000 deaths and for at least 35,000 new cases of illness.

Nationally, as well as in New York State, success in reducing work-related illness has remained elusive. Cancer mortality appears to be increasing, and occupational exposures may account for at least part of this trend.[42] Death rates in underground miners have increased.[42] Asbestos, although used less frequently than in the past, remains widely dispersed; approximately 10,000 asbestos-related deaths are expected to occur in the United States each year for the remainder of the century.[44] Silicosis, a disease recognized since antiquity, is still common among miners and foundry workers;[45] a recent review of OSHA inspection records indicates that the level of silica exposure in 43% of American foundries remains above legally mandated standards.[46] These factors led the American Public Health Association to conclude in 1984 that "occupational disease is at epidemic proportions in the United States."[47]

Prevention of occupational disease both in New York State and nationally requires a comprehensive and unified plan. Appropriate medical diagnostic and industrial hygiene services need to be made available. Physicians and other health providers must be trained adequately to recognize work-related problems. Surveillance efforts, although praiseworthy at present, are limited in scope and resources and need urgently to be expanded and made more effective. Comprehensive plans must be made available for providing information to workers on the nature of the exposures that they encounter at work and on the work relatedness of the diseases that they suffer as the result of those exposures.

In order that a start be made toward accomplishing these goals, we recommended that New York State strengthen its efforts to protect the health and safety of its workforce by expanding the capacity of the health care system to diagnose and treat workers with occupational diseases. Complementary efforts to enhance professional training and to strengthen ongoing surveillance, evaluation, and planning with respect to occupational disease are also vital.

1. We recommend that the State of New York initiate and fund a demonstration project to establish a statewide network of occupational health clinical centers coordinated through a network office.

The central goal of these centers is to provide accessible diagnostic, preventive, and treatment services for all workers in New York State with occupational diseases or with exposure to occupational hazards. Introduction of this network in New York State will entail: (1) transformation of existing facilities with limited programs into comprehensive occupational health centers; (2) establishment of additional centers in those parts of the State that currently lack even limited occupational health services; and (3) creation of a network office to coordinate network activities. The resulting integrated system will make occupational health care services available to all workers and employers in the state.

The proposed occupational health clinical centers will concentrate on the diagnosis and treatment of occupational diseases. However, a commitment to prevention at primary, secondary, and tertiary levels additionally requires the integration of industrial hygiene, educational, and social work services into a traditional medical model. The diagnosis of occupational disease in an individual can be exploited to ameliorate unsafe conditions in the workplace, to prevent coworkers from becoming ill, and to detect disease early in exposed coworkers.

Development of a clinical center network might best be accomplished by a 5-year demonstration project financed primarily by the State. The 5-year demonstration period would consist of two major components: a planning phase and an implementation and evaluation phase. The length of the planning process would vary among network components. Expansion of existing facilities will require 6–12 months of planning, depending on the present level of development of each center. Twelve months of planning will be needed before new centers in currently unserved regions of the State can reasonably be expected to be operational. Organization of the network office will also require a 12-month planning period.

Funding of the demonstration project should be provided by the State. One appropriate source of funds for the provision of medical services for patients with occupational diseases could be the workers' compensation system, that is, insurance premiums. The need for funding during the later years of the operation of the clinical centers will be partially decreased by revenues from patient care and consultations.

The total costs estimated for the demonstration project as currently envisioned will be approximately 2 million dollars for the first year and 4–5 million dollars for each of the subsequent 4 years. These figures represent the ceiling funding levels that will be required. The total funds needed will in fact be lower by the amount of revenues generated by the project's operations. These revenues can be estimated to increase from 10% of the operating expenses of the clinical centers in year 2, to 20–30% of operating expenses in years 3 and 4, to 40–50% of expenses by year 5 of the demonstration project. These figures represent, at a maximum, 0.8% of the annual costs of occupational disease in New York State.

In April 1987, the New York State Legislature appropriated 1 million dollars for the planning and partial implementation of six occupational health clinical centers in New York State. Six institutions, including four medical schools, a health maintenance organization, and a free-standing clinic, received grants ranging from $100,000 to $225,000 in 1987 to establish the clinic network suggested by this study. The program is being administered by the New York State Department of Health. Three million dollars has been requested for funding of this network in the second year, when all centers will become fully operational.

2. We recommend that the State Departments of Health, Labor and Environmental Conservation coordinate and expand existing occupational disease and hazard information systems in order to create a comprehensive, coordinated surveillance system.

In New York State as well as at the federal level there is an urgent need for the various agencies with responsibilities in occupational health and safety, including the Department of Health and Human Services, the Department of Labor, and the Environmental Protection Agency, to work together in a coordinated fashion to improve disease and hazard surveillance, environmental health research, and regulation.

3. We recommend that the State Board of Regents and the State University of New York establish requirements mandating that all schools of health professions such as schools of medicine and nursing enhance the training of all health professionals in occupational and environmental health.

Health professional schools throughout the nation are sorely lacking in appropriate and ample instruction in occupational health and safety. The average medical student in the United States receives only a few hours of instruction in occupational medicine.[48] This lack of training occurs despite the recognized need for and lack of qualified professionals in all of the disciplines encompassed by the field. An expansion of the funding for NIOSH-supported Educational Resource Centers and an incentive program for health professional schools to introduce occupational health and safety in the curriculum are effective ways to begin to increase the supply of occupational health professionals.

SUMMARY

The data from our study indicate that the magnitude of occupational disease in New York State is considerable, and that a detailed and comprehensive plan must be initiated and implemented if occupational disease is to be controlled. New York State contains slightly less than 10% of the nation's workforce. A direct linear extrapolation of findings in New York State cannot be made to derive estimates of the national burden of work-related illness. Nevertheless, a crude estimate of the national magnitude of occupational disease can be derived from the New York experience. Such extrapolation provides a crude estimate of 50,000–70,000 deaths each year from occupational disease and of 350,000 new cases of occupational illness. These numbers are distressingly similar to the annual estimates of 100,000 deaths and 400,000 cases of occupational illness developed almost 15 years ago by Ashford.[1] Clearly substantial progress remains to be made.

REFERENCES

1. ASHFORD, N. A. 1976. Crisis in the Workplace; Occupational Disease and Injury. MIT Press. Cambridge, Massachusetts.
2. Occupational Illness Data Collection: Fragmented, Unreliable, and Seventy Years Behind Communicable Disease Surveillance. Sixtieth Report by the Committee on Government Operations. House Report 98–1144, October 5, 1984.
3. FOEGE, W. H., J. D. MILLAR & J. M. LASTE. 1971. Selective epidemiologic control in smallpox eradication. Am. J. Epidemiol. **94:** 311.
4. FRANK, J. A., W. A. ORSENSTEIN, J. R. BART, et.al. 1985. Major impediments to measles elimination. The Modern Epidemiology of an Ancient Disease. Am. J Dis. Child. **139:** 881–888.
5. DOLL, R. & R. PETO. 1981. The causes of cancer: Quantitative estimates of avoidable risks of cancer in the United States today. J. Nat. Cancer Inst. **66:** 1191–1308.
6. BRIDBORD, K. et al. Estimates of the Fraction of Cancer in the United States Related to Occupational Factors NCI/NIEHS/NIOSH, September 15, 1978.
7. DAVIS, D. L., K. BRIDBORD & M. SCHNEIDERMAN. 1981. Estimating cancer cases: Problems in methodology, production and trends. In R. Peto and M. Schneiderman, eds. Quantification of Occupational Cancer, Banbury Report #9. Cold Spring Harbor Laboratory, NY.
8. STALLONES, R. A. & T. A. DOWNS. 1981. A critical review of Bridford, K. et al. Prepared for the American Industrial Health Council, 1979. Cited in S. S. Epstein and J. B. Swartz. Fallacies of Lifestyle Cancer Theories. Nature. **289:** 127–130.
9. On Occupational Cancer Estimation: Report of the Occupational Cancer Risk Subcommittee of the Department of Health and Human Services Committee to Coordinate Environmental and Related Programs November 4, 1983. Report prepared by the U.S. Department of Health & Human Services, Washington, D.C.
10. WYNDER, E. L. & G. B. GORI. 1977. Contribution of the environment to cancer incidence: An epidemiologic exercise. J. Nat. Cancer Institute **58:** 825–832.
11. ROSENMAN, K. D. 1979. Cardiovascular disease and environmental exposure. Br. J. Indus. Med. **36:** 85–97.
12. Leading Work-Related Disease and Injuries—United States: Cardiovascular Diseases. 1985. Morbid. Mortal. Weekly Rep. **34:** 219–222.

13. Leading Work-Related Diseases and Injuries—United States: Occupational Lung Diseases. 1983. Morbid. Mortal. Weekly Rep. **32:** 24–26, 32.
14. LANDRIGAN, P. J. *et al.* 1984. The work-relatedness of renal disease. Arch. Environ. Health **39:** 225–230.
15. New York State Department of Health, Bureau of Cancer Control.
16. State of California Department of Industrial Relations, Division of Labor Statistics and Research, Occupational Disease in California 1983. San Francisco, California, September 1985.
17. FROINES, J., C. DELLENBAUGH, & D. WEGMAN. 1986. Occupational health surveillance: A means of identifying work-related risk. Am J. Pub. Health **76:** 1089–1096.
18. FROINES, J., C. DELLENBAUGH, S. SEABROOK & D. WEGMAN. 1984. A profile of the occupational health experience in Los Angeles County. September 28. Los Angeles: Southern Occupational Health Center, Univ. of California (Unpublished report to the Department of Health Services, State of California).
19. PEDERSON, D., R. YOUNG & D. SUNDIN. 1983. A Model for the Identification of High Risk Occupational Groups Using RTECS and NOHS Data. NIOSH Technical Report 83-117. US Government Printing Office. Washington, DC.
20. NIOSH. 1977. National Occupational Hazard Survey, Volumes 1–3. DHEW Publication No. 74-127, May 1974. DHEW Publication No. 77-213, July 1977. DHEW Publication No. 78-114, December 1977. Cincinnati, OH. National Institute for Occupational Safety and Health.
21. NIOSH. Registry of Toxic Effects of Chemical Substances, 1980 Edition. DHHS Publication No. 81–116, February 1982. Cincinnati, OH. National Institute for Occupational Safety and Health.
22. HODGSON, T. & M. MEINERS. 1982. Cost of illness methodology: A guide to current practices and procedures. Milbank Mem. Fund Q./Health and Soc. **60:** 429–462.
23. SCITOVSKY, A. 1976. Estimating the direct cost of illness revisited. Soc. Sec. Bull. (February): 21–36.
24. RICE, D. P. 1966. Estimating the Cost of Illness. Health Economic Series, No. 6. U.S. Public Health Service. Washington, DC.
25. COOPER, B. S. & D. P. RICE. 1976. The economic cost of illness revisited. Soc. Sec. Bull. February: 21–36.
26. RICE, D. P., T. A. HODGSON & A. N. KOPSTEIN. 1985. "The Economic Costs of Illness: A Replication and Update," *Health Care Financing Rev.* 7 (Fall): 61–80.
27. PARSONS, P. E., R. LICHTENSTEIN & S. E. BERKI. 1986. *Costs of Illness, United States, 1980.* National Medical Care Utilization and Expenditure Survey. Series C, Analytical Report No. 3. DHHS Pub. No. 86-20403. National Center for Health Statistics, Public Health Service. Washington, DC.
28. Institute of Medicine. 1981. Costs of Environment-Related Health Effects. National Academy Press. Washington, D.C.
29. HARTUNIAN, N. S., C. N. SMART & M. S. THOMPSON. 1981. The Incidence and Economic Costs of Major Health Impairments. Lexington Books, D. C. Heath and Company. Lexington, MA.
30. Bureau of Labor Statistics, Consumer Price Index, Medical Care Component.
31. DAVIS, C. K. 1983. Statement of the Administrator, Health Care Financing Administration, Before the Subcommittee on Health and the Environment, Committee on Energy and Commerce, U.S. House of Representatives. Washington, DC. October 17.
32. STRAUSS, M. J., D. CONRAD, J. P. LOGERFO, L. D. HUDSON & M. BERGNER. 1986. Cost and outcome of care for patients with chronic obstructive lung disease. *Med. Care* **24:** 915–924.
33. Marquis Who's Who. Directory of Medical Specialists, 1985–1986, Volume 2.
34. Medical Society of New York. Medical Directory of New York State, 1986–1987, Volume LX.
35. American Medical Association. 1985. Directory of Physicians in the United States, Volume 3, 29th Edition. Chicago.
36. American Industrial Hygiene Association. Membership Directory, 1985–1986. Akron, Ohio.

37. KORNREICH, L. 1983. CIH, President, Metropolitan New York Chapter, AIHA, November 19. Personal communication.
38. SETA, J. & D. S. SUNDIN. 1984. Trends of a decade—A perspective on occupational health surveillance, 1970–1983. Morbid. Mortal. Weekly Rep. **34** (2SS): 15SS–24SS.
39. GUIDOTTI, T. L. & B. H. KUETZING. 1985. Competition and despecialization: An analytical study of occupational health services in San Diego, 1974–1984. Am. J. Indust. Med. **8**: 155–165.
40. ZOLOTH, S. et al. 1986. Asbestos disease screening by non-specialists: Results of an evaluation. Am. J. Pub. Health **76**: 1392–1395.
41. CROWLEY, A. E. & S. ETZEL. 1986. Progress against cancer? New Engl. J. Med. **314**: 1226–1232.
43. WEEKS, J. L. & M. FOX. 1983. Fatality rates and regulatory policies in bituminous coal mining, United States 1959–1981. Am. J. Public Health **73**: 1278–1280.
44. NICHOLSON, W. J. 1985. Cancer from occupational asbestos exposure: Projections 1965–2030. In Disability Compensation for Asbestos-Associated Disease in the United States. I. J. Selikoff, Ed. Mount Sinai Press. New York.
45. LANDRIGAN, P. J. et al. 1986. Silicosis in a grey iron foundry: The persistence of an ancient disease. Scand. J. Work Environ. Health **12**: 32–39.
46. OUDIZ, J. et al. 1983. A report on silica exposure levels in United States foundries. Am. Indus. Hygiene Assoc. J. **44**: 374–376.
47. American Public Health Association Policy Statement 8329. 1984. Compensation for and Prevention of Occupational Disease. Am. J. Public Health **74**: 292–295.
48. LEVY, B. 1985. The teaching of occupational health in United States medical schools. Am. J. Public Health **75**: 79–80.

Occupational Diseases: New Workforces, New Workplaces

BRUCE A. FOWLER[a] AND ELLEN K. SILBERGELD[a,b]

[a]*Toxicology Program and the Department of Pathology*
University of Maryland Medical School
Baltimore, Maryland 21201

[b]*Environmental Defense Fund*
Washington, D.C. 20036

A conference on the subject of occupational medicine is a timely opportunity to establish rational plans for reforming strategies and to determine what issues are likely to arise in the near future. This report deals with the impact of three rapid changes in occupational health in the future and with new techniques for recognizing and dealing with health effects in the workplace. The three changes, which are in process right now, relate to the workforce, the workplace, and the definition of adverse health effects in working populations. It is the thesis of this report that periods of change, like the present, provide opportunities to learn from the past in order to more effectively prevent occupational disease in the future.

Two major changes in the workplace as well as new developments in biomedicine will greatly influence the types of occupational diseases that are likely to occur over the next decade. First, demographically, the U.S. workforce is becoming less homogenous as a result of several socioeconomic factors. The second change is technologic, with new substances and new uses of old materials being exploited in new industries and organized in novel workplace structures. The third factor concerns the fact that new approaches to detect and assess the significance of early chemical-specific events in the progression of cell response and injury will challenge present concepts of disease and definition of toxicity. It should be a goal of all the sciences, clinical disciplines, and regulatory authorities associated with occupational health policy to marshal this new knowledge into an efficient and responsive program that will permit early detection of insidious chemically induced systemic organ damage before overt clinical toxicity occurs in new groups of workers exposed to new classes of chemical toxicants found in new industries or new settings of work.

CHANGES IN THE WORKFORCE

The U.S. workforce has undergone significant demographic changes over the past decade. Women, a broader range of racial and ethnic groups, and a wider age range of workers are now employed. More than half of all women between 18 and 65 now work outside the home; many teenagers work at least part-time, and many persons, for economic reasons or by choice, prolong employment beyond the legal retirement age of 62. Large shifts in the U.S. population over the last two decades have increased the percentage of Hispanic and Asian ethnic groups in the working and general population. Moreover, many of these groups are now employed in occupations formerly closed to them.

These changes will have many impacts on American society. Within the context of this report, diversification of the U.S. workforce raises concerns about the validity of current occupational health standards based on a reference population of young white males.[1] Although we cannot, on the basis of present knowledge, incorporate considerations of genetic or phenotypic heterogeneity into occupational health policy or clinical medicine, the increased diversity of the working population should be a basis for assuming a wider range of responses to chemical exposure (as in immunology and aging[2]).

In one obvious area, assuming a homogenous workforce limits the detection of effects that may occur in the modern workforce. For example, reproductive toxicology has historically not been a major occupational health concern when it could be assumed that workers—particularly in the chemical industry—were male. This assumed—without extensive scientific foundation—that relatively few toxins affect the male reproductive system to reduce fertility or to affect the fetus.[3] However, exposure to chemicals such as kepone, dibromochloropropane, and ethylene dibromide has induced infertility in men.[4] With the entry of women into employment in which chemicals potentially toxic to reproduction are such, all three organisms of reproductive importance—male, female, and the fetus—may be present in the occupational environment. The social response to this change over the past decade has been repressive: directly perceived risks have been reduced by restricting the opportunities for women's employment rather than by reducing the presence of the toxins in the workplace environment.[5] As women became increasingly represented in such occupations, this policy was legally ruled in some instances as blatantly discriminatory. It is critical that we do not repeat this pattern of protecting the workplace from the worker, rather than the other way around, until accurate methods are validated that permit within the working population the identification of subgroups with critical differences in responsiveness to toxic chemicals.

Second, workers are now being employed in different settings from those where opportunities for chemical exposure have traditionally occurred. As will be discussed, many new technologies evolve as small entrepreneurial businesses—some even starting in garages—in small scale operations in which unionization rarely succeeds and in which the size of the operation is insufficient to support corporate medical departments, epidemiologic services, toxicology research, or other activities that facilitate—but do not guarantee—early detection and long-term followup of occupational diseases. The size of the workplace may fall below that which triggers inspections or reporting requirements. Very broadly speaking, exposures to new chemicals or novel operations of the present or future in which contact with new hazards may occur will most likely involve these new companies. In the absence of unionization, worker rolls for retrospective epidemiologic/clinical studies will not be available; in workforces with high dependence on part-time or contractual workers, there may be no medical record keeping. It will be difficult even to use hospital records or admissions for surveillance purposes.[6]

NEW TECHNOLOGIES AND WORKPLACES: EXAMPLES

Hazardous Waste Management

One occupational category that has grown in response to new obligations in environmental policy concerns waste management and hazardous waste cleanup. This latter activity is now budgeted at 12 billion dollars over the next 5 years of

CERCLA, the national Superfund law. In addition to these federally authorized activities, private sector waste management and remedial actions will involve further multibillion dollar resources. The need to develop new worker education and protection methods in these novel situations has been recognized. NIOSH has been authorized under the Superfund amendments to develop model training and education programs for hazardous waste workers.

Hazardous waste management and cleanup are remarkably diverse activities. They include decontamination of buildings and other facilities, detection of hidden wastes, removal and storage of wastes, application of detoxification and destruction technologies, and construction of barriers between wastes and environment. Hazards of such activities include dangers of explosion and fires and contact with highly corrosive agents and with materials of unknown toxicity in highly complex mixtures, presenting in all potential routes of exposure. At most sites where wastes have been poorly managed, there is little information as to the specific materials on site, their amounts, or the degree to which they have already been released from drums or other containers.[7] Many well-known toxic materials, including halogenated hydrocarbon solvents, pesticides, and metals, have frequently been detected at hazardous waste dump sites. Experience has shown that under such circumstances, workers can become exposed to hazardous substances in waste, as reported in a study by Baker et al.[8] on PCB uptake by sewage treatment workers.

Because of the range of uncertainty concerning hazards involved in these occupations, most workers are required to wear a high level of personal protective gear, including a complete covering with impermeable material and an enclosed breathing apparatus. In addition, many operations have set up medical monitoring and continued surveillance as requirements for cleanup crews. The experience of New York State with decontamination operations at the Binghamton State Office Building exemplifies a strategy developed to deal with these uncertainties. At Binghamton, a program for clinical monitoring and followup, past the time of completion of employment in this job, was instituted. Workers' blood was periodically sampled and assayed for the presence of PCBs and for certain endogenous materials thought to be biologic markers for exposure to PCBs and related compounds, specifically plasma triglycerides and serum enzymes of liver cell origin. A preemployment clinical examination was developed to derive a "baseline" health status record against which postemployment exposure and medical history could be tracked. To date, no indication of overexposure has been found.[9]

Semiconductor Manufacture

During the past decade there has been a marked growth in the semiconductor microelectronic industry with increases in the use of some novel organic, inorganic, and organometallic compounds. In particular, expanded development of III–V semiconductors, such as gallium arsenide (GaAs), has introduced a number of new compounds and, most importantly, new manufacturing procedures into the workplace. The toxicologic data base for these agents is currently extremely limited or nonexistent, so that it is extremely difficult to predict potential risks to workers in this industry. It is worth noting, however, that women comprise approximately 50% of this rapidly turning over workforce. As just noted, this demographic pattern raises special concerns with regard to noncarcinogenic endpoints in this working population. A widely publicized scientific study at the University of Massachusetts reported increased rates of adverse reproductive outcome in women at a microelectronics facility; however, to date, these findings have not been confirmed.

Biotechnology

Biotechnology is another new and rapidly developing industry with enormous potential. Again, it uses unusual chemical reagents and biologic entities in unique ways. At present, the toxicologic potential of many of these agents has not been completely evaluated from the perspective of product safety, occupational health, or environmental consequences. This rapidly expanding field hence represents a special challenge to toxicologists, occupational health physicians, and regulatory agencies, because it will require the development of new approaches for detecting exposures and assuring the safety of both this new technology and its products.

Service and Office Sectors

The U.S. economy is widely recognized as shifting base from basic industries to one in which most jobs will be in the service industry and office work.[10] Such workplaces are not usually thought of as involving exposures to hazardous substances, although they must be stressful.[11] However, the service sector includes opportunities for contact with cleaners and fumigants, some of which are mutagenic and otherwise toxic. Office workers increasingly work with computers, and health concerns over VDTs remain unanswered. Moreover, the physical structure of these workplaces may itself have an impact on workers' health; the "sick building syndrome" has been described as a condition of office workers resulting from exposure to chemicals released from synthetic materials in office products and furniture, which become concentrated in the air because of the low-ventilation rate of modern office buildings (AVPH).[12] Experience with formaldehyde demonstrates how deleterious such exposure can be. Formaldehyde is released from a variety of wood products made with urea-formaldehyde resins and from urea-formaldehyde foam insulation materials; concerns over the possible carcinogenic properties of formaldehyde have curtailed its use in the United States.[13] Reports on neuropsychologic dysfunction in workers exposed to formaldehyde vapors in enclosed spaces, however, clearly show its toxic effects. In a study of workers in a Danish nursery school, in which formaldehyde-treated pressboard was used extensively, a range of sensitization-like and neuropsychologic problems, including nausea, headaches, muscle aches, and itching, was reported by workers.[14]

CHANGES IN BIOMEDICAL UNDERSTANDING OF OCCUPATIONAL DISEASES

The advent of new approaches for assessing preclinical toxicity from low-dose exposures to chemical mixtures in recent years has the potential for markedly improving our ability to detect and to specify the chemical species responsible for an observed biochemical or physiologic change. This area of research, on biologic markers, will change the manner in which we define both exposure and effect.[15] It is envisaged that as analytic methods are refined, and more precise relationships further established between biologic indicators and cell injury, these tools will provide a new foundation for risk assessment and regulation. Even in the absence of validating studies on the predictive power of such markers (e.g., long-term prospective followup), the detection of such alterations, in the context of ever more biochemically oriented medicine, will continue to stimulate debates as to the appropriateness of reducing exposures.

Some specific examples of these biomarker approaches are as follows:

a. Chemical-Induced Alterations in Heme/Porphyrin Metabolism: The heme biosynthesis pathway is highly sensitive to a wide variety of both organic and inorganic chemicals.[16] Chemically induced selective inhibition of enzymes in the

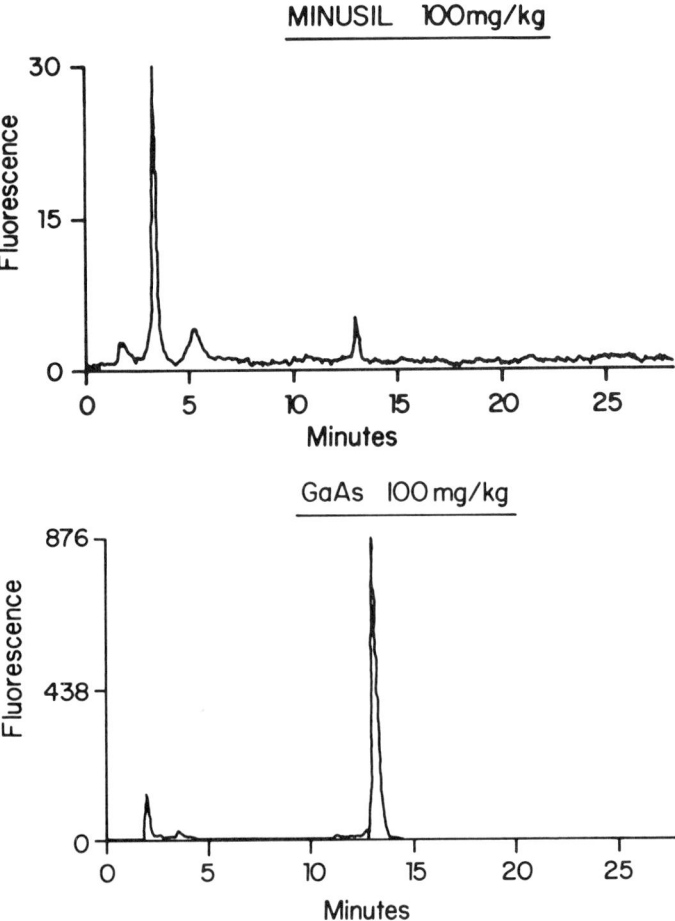

FIGURE 1. Higher performance liquid chromatography analyses of urine samples from silica particle (minusil) control (*top*) and gallium arsenide (*bottom*) at 7 days following a single intratracheal instillation of 100 mg/kg of either agent. Note the increase in relative fluorescence scale on ordinate in gallium arsenide–treated animals.

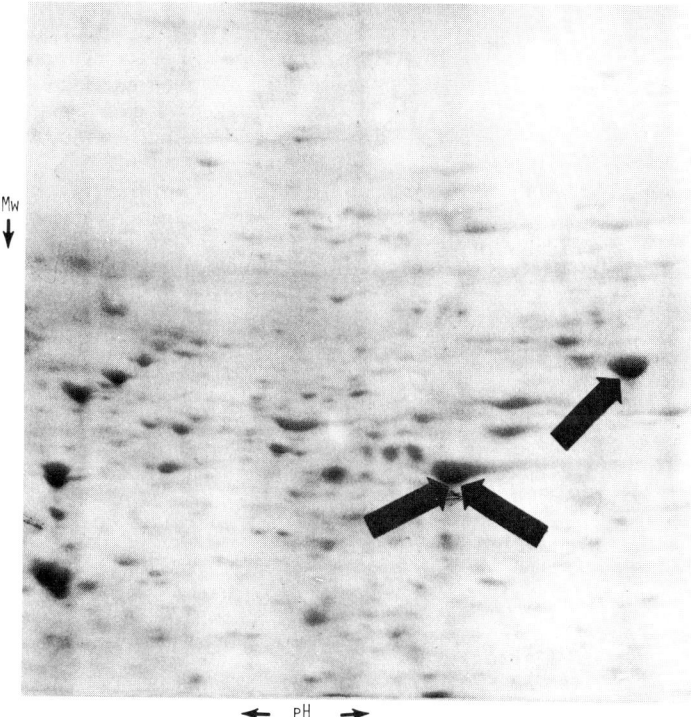

FIGURE 2. Coomassie-Blue stained two-dimensional gel map from a control rat kidney, showing normal gene expression pattern. Molecular weight (Mw) and pH axes are indicated. The marker proteins tubulin (*single arrow*) and actin (*double arrow*) are shown.

pathway, with resultant urinary excretion of specific porphyrin/heme precursors, has been effectively used for decades to monitor the *in vivo* bioavailability of major toxicants such as lead. This class of biomarkers was recently expanded, in experimental systems, to include III–V semiconductors such as gallium arsenide[17-21] (FIG. 1) and, as such, offers great promise for detecting ongoing cell injury at intermediate dose levels, *before* overt clinical manifestation of toxicity. The point here is that well-established and well-understood classes of biomarkers with a long history of both clinical and experimental usefulness may also be readily applied now to new classes of chemical toxicants.

b. Two-Dimensional Gel Electrophoresis of "Stress Protein" Induction Patterns: There are several techniques that hold great promise in the early detection of biologic changes at the biochemical level. One of these is the advent of computerized image analysis of two-dimensional gel electrophoretograms (FIG. 2) for monitoring "stress protein" induction patterns in target tissues that represent early genetic responses to chemical insult. With further refinement, these techniques may provide new levels of sensitivity for "fingerprinting" chemical insults at the genetic level of biologic organization.[22,23]

c. *In Vivo* Nuclear Magnetic Resonance (NMR) Spectroscopy of Tissue ATP Concentrations or Altered Metabolic Products: *In vivo* NMR is another technique that has recently been extended to nonmammals to measure changes in cellular energy metabolism (e.g., ATP levels) after acute exposure to toxicants that disrupt this essential cellular function[24] (FIG. 3). Again, with refinement and further development of correlations with other morphologic or biochemical parameters of cell injury, this technique may be used as a biomarker for monitoring injury *in vivo*. Other investigators[25] have used proton NMR for monitoring changes in urinary excretion of metabolic products or for imaging analysis.[26]

d. *In vivo* X-Ray Fluorescence for Lead Deposition in Bone: *In vivo* x-ray fluorescence was recently used to evaluate bone stores of metals such as Pb which are extensively deposited in the skeleton.[27] They may be later mobilized from these stores, resulting in episodic exposure conditions that occur decades after occupational exposure has ceased.[28] Again, with further refinement, this technique could be used for monitoring skeletal deposition of not only lead but also perhaps other bone-seeking elements.

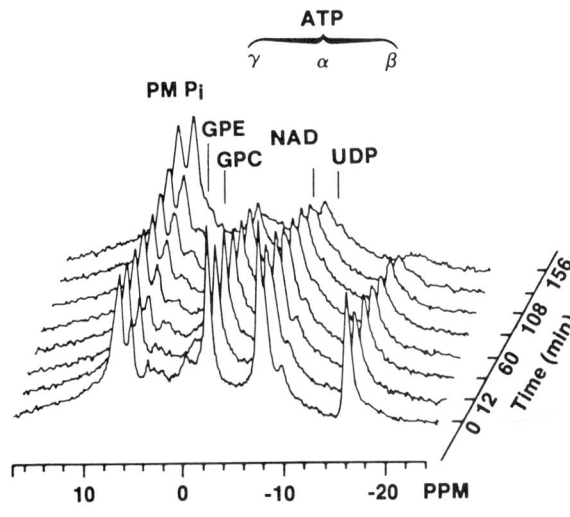

FIGURE 3. Time course of rat hepatic ^{31}P NMR spectra via *in vivo* surface coil technique, showing less ATP following a single intraveneous injection of sodium arsenite (As^{3+}). (From Chen *et al.*[24] 1986.)

CONCLUSION

The changing aspects of the workplace and the workforce, coupled with changes in methods available for assessing chemical changes, need to be accommodated within new strategies for preventing occupational disease. Fundamentally, all these changes are likely to make disease detection and prevention more complex. To avoid repeating the past, several changes in health policy and strategy are clearly necessary. First, we should more strategically anticipate the introduction of new substances or, in the case of biotechnology, new organisms into the workplace and provide for the timely accumulation of the necessary toxicologic data for assessing likely risks. This is currently not done in anything like an appropriate fashion, and it is imperative that state, federal, and international agencies begin taking *prospective* approaches to these new industries or processes. For example, with the deployment of the recent extraordinary advances of superconductivity application, we can already anticipate that some very exotic organometals will be put into production; ytterbium and yttrium compounds have already been shown to support superconductivity. We know nothing about the toxicity of these metals or of the organocomplexes used in superconductivity experiments. Yet it is reasonable to anticipate that such organometals may well be biologically active; the nondegradability of metals as elements means that, once released, they will probably accumulate within the environment over time, as experience with lead, mercury, manganese, and cadmium have already shown.[29] It is critical to activate the information-forcing principles of Section 5 of the Toxic Substances Control Act to obtain the necessary information to reach reasonable decisions about risk *before* such compounds become widely dispersed in commerce and the environment. For materials that are not new but are newly exploited in new technologies, it is important that the powers of the "significant new use rule" in TSCA be expanded and implemented to catch these changes in potential exposure before they occur.

REFERENCES

1. CASTLEMAN, B. & G. ZIEM. 1988. Corporate influence on threshold limit values. Am. J. Ind. Med. **13:** 531–559.
2. NAGEL, J. E. & W. H. ADLER. 1987. Effects of aging on immune function and reserve capacity. *In* Environmental Chemical Exposures & Immune System Integrity. E. J. BURGER, R. G. TARDIFF & J. A. BELLANTI, eds.: 195–203. Princeton Scientific Pub. Co. Princeton, NJ.
3. SCIALLI, A. R. 1988. Editorial. Reproduc. Toxicol. 1: 91–92.
4. BARLOW, S. M. & F. M. SULLIVAN. 1984. Reproductive Hazards of Industrial Chemicals. Academic Press, London.
5. BERTIN, J. E. 1986. Reproduction, Women, and the Workplace: Legal Issues. Occupational Medicine. State of the Art Reviews. Vol. 1, No. 3. Hanley-Belfus, Inc. Philadelphia, PA.
6. LANDRIGAN, P. J. 1983. Toxic exposure and psychiatric disease: Lessons from Epid. of Cancer. ACTA Psychiatric (Scand.) 67 (Suppl. 303): 353.
7. PHILLIPS, A. M. & E. K. SILBERGELD. 1985. Health studies at hazardous waste sites: Where are we now? Am. J. Ind. Med. **8:** 1–7.
8. BAKER, E. K., P. J. LANDRIGAN, C. J. GLUECK, M. M. ZACK, J. A. LIDDLE, V. W. BURSE, W. J. HOUSEWORTH & L. L. NEEDHAM. 1980. Metabolic consequences of exposure to PCBs in sewage sludge. Am. J. Epidemiol. **112:** 553-563.
9. FITZGERALD, G. F., F. STANDFAST, L. YOUNGBLOOD, J. MELIUS & D. JANERICH. 1985. Assessing the health effects of pollution exposures to PCB's, dioxins and furans from electrical transformer fires: The Binghamton State Office Building Medical Surveillance Program. Arch. Env. Health **41:** 368–376.
10. U.S. Department of Labor, Bureau of Labor Statistics, *Employment and Earnings*, 1988.
11. STEIN, Z. A., M. W. SUSSER & M. C. HATCH. 1986. Work during pregnancy: Physical and psychosocial strain. Occup. Med. State of the Art Reviews **1:** 405–410.
12. STOLWIJK, J. Impact of new developments in shelter on human health. Paper presented at "Environmental Health in the 21st Century," NIEHS, 1988, Environmental Health Perspectives. In press.
13. HILEMAN, B. 1984. Formaldehyde: Assessing the risk. Environ. Sci. Technol. **18:** 216A-221A.
14. OLSEN, J. H. & M. DOSSING. 1982. Formaldehyde-induced symptoms in day care centers. Am. Ind. Hyg. Assoc. **43:** 336–370.
15. NRC, Committee on Biological Markers, 1987. Biological markers in environmental health research. Environ. Health Perspec. **74:** 309.

16. SILBERGELD, E. K. & B. A. FOWLER, Eds. 1987. Mechanisms of Chemical-Induced Porphyrinopathies. Ann. N.Y. Acad. Sci. **514**: 1–352.
17. WOODS, J. S. & B. A. FOWLER. 1978. Altered regulation of mammalian hepatic heme biosynthesis and urinary porphyrin excretion during prolonged exposure to sodium arsenate. Toxicol. Appl. Pharmacol. **43**: 361–371.
18. WEBB, D. R., I. G. SIPES & D. E. CARTER. 1984. *In vitro* solubility and *in vivo* toxicity of gallium arsenide. Toxicol. Appl. Pharmacol. **76**: 96–104.
19. GOERING, P. L. & B. A. FOWLER. 1987. Mechanism of urinary excretion of δ-aminolevulinic acid following intratracheal instillation of gallium arsenide. Ann. N.Y. Acad. Sci. **514**: 330–332.
20. GOERING, P. L., R. R. MARONPOT & B. A. FOWLER. 1988. Effect of intratracheal administration of gallium arsenide on δ-aminolevulinic acid dehydratase in rats: Relationship to urinary excretion of aminolevulinic acid. Toxicol. Appl. Pharmacol. **92**: 179–193.
21. BAKEWELL, W. E., JR., P. L. GOERING, M. P. MOORMAN & B. A. FOWLER. Arsine and gallium arsenide-induced alternations in heme metabolism. Proceedings of the 27th Annual Meeting, Society of Toxicology, Dallas, TX, February 1988.
22. MISTRY, P., C. MASTRI & B. A. FOWLER. 1987. Lead-induced alterations of renal gene expression within cellular compartments. The Toxicologist **7**: 78.
23. ANDERSON, N. L., F. A. GIERE, S. L. NANCE, M. A. GEMMELL, S. L. TOLLAKSEN & N. G. ANDERSON. 1987. Effects of toxic agents at the protein level: Quantitative measurement of 213 mouse liver proteins following xenobiotic treatment. Fund. Appl. Toxicol. **8**: 39–50.
24. CHEN, B., C. T. BURT, P. L. GOERING, B. A. FOWLER & R. E. LONDON. 1986. *In vivo* ^{31}P nuclear magnetic resonance studies of arsenite-induced changes in hepatic phosphate levels. Biochem. Biophys. Res. Commun. **139**: 228–234.
25. NICHOLSON, J. K. & K. P. R. GARTLAND. 1986. A nuclear magnetic resonance approach to investigate the biochemical and molecular effects of nephrotoxins on cells, membranes, and disease including renal. E. REIN, G. M. W. COOK & J. P. LUZIO, Eds.: 397–408. Plenum Press. New York.
26. ANDREASEN, N. C. 1988. Brain imaging: Applications in psychiatry. Science. **239**: 1381–1388.
27. CHRISTOFFERSSON, J. O., A. SCHUTZ, L. AHLGREN, B. HAEGER-ARONSEN, S. MATTSON & S. SKERFVING. 1984. Lead in finger bone analyzed *in vivo* in active and retired lead workers. Am. J. Ind. Med. **6**: 447–457.
28. SILBERGELD, E. K. 1986. Maternally mediated exposure of the fetus: In utero exposure to lead and other toxins. Neurotoxicology **7**: 557–568.
29. NRIAGU, J. O. (ed.) 1984. Changing Metal Cycles and Human Health. Life Sciences Research Report 28. Springer-Verlag. Berlin.

Discussion: Part I

M. A. EL BATAWI (*World Health Organization, Geneva, Switzerland*): The opening presentation made an attempt at defining occupational disease. The World Health Organization has published a book on the interaction between work and health demonstrating the different levels at which work may influence health. For example, the occupational disease of lead poisoning cannot be caused by carbon monoxide; it has to be caused by lead exposure. That is a cause/effect relationship—one cause, one effect. Other such relationships include carbon monoxide–carboxyhemoglobin, asbestos–asbestosis, and silica–silicosis. These can be called the "hundred percent" relationships.

Beyond those few relatively straightforward examples, however, we consider many of the diseases that affect the working population and human beings as a continuum: a person has his work; he interacts with so many pollutants in food and air and water; he undergoes stress at work and stress at home; and all these things add up to the well-named diseases of multifactorial causes. Now, I am distinguishing between the terms "occupational" and "work-related," which implies a partial relatedness. Here we do not find causes, we find risk factors. And there is a difference between a cause and a risk factor. For example, if you discuss chronic obstructive pulmonary disease (COPD) or occupational asthma, smoking plays a very important role in causation as does pollution in the work environment and irritants from the atmosphere. Multiple factors play a role in COPD, yet when you diagnose a case of chronic obstructive pulmonary disease in a person exposed to dust, you are faced with the question of compensation. Do you compensate this person and declare the condition an occupational disease? Or is the disease only partly work-related? To what extent is it related to occupation?

Epidemiologists are facing a crucial and a very important matter in assessing the role that work may play in the causation of such general diseases as the low back pain syndrome, hypertension, cardiovascular diseases, and stress-related conditions. Unless you consider the person in his or her totality, you will never be able to pin down the causative factors or the risk factors towards which you aim to direct the control measures.

IRVING J. SELIKOFF (*Mt. Sinai School of Medicine, New York, N.Y.*): Dr. Fowler, of the 100,000 or so workers now in these high-tech industries, have baseline surveillance mechanisms been set up to see what the problems are going to be?

BRUCE A. FOWLER (*University of Maryland Medical School, Baltimore, Md.*): There is a great concern in the semi-conductor industry about these issues. They are moving very rapidly in the direction of setting up good surveillance procedures. In this case, it is the large manufacturing companies that are very concerned about their workers, who represent a highly trained work force, and it is in everyone's best interest that these workers be maintained in the best of health. However, the greater concern is with the smaller companies, those with fewer than 50 or 100 employees. These workers may not get enough attention and may fall through the cracks of a surveillance system that is being set up mainly by the larger companies.

MORTON CORN (*The Johns Hopkins University, Baltimore, Md.*): As you may know, at the Johns Hopkins School of Hygiene and Public Health we have designed and proposed epidemiologic studies for certain of the larger semiconductor companies. I would not want the impression to be left that the exposures in that industry at the leading edge of chip manufacture are of a magnitude that would require the adoption of porphyrin testing. Porphyrin testing would require massive exposures if the doses demonstrated by Dr. Fowler were present but they are not. Therefore, that technique will not serve to answer the allegations of adverse reproductive outcomes in front-end workers. The method is exciting, but it is a technology suitable for massive exposures. The other technology, the one that lends itself to imaging, has promise. The industry is anxious to determine whether these effects are indeed occurring. However, the technology for surveillance referred to by Dr. Selikoff does not yet exist to the point where it could be immediately applied among thousands of workers.

SELIKOFF: Dr. Corn, are biological samples from these workers being frozen, so that later on, as technologies improve, they will be available for examination and for possible subsequent analysis of parameters that will emerge from the testing of these new technologies?

CORN: To my knowledge that is not being done at this time.

PAUL D. BRANDT-RAUF (*Columbia University School of Public Health, New York, N.Y.*): I want to note, in reference to this issue, that at the November 1987 semiconductor meeting in Boston two papers were presented on the issue of arsenic screening in workers exposed to gallium arsenide. They showed that the exposures, even in the worst cases, are probably very low; these studies were done in Japan and Canada.

The suggestion by Dr. Corn that these very low doses may not affect the enzyme systems may or may not be true. I am sure you are familiar with Dean Carter's study in Arizona that supports Dr. Fowler's results and suggests that, even at low-dose levels in animals, there is a coproporphyrin peak in the urine. I think, therefore, that the possible utility of biological markers in this industry should be viewed as unsettled. I think that the Japanese may be banking specimens in their studies.

CORN: My point was not that it is settled. I came away from that meeting detecting a very optimistic note for the gel system, but I believe that there is no evidence at this point that optimism is justified. It would be wonderful if the technique proves to be sufficiently sensitive, but I am aware of the exposure levels in the sector I specifically pinpointed, and I am not optimistic for this particular method.

FOWLER: I agree with you in part, Dr. Corn; that is the reason for the second set of indicators. Not one of these tools is a panacea. However, it is important to emphasize that our ability to measure these changes is improving too; that is really the point in showing that the limits of detection for these indicators, like limits of detection for other kinds of analyses, are improving all the time. Soon we may be able to sort this out, particularly at moderate to elevated exposure levels. Perhaps the stress proteins may prove to be an even better biological marker than the porphyrins.

BRANDT-RAUF: In connection with that, have you looked at heat-shock proteins?

FOWLER: That is basically what we are doing now. If you spend some time in the sun or burn your hand, heat-shock proteins are released into the blood stream by injured cells. The cells respond to that stress by turning on several genes which encode protein products called heat-shock proteins.

Since 1971, investigators have begun to examine other chemically induced stress proteins. We have been working on stresses caused by metals. Dr. Norman Anderson had a paper published last fall in *Fundamental and Applied Toxicology* on proteins stimulated by a number of organic chemicals and drugs. Given the large number of possible spots on the gels with the computerized image analysis, he is able to sort out each chemical. In other words, he can get a fingerprint, if you will, for the genetic response corresponding to a given chemical. My point in showing these data is to try to generate some optimism. We are confronted with a situation of having a new class of individuals in the workplace who are exposed to new chemicals in large numbers. Thus we have some new problems, and we must move as quickly as possible to address them. There is no other choice, and no time for the luxury of pessimism.

BRANDT-RAUF: I would like to pose one other technical question. The conventional wisdom has been that gallium and gallium salts are not toxic because they are not absorbed. That point has been supported by studies of gallium arsenide. Do you believe differently?

FOWLER: The point in Dean Carter's paper was that he was able to follow the biological effects of arsenic using the porphyrins. He was not able to measure gallium, which is very difficult to measure by conventional atomic absorption techniques and was always below his detection limit. That did not mean that it was not there; he just could not measure it. With regard to the enzyme delta-amino levulinic acid dehydratase, we found that indium is a very potent inhibitor, as are other elements in the group 3 category.

FRANKLIN MIRER (*United Auto Workers' Union, Detroit, Mich.*): I have several comments of a policy nature. The first is with regard to large versus small industry. Conventional wisdom has it that the big plants are safer and have lower exposure levels than in the little plants, but this has not been borne out, especially in the foundries. The same observation was true in the case of safety and fatalities within the auto industry.

The second point is that high-tech products do not necessarily result from high-tech production, particularly in the electronics industry. Often such materials are the products of small assembly work that can be easily shipped out to Thailand or Singapore, rather than being performed with well-educated workforces.

The third point is that a scattershot approach to screening, where the effects have not been well defined in advance, often represents a cosmetic effort which consumes a lot of money. It looks like it is doing something, but is actually not a good use of resources.

The last point is that a lot of the surveillance activity in the microelectronics industry was stimulated by the DEC study which reported reproductive effects in exposed women. From the public policy point of view, with respect to the electronics industry, you have to look at which slices of the process are contained in various sectors of the industry. We do not want to define semiconductors as a problem, when it is really an electronics assembly or circuitboard problem.

FOWLER: I generally agree with most of those points, Dr. Mirer. The issue here, from the point of basic science, is that once some of the scientific questions are addressed, and the relationships between exposures and changes in indicators and in toxic endpoints are delineated, then some of these tests should be tried in the workplace. I would not advocate trying them out now, but I would let you know that basic science is not standing still. These tools are being developed and it might not be unwise to think about banking specimens.

STUART SHALAT (*Yale University, New Haven, Conn.*): Technology is changing very rapidly in the semi-conductor industry. If you went into a plant today, and then went back in a month or two, the techniques and the chemical exposures may have changed very radically. Dr. Fowler, how will some of these approaches be useful in terms of having a broad-based ability to look at the biological effects of completely different compounds?

FOWLER: A point worth mentioning here in regard to the porphyrins is the system's sensitivity to a wide range of organic solvents and organic chlorinated compounds; I refer you here to Volume 514 of *Annals of the New York Academy of Sciences*.[a]

Another point to bear in mind is that people make mistakes. Episodic exposures and accidents are not completely farfetched in the high-technology industries, which deal with large amounts of chemicals. In 1981, approximately 30 tons of gallium were going into semiconductor manufacturing, and that was before this process started to grow. Consequently we need to be constantly on the alert for new and more sensitive tools to bring to bear on these problems. As the technology changes, accidents and sentinel exposures are going to give us examples of where exposures can occur even though they are not supposed to, such as the case in Bhopal. I hope that in the discipline of toxicology we will think in an anticipatory mode. We are going to try to get ahead of some of these problems and to be vigilant.

JACQUES DUNNIGAN (*Québec Asbestos Institute*): My question relates to the presentation by Dr. Ozonoff and relates to the ambiguity in identifying and defining quantitatively the causal agent. Why is it that at this scientific meeting in 1988 we are still using the word *asbestos*, which is a commercial rather than a scientific term? Why are we still talking about asbestos-related disease, when we should be talking about chrysotile, amphiboles or even more specifically crocidolite, amosite and so on? When we do not specifically identify the type of asbestos, it means that we do not have much of a feel for the exposure. I would like to touch on the use of another expression, "work-related disease." I agree that there are very clear work-related injuries or accidents when you are talking about a machine or the malfunctioning of a machine, but that expression is not useful as it relates to dust or volatile agents. For those I would rather use the expression "exposure-related" disease because we are aware that there are work situations where there are low exposures and there are no diseases. What do you call these diseases then? To sum up, I would much prefer using the specific words for the causal agents and to talk about exposure-related disease rather than work-related disease.

ARTHUR UPTON, CHAIRMAN (*New York University Medical Center, New York, N.Y.*): Thank you for your remarks. I think your question was more rhetorical than interrogative, and we accept your recommendation to be more precise.

JEFFREY LEE (*University of Utah, Provo, Utah*): Mr. Cheek in his presentation commented on the need to show an increase or doubling of relative risk in order to establish a preponderance of evidence that any individual's disease is attributed to a particular cause. Then he went on to talk about the High Risk Worker Notification bill. I would like to know whether or not he is implying that a doubling of relative risk is necessary to trigger the provisions of such a bill.

DR. WILLIAM NICHOLSON: I will answer that because Mr. Cheek has left. The doubling provision is not part of the high-risk bill. However, I would like to comment on the implications of the doubling provision for compensation. Consider the example of asbestos, and specifically the examples of chrysotile asbestos and amosite asbestos, each of which has been shown in some worker groups to produce a ten-fold excess risk of lung cancer over that of persons not exposed. We are talking about a very high-risk agent. If one looks at the distribution of

---

[a] Mechanisms of Chemical-Induced Porphyrinopathies. Edited by Ellen K. Silbergeld and Bruce A. Fowler. *Annals of the New York Academy of Sciences* **514**: 1–352 (1987).

exposures to asbestos in past work circumstances, including shipyards and others, the vast majority of workers, such as shipyard workers employed for short periods of time, were exposed to asbestos at levels that gave rise to a risk of less than two. If you calculate the number of persons who would be compensated, including those who would have developed lung cancer by happenstance with a relative risk greater than two, the total number is about 25% of the actual number of cases of lung cancer that are asbestos-related in the entire exposure circumstance. In other words, in the case of asbestos, the requirement of a doubling provision would compensate in only 25% of the cases of disease that was produced by asbestos. Thus, in looking at these circumstances, one must consider that in most occupational settings, the risk will be less than two-fold.

In terms of compensation, one must look then at appropriate mechanisms of dealing with that feature: either have compensation criteria—all or none—at a lower than two-fold risk, or have proportionate pro-rated payments. My point here is that a doubling criterion places an extreme limitation on workers' compensation were it to be strictly applied.

BRANDT-RAUF: The House version of the High Risk Worker Notification bill had a cut-off of 30%, that is, high risk was defined as a rate 30% greater than that of the comparable population not exposed by virtue of a hazardous occupation. That was the original Gaydos bill. Later, the criterion was changed to "significant excess."

DOROTHY WIGMORE: I am an occupational hygienist with the Manitoba Federation of Labour Occupational Health Center. Obviously we are concerned about work-related disease and so I have looked at implementation through legislation of a full occupational hygiene program that includes not only identification of hazards and health surveillance, but also an attempt to measure and control the problems. I noted one thing missing from Dr. Landrigan's talk, however, and that is a recommendation for enforcement by government agencies of appropriate standards. If you go back to some of the questions raised earlier by Dr. Selikoff about who is responsible, it is very obvious, in your country as well as in mine, that inspections are not being done. You cannot do a proper job in your prevention program if you do not have enforcement and inspection. I am wondering, therefore, what you recommend be done once a problem arises.

PHILIP LANDRIGAN (*Mt. Sinai School of Medicine, New York, N.Y.*): You are absolutely correct that OSHA field inspections are few and far between. Too many inspections take place at a desk where an inspector reviews safety records and then tries to derive a judgement about health hazards without making an actual visit to the factory. This approach is contrary to the best dictates of what constitutes preventive medicine in occupational health and is a national disgrace. It is clear that one of the important recommendations that will emerge from this workshop will be a call for more vigorous enforcement of the Occupational Safety and Health Act.

Also, we have to address the fact that funding for training programs in occupational health has been cut by more than 50% since 1981 and thus the number of doctors, industrial hygienists, and occupational health nurses now in training programs is less than half of what it was at the beginning of the decade. Unfortunately, therefore, the current situation will not be reversed overnight. It is important, however, that we begin to think constructively.

UPTON: In closing I would like to share a couple of the high points as I have seen them. We began with the theme of the meeting: how do we develop a platform in occupational health in the 1990s for the prevention of disease associated with workplace exposures? What is it we are trying to prevent? We have heard that the definition of the problem depends on the area you come from, and whether you view the problem as a lawyer, a physician, a worker, or as a sociologist: there does not seem to be one, clear, unifying definition. We do not have a clear idea at the outset of what we are trying to prevent. Obviously, then, there are going to be problems.

A further difficulty relates to scientific uncertainty. We are looking at a moving target. Twenty-twenty hindsight allows us to see a problem in retrospect, but we must be able to anticipate new diseases and new risk factors. I particularly enjoyed Dr. Selikoff's reference to mesothelioma and his point that only a few decades ago there was serious question as to whether such a disease even existed.

So we are going to have to rely on all of the tools at our disposal, using laboratory as well as epidemiologic evidence. However, we cannot rely solely on the epidemiologic evidence for it is a less sensitive factor and it comes too late for effective prevention. Additionally we have to consider the interactions of multiple factors. There are some obvious occupational injuries where we know the cause, yet much of the time we are dealing with causal contributions of differing importance. There is also the problem of latency, and the whole question of dose-effect relationships. Is there a low enough level of asbestos, of radiation, or of ethylene dibromide that is essentially without risk under any circumstances, irrespective of what other agents or risk factors may enter the picture?

I am reminded of a picture that I saw on a colleague's wall. It shows a pile of jackstraws, all of which are tan-colored except one, which is maroon. The caption reads, "Every new idea begins as a minority of one." The evidence with which we deal is frequently very fragmentary and controversial, certainly in its early stages. So the definition becomes, to some degree, judgmental. It is clear from what we heard that we have not begun to apply the knowledge we have. That is a real tragedy. Much better surveillance, record-keeping, compliance incentives, and legal and economic measures are needed. We have heard that the big industries are not necessarily the best, although they have the resources, one would think, to deal more effectively with these problems.

And finally, of course, we have heard much about the need for dedicated individuals to work on the problems at every level.

PART II. WORKPLACE REGULATION AND DISEASE PREVENTION

Workplace Regulation Gone Wrong

EULA BINGHAM

Department of Environmental Health
University of Cincinnati College of Medicine
Cincinnati, Ohio 45267

Although the title of this presentation implies a problem, it must be pointed out that many interest groups in this country do not believe there is anything wrong. A deregulatory movement—political, well-organized, and well-funded—prefers fewer standards to cover workplaces, a smaller enforcement activity, and generally a reversion to the voluntary effort that characterized workplace safety and health activities before passage of the Occupational Safety and Health Act of 1970.

Prevention of occupational disease requires control measures in the work environment that either eliminate the physical or chemical agent or reduce the level to a point where men and women can work without incurring disease. This concept of prevention is at the heart of the Occupational Safety and Health Act. A diagram of the concepts is presented in FIGURE 1. The identification of disease and contaminants responsible for the disease is the research activity of the academic community, National Institute of Occupational Safety and Health, other NIH institutes, industry, and labor. The result of such activity all too often ends after the first step: the identification of disease. However, the route to determining mechanisms of action that pinpoint the specific biochemical lesion may be a high-priority activity and consume everyone's attention. An excellent example of this approach has been the case of lead. The ill effects of lead exposure have been recognized for several hundred years, and while there has been a relentless pursuit of the biochemical lesions and their sites of occurence, little attention was paid to control of lead in the workplace until the OSHA lead standard was promulgated in 1979. It must be admitted that the pursuit of the molecular level mechanisms of toxicity has driven the recognition that more protective standards are necessary. However, the lag between identification and control, as well as the lag between understanding certain biochemical effects and control, has meant that "prevention" did not occur for thousands of workers or their families. (Do we need to be reminded that even now there are documented cases of children whose blood lead levels are excessive because of contamination by parental clothing?) Embodied in the Act is the notion that objective measures ensuring the control of physical and chemical agents shall be instituted. One set of "objective measures" is clearly spelled out as "Standards" in the Occupational Safety and Health Act. Included are the procedures (Enforcement) for ensuring that those standards are met.

If we accept the notion that there are enormous numbers of workers still at great risk of disease, injury, and death, then it may be worthwhile to analyze the record on standards promulgation for clues regarding the factors that either promote or inhibit the promulgation of standards. This record represents only one aspect of regulation, but it provides insight into understanding what is wrong—or right—with the current approaches.

Examination of the health and safety standards record of the Occupational Safety and Health Administration makes it obvious that the productivity is very

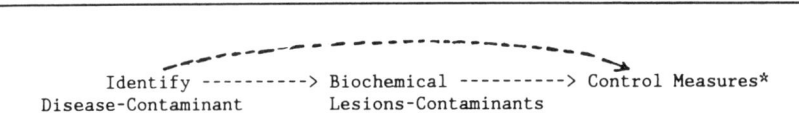

FIGURE 1. Paradigm for prevention of occupational disease.

low. TABLE 1 provides a list of the health standards since the Act was passed in 1970.

The first and most striking observation regarding the small number of standards is that during the first 10 years of the Act, between 1971 when the Act became effective and January 1981, 14 health standards were issued and 10 of those 14 were in the four years between 1977–81. The last seven years have produced six additional or updated standards. Clearly there is a factor that may be referred to as "political." This factor is listed in TABLE 2 along with several other factors that are "inhibiting."

TABLE 3 lists factors influencing the promulgation of standards. These factors are "promoting." Several of the factors listed in both TABLES 2 and 3 are mirror images. For example, the political factor represents ideological differences such that the leadership will encourage (promote) promulgation of standards or discourage (inhibit) their issuance. Another example is "advocacy," which can be *pro* or *con* for standards. For example, the well-organized, well-financed resis-

TABLE 1. Health Standards Record of 1971–1987: Occupational Safety and Health Administration

Areas of Regulation	Year of Standard Issue
Asbestos	1972
Carcinogens—14 substances	1974
Vinyl chloride	1974
Coke oven emissions	1976
Diving operations	1977
DBCP (1,2-dibromo-3-chloropropane)	1978
Acrylonitrile	1978
Benzene	1978
Arsenic	1978
Cotton dust	1978
Lead	1978
Carcinogen policy	1980
Access to medical and exposure records	1980
Noise abatement–hearing conservation	1981
Hazard communication	1983
Ethylene oxide	1984
Formaldehyde	1987
Field sanitation	1987
Asbestos	1987
Benzene	1987

TABLE 2. Factors Inhibiting Standard Promulgation

1. *Political.* There is often a high priority within an administration to deregulate (that is, to not issue standards)
2. *Lack of urgency.* The media and interest groups are slow to act.
3. *Advocacy.* Organized, well-financed resistance by the private and industrial sectors (e.g., the Institutes for Chemicals) work against regulation.
4. *Multisector coverage.* A noise standard, for example, affects chemical industries, the manufacturing sector, wholesale and retail operations, etc., and not just one industrial sector.
5. *Legal challenges.* Extensive and lengthy court action causes delays.
6. *Agency characteristics.* Low morale, frustration, and inadequate technical and legal resources within the regulating agency are another factor that impedes regulation.
7. *Red tape within the government.* Executive orders and OMB control, for example, also work against the promulgation of standards.

tance of the private industrial sector is an obvious roadblock to an agency's and/or administration's decisions to issue new standards. Conversely, the recent industrial pressure to issue a federal Hazard Communication Standard as a countermeasure to numerous state and local regulations was clearly significant in the Reagan Administration's decision to move forward even though the Office of Management and Budget (OMB) and the Bush Task Force on Regulatory Relief had delayed the standard's release.

Advocacy groups can promote the promulgation of standards through labor unions and public interest groups. There was a long delay in issuing the Cotton Dust Standard, but the legal intervention of several organizations (public interest and labor) was clearly instrumental in the eventual promulgation of the standard. The same scenario has occurred in the cases of field sanitation and exposure to formaldehyde and ethylene oxide.

If many industrial sectors are covered with a single rulemaking, the process becomes so enormous and complicated that the standard may languish (as with the noise standard). However, a very targeted or narrow standard, at least in terms of the number of industrial sectors and number of companies affected, results in a relatively smooth rulemaking (such as that of dibromochloropropane). This issue is particularly pertinent in view of the many recommendations that have been made for a greater number of generic standards.

Especially influential inhibiting factors are governmental red tape and inadequate resources (TABLE 2). The use of governmental red tape to slow the standards process was begun during the Ford administration, when an executive order required an economic impact analysis. The amount of red tape was alleviated

TABLE 3. Factors Promoting Standard Promulgation

1. *Political.* An administration places a high priority on the issuance of standards.
2. *Public outcry.* The media, environmental movement, and community groups are alerted to the problem and actively move to solve it.
3. *Health crises.* Examples include HIV transmission to health care workers or sterility among pesticide (DBCP) workers.
4. *Narrow sector regulated.* A highly targeted standard covering a few plants in one industrial sector.
5. *Adequate technical and legal resources.*

somewhat in the Carter Administration. However, OSHA staff still was required to present to an economic council a defense of the regulatory plan for compliance outlined in various standards. Interference from outside the Environmental Protection Agency escalated in the Reagan era by virtue of a new rule that required the Agency to defend its health conclusions regarding levels of exposure as well as preventive measures and compliance procedures to the superagency, the Office of Management and Budget. It is important to note that the OMB controls the Agency's budget and staffing levels so that the positions and edicts of the OMB really are not negotiable. This escalation in demands has been very successful in inhibiting both the number of standards and their content. An excellent example of this was the failure of OSHA to issue a short-term exposure limit (STEL) for ethylene oxide until a lawsuit was filed. As was mentioned before, the OMB inhibitors were overcome by a well-organized, influential, outside interest group, the industrial sector, when it urged the release of the Hazard Communication Standard (Labeling). Passage at state and local levels of numerous labeling standards made it in the best economic interest of industry to urge promulgation of the Hazard Communication Standard. Depending on the circumstances, a well-organized interest group can exert an almost irresistible pressure. A threat of a picket at the U.S. Department of Labor in 1975 by a union undoubtedly resulted in the formation of the Standards Advisory Committee for Coke Oven Emissions and the eventual standard.

The legal processes involved with promulgation can be prolonged so extensively that standard issuance is delayed for months or years. On the other hand, even when there are numerous "inhibitors," a court decision to require the Agency to issue a standard will eventually produce the standard, as was notably the case with cotton dust, field sanitation, and ethylene oxide.

In my mind there is another very persuasive promoting factor listed in TABLE 3—health crises. Such crises often bring outrage from the citizens, and various organized groups can be an enormous stimulus for passage of a specific standard, notably with asbestos and DBCP. The fact that the media was heavily involved in reporting episodes involving DBCP and asbestos clearly served as pressure to regulate. The nature of the illness can also impart a sense of urgency to the Agency, as is the case with irreversible diseases (such as cancer or neurological disease) or an outcome such as reduced reproductive potential (as caused by DBCP). The counterpoint or "inhibitor" here is not the lack of health crises or problems, but rather the failure to talk and read about the episodes. Lack of recognition by the public that there are still tragedies comparable to those associated with kepone and DBCP is due to the federal agencies' policies of "no comment" on such incidents, cutbacks in recordkeeping, and probably general apathy among the media regarding such episodes.

A willingness on the part of NIOSH and OSHA to report publicly such events, along with a concerned Congress, leads to demands for action. The data in the paper by Landrigan's group are significant because they indicate that during the last few years, when there was little media focus on occurrences of occupational disease, a false sense of security developed.

A task force supported by public and/or private institutions could develop data on five or six states so that more accurate projections can be made. The recommendations of the NAS report entitled Counting Injuries and Illness in the Workplace (1987) must be acted upon.

A series of strategies for change must occur. Consultation is alive and well, but the funding for it has not kept up with inflation. One can argue, however, that employers, almost 20 years after the Act was passed, should begin to pay for this service.

Criminal sanctions must be explored as a means of dealing with the most flagrant criminal acts in the workplace. This enforcement tactic is one that many public health professionals avoid. Yet the public demands strong criminal sanctions in death and injury cases resulting from drunk drivers, so how can one argue against such sanctions in the case of *People* vs. *Steven O'Neil, Film Recovery Systems, Inc.?*[a] While the courts and Congress settle the issue of preemption, OSHA can provide the technical assistance to local law enforcement agencies. Los Angeles County has a team to deal with such possible criminal violations—why shouldn't other big cities have the same?

Medical removal protection, as a critical aspect of the lead standard rules, has been credited with reducing exposures at a more rapid pace than skeptics considered possible. What other standards can be leveraged by this mechanism?

Alternative technologies must be considered as a means of eliminating hazards. NIOSH in concert with other federal agencies, academia, and industry could provide the leadership for such a new initiative. Substitutions for sand, certain solvents, and certain dyestuffs and intermediates could be addressed and recommendations made immediately. In 1912, a tax on matches made with white phosphorus forced an extremely hazardous operation to cease. Can this generation not be as creative? The free marketplace needs a nudge!

A series of recommendations from the labor movement have urged mechanisms to relieve the acute shortage of compliance officers. Consideration of an arrangement for on-site inspectors and local deputies must be made.

If you subscribe to the notion that something is wrong with workplace regulation, then what is it?—a lack of will and resolve at the highest political levels, money, American industry, leadership in the public health service and OSHA? We have heard, and will hear at this workshop, of state and local achievements that are dependent upon the isolated efforts of a few individuals, but these efforts need to be translated nationwide if we are to prevent disease in the next generation. This can best be done by federal leadership to bring the most innovative preventive measures from individual states to the whole country.

There are gaping holes in the standards list. A survey of bridge painting operations will provide the data that acute lead poisonings still occur all over this country, but we need not wait for the results to begin to issue a lead standard for the construction industry. Generic standards may be the most difficult to promulgate, but they provide an important approach. The first generic standards actually promulgated by OSHA were the Access to Medical and Exposure Records and the Carcinogen Policy Standards in 1980. Training, medical surveillance, solvents, and pesticides (manufacture), for example, all are possible areas for generic standards that cover larger groups of workers.

New source performance standards have long been a strategy at the EPA. What about a requirement for improved noise abatement and reduced solvent exposure releases in all new industrial facilities?

Recent revelations regarding working conditions in the meatpacking industry have caused many of us to recall Upton Sinclair's *The Jungle*, written in 1906, and we see that in this industry workers are still using 19th-century techniques in the "high tech" America of 1988. Recent comments from the industry indicate that

---

[a] Nos. 84C5064 and 83C11091 (Circuit Court, Cook County, Illinois, June 14, 1985).

competition is so great and profit margins so narrow that it is impossible to slow down the line and alleviate the ergonomic problems. It is ludicrous that a society so advanced in space and military technology cannot muster a collaborative industrial, federal, and academic effort to solve an antiquated assembly-line problem that is maiming hundreds of workers. I call such impotence a lack of leadership, a lack of vision, and a fundamental disregard for the workers.

Public Funding for Worker Education in Occupational Health and Safety

BARBARA BERNEY[a] AND DEBORAH NAGIN[b]

[b]Public Health Institute
New York, New York

This paper discusses the need for worker education in occupational health and safety, and presents models for publicly funded worker education programs within several states. The funding mechanisms and program designs are discussed and evaluated.

Occupational health education and training for workers and employers is an integral part of any effective program to control hazards at the workplace. Quality programs provide information to workers and employers on their rights and responsibilities under the law as well as specific information on hazards and their control, including organizational and administrative approaches to achieving compliance with laws and regulations.

Education also helps to build a constituency for maintaining occupational health and safety programs as well as regulation, enforcement, and new legislation. Constituencies may include workers and their labor union representatives, health and safety professionals, and safety conscious employers and their trade associations.

When the Occupational Safety and Health Act (OSHA) was passed in 1970, these constituent groups hoped that the law would result in the systematic reduction and elimination of hazards in American workplaces. It rapidly became apparent that OSHA, with its limited inspection force, was unable to accomplish this mammoth task. Instead, workers and others at the workplace who supported safer workplaces would have to take on the responsibility for getting workplace hazards corrected. For them to be effective, occupational health training was required. Acknowledging this need, federal OSHA, under the direction of Dr. Eula Bingham, Assistant Secretary of Labor in the Carter Administration, initiated the New Directions program. It represented the model for publicly funded worker education. The New Directions program funded unions, nonprofit organizations including local Committees on Safety and Health (COSH groups), universities, and trade associations to provide occupational health and safety education to workers and employers. (COSH groups are coalitions of local labor unions, health and safety professionals, and others concerned with occupational health. They often provide training and technical assistance to workers and unions on health and safety issues as well as putting pressure on unions, government, and employers to improve safety and health conditions.)

New Directions funds enabled organizations to develop and expand worker-education programs and hire professionals to carry out these programs. It seeded the development of innovative materials and teaching techniques. When funds were cut, these groups looked for new funding sources and acted to create programs at the state level.

---

[a] Address for correspondence: 3817 Upton Street, N.W., Washington, D.C. 20016.

The experience in several states, including Connecticut, Maine, Massachusetts, Michigan, and New York, suggests a range of such programs and provides lessons on how to finance and organize them. Each state program will be briefly described and the lessons discussed.

In Connecticut, legislation for the state-funded program was crafted with the help of the State AFL-CIO, many local unions, and the Connecticut COSH in collaboration with the Workers' Compensation Commission, and made part of labor's legislative package. The Connecticut Citizen Action Network also helped build grassroots support and lobby for the bill. With bipartisan support, it passed both houses unanimously.

The legislation's language provided for salaried staff and allowed, but did not require, grant giving.[1] The existing program, funded by an 0.2% assessment on workers' compensation premiums, collected approximately $500,000 in 1986. It gives virtually no grants for educational programs. The in-house staff focuses largely on how to obtain workers' compensation rather than on providing health and safety training.

The Michigan program is part of the original state OSHA plan (MiOSHA) passed in 1975 and is one of the oldest state programs.[2] MiOSHA established the Safety and Education Training Division supported by a tax of between 1/2 and 3/4 of 1% on workers' compensation income benefits. Although the fund builds up a significant sum—indeed the tax was suspended for 1 year because the fund was running such a large surplus—only a limited amount is used for grants. In 1987 only $500,000 was divided among 10 grantees. The state program supports about 20 professional staff who focus largely on providing consulting services to employers.

The Maine program is funded by an assessment of up to 1/4 of 1% on workers' compensation income benefits paid out and has been in place since 1985.[3] The worker training fund was created in part as a trade-off for cuts in workers' compensation benefits. In 1987, it gave out $25,000 each quarter, largely for developing new programs or materials. The grants are relatively small ($10,000 maximum) and have gone to a variety of groups including industry trade groups, clinics, the Lung Association, and the Maine Labor Group on Health (a COSH). Being funded by the state has given nonprofit groups increased visibility and broader access to workers and workplaces. In addition to providing grants, the state supports staff and has purchased industrial hygiene and educational equipment. The program also funds the state right-to-know program and collects data on occupational disease and injuries.

The New York program gets its funds from an 0.5% tax on workers' compensation premiums.[4] The assessment has provided $4.8 million annually since 1985. The funds are awarded by an independent board composed of representatives of labor, management, and the public. The program is administered by the Department of Labor. It has funded well over 100 organizations including all the state's COSH groups. The program has only one professional staff person with training in safety in safety and health, so evaluation and technical assistance are severely limited. Additional personnel may be hired in 1988. The legislation was supported not only by labor, but also by school boards throughout the state, the Association of Counties, and the Safety Council affiliates. The year that it was passed, it was very high on labor's legislative agenda.

Massachusetts has a two-part program. The first, located in the Public Health Department, grew out of a 1985 conference on Women and the Workplace, where Governor Michael Dukakis promised a programmatic response to problems highlighted by the conference. The 1,200 participants and the groups that put the conference together, including Massachusetts COSH, pressured the Governor and in 1987 won $100,000 for the Working Women's Health Project to provide training in office technology, reproductive hazards, and hazards in the health care industry.

The second part of the program was created by a 1985 change in the workers' compensation law that created an Office of Safety to train employers and employees.[5] The first funds for this 3-year-old program were allocated for the 1988 fiscal year. Additional funds and larger grants and a workshop for organizations on how to apply for funds have been promised for 1989. However, because funds must be appropriated through the budget process, there is no guarantee that they will be forthcoming.

Using workers' compensation as a mechanism to fund occupational health and safety education, as was done in Connecticut, Maine, Michigan, and New York, has several advantages. Many legislators see tying prevention through education to workers' compensation as a natural, logical, and equitable extension of these programs. It also appeals to legislators' and the public's sense of justice insofar as the companies paying the highest premiums (and certainly payouts) have historically been the least safe. Insofar as workers' compensation is more likely to pay for injuries than work-related disease, this system is certainly imperfect, but at least in theory, the funding mechanism is designed to make those companies contributing most to the problem contribute most to its prevention. Moreover, the funding mechanism has a built-in "sunset provision" in that decreasing accidents and illnesses resulting in fewer successful compensation claims and lower premiums will reduce the size of the education fund as the need for it decreases.

Budget-conscious legislators like it because it does not tap the general fund and is not generally perceived as a new tax. The percentage of premium or payout set aside is small, but the sums raised are considerable. In the states where the monies are derived from workers' compensation and the rate is suggested in the law (Michigan, Maine, and Connecticut) and become part of a fund, they are extremely stable and insulated from the political vagaries of the appropriations process. In New York where the provisions for funding are somewhat less explicit, the funds are less secure, but still somewhat removed from the appropriations process. Nevertheless, experience has shown that continuing political pressure is necessary to maintain constant levels of support or to increase funds for an expanded program.

Some worker advocates have argued against using the workers' compensation systems for funding education. They argue that it creates a new constituency for the state system when what is needed is to replace the varied state programs with a single federal compensation system. Others point out that worker education programs have been used, as in Maine, to sweeten the loss of other benefits in the compensation system. Although there is some merit in these concerns, the possibility of a federal system seems extremely remote, and the critical need for worker education would appear to outweigh these concerns.

The goals of the programs described are to provide workers with information on the hazards they face, available control technology including work practice and administrative controls, and worker and employer rights and responsibilities under existing law in the hopes that workers will be able to use this information to improve conditions on the shop floor, thus reducing accidents and illness. In addition to learning specific means to protect themselves against hazards, occupational health education is often designed to increase worker consciousness and activism. The educational process also builds a constituency for occupational health and safety legislation, regulation, enforcement, and continuing educational programs. Funded programs also encourage the continued existence and growth of institutions and professionals committed and competent to provide educational and technical assistance services to both workers and employers.

The activities undertaken to implement these goals have varied from state to state. The programs in New York and Maine are essentially grant-based programs. The Michigan program gives out a few grants, but it is basically a staff program. The Connecticut program, while having the option of providing grants, is currently conducted by state employees.

The grant programs have been more successful in generating interest in worker education and have addressed a wider range of topics than have the staff-only programs. The programs carried out by grantees tend to be much more specific to the needs of the groups being served and more varied than those carried out by staff of state programs. For example, the Connecticut program is basically in-house and has concentrated on teaching workers how to obtain workers' compensation. The programs in Maine and New York, however, have provided grants for programs aimed at identifying toxins, preventing back injuries, or teaching safe asbestos removal procedures to groups uniquely concerned with these particular problems. The programs are tailored to the needs of the particular audience. Moreover, grant-giving programs that support training by unions, COSH groups, small business associations, safety councils, clinics, and the like create a wide constituency and political support for the program and for occupational health and safety in general. It is important to have clear guidelines for evaluating both proposals and funded programs to insure fairness and that all grant programs meet minimum standards.

Although services provided by grantees are extremely useful, experience suggests that sufficient professional staff is an important asset to programs. One staff function is to provide technical assistance to grantees and to evaluate their programs. Another function of program staff is to develop and implement generic training for shop stewards and health and safety committee members, programs for small businesses, and special groups of workers who might otherwise be without services. State program staff can also develop a statewide approach, collect epidemiologic data, and put pressure on federal and state OSHA for increased enforcement and regulation. Staff can also encourage unions and corporations to develop health and safety programs of their own. Thus, the best program seems to be one with adequate professional staff to perform these functions and an active, varied grant program.

The role and goals of program staff and grants can be clearly expressed in the legislation or left vague and be determined by the program director and other state officials once the program is operational. Only the New York law specifically requires grants. Only the Connecticut law spells out the need for salaried staff. The New York program is short on professional staff with training in safety and health, and Connecticut gives no grants. The Michigan and Maine laws do not describe how the programs will be set up; the former, although it gives grants, is largely a staff-based program, whereas the latter is largely the reverse.

Getting these programs enacted has required active efforts by labor and support from other interested groups. Experience in several states has shown that the key to getting such a program through the state legislature is to make it high on labor's legislative agenda. The work of COSH groups in mobilizing local unions and organizing letter-writing campaigns to state legislators has been crucial. It is also critical to have support beyond the labor community. Small businesses, universities, and clinics have testified in support of these programs in New York, Maine, Massachusetts, and Connecticut, in part because they anticipate getting funding or services through them.

Worker education can make a difference in achieving safer workplaces and building support for continued public regulation of workplace hazards. Experience indicates that a small assessment on workers' compensations premiums can provide funds for successful worker education programs in occupational health and safety carried out through grants to groups experienced in training workers aided by sufficient professional staff to provide direction, evaluation, and technical assistance. These programs can be advanced by coalitions of labor, occupational safety and health professionals, and other concerned organizations as well as by employers anxious to receive services that will help them comply with federal and state health and safety and right-to-know laws. They provide an economic foundation for groups concerned with occupational health and safety and provide a basis for interesting groups that might otherwise only be marginally involved in occupational health to take on the issue. Through the grant-giving and educational process, the programs enhance and expand the constituency for further education in occupational health and for better legislation and enforcement as well.

REFERENCES

1. General Statutes of Connecticut. 1987. Section 31-283g and 31-283h.
2. Michigan Statutes Annotated. 1987. Section 17.50(55) *et seq.*
3. Maine Revised Statutes Annotated. 1985. Labor and Industry, Title 26, Section 61.
4. New York Labor Law. 1987. Section 884 *et seq.*
5. Massachusetts General Laws. 1987. Section 152:1 *et seq.*

Discussion: Part II

MOLLY COYE (*State of New Jersey Department of Health, Trenton, New Jersey*): I would like strongly to endorse the notion of establishing independent funds for the support of research and training in occupational health. You will recall that the Latin word *fundus*, the root of the English word *fund*, refers to the foundation, something that goes deep into the earth and renders stability to an enterprise. That is the essence of an independent fund. If we are able to create independent funds for the support of training and research in occupational health, then we provide a stable long-term basis which insulates the enterprise from the vagaries of the political process. The notion of supporting these funds through a revenue-generating mechanism independent of general taxation is very intriguing.

FRANKLIN E. MIRER (*United Automobile, Aerospace and Agriculture Implement Workers' Union, Detroit, Michigan*): This may seem a little self-serving, but I want to note that very few workers are here at this workshop. In Nashville a couple of months ago, more than 800 local union representatives attended the AFL-CIO Health and Safety Conference, setting a future agenda a lot like this one. We had 300 from the U.A.W. alone in Washington last May, and we will have another 300 at Black Lake in a month or so, so there is quite a bit of activity in unions. We obviously can do more, but interest is broadening within the union movement, not declining, even in the absence of New Directions funding.

With regard to standard-setting, I believe that steel workers have really taken the lead on this in the labor movement, although the most recent effort over formaldehyde was principally our show. For all its time-consuming nature, the current 6(B) process, including the informal rule-making hearings, really turns on feasibility issues. These issues are more complicated because more industries are involved, and thus the feasibility issues become more complex. Those hearings are the only place where industry can be made to step forward, to describe the health problems as they are, to face questions about these problems, and to present their data on what is feasible and what is not. By considering the hazards and controls at the same time, we narrow the gap in the contended issues. I do not see a way that we can completely turn around the way a major industry does business, as was done with the lead standard, unless there is that kind of exhaustive process.

EULA BINGHAM (*University of Cincinnati Medical Center, Cincinnati, Ohio*): I agree with that. I have no problems with confrontational engagement at the hearing process. I am still one of those persons who believe in a Standards Advisory Committee and would like to see OSHA put together several of them. Some of the issues can be delineated, some of the lines drawn, and some of the problems laid out before the Agency issues a proposal and spends all the money on the economic analysis that they have to do. Even if they are not doing cost–benefit analysis, they have to do economic analysis for feasibility. I am much in favor of dialogue; I agree with you that the process should remain in place. However, we have to put more will behind the process, and more technical and legal resources behind the process. Policy-setters could do a better job if there were *will* at the top, and if resources were reallocated. I am not suggesting big spending: I think that one could reallocate present resources and still accomplish much.

COYE: I invite Eric Jannerfeldt to comment about the Swedish Work Environment Fund experience and standard-setting in terms of worker education.

ERIC JANNERFELDT (*Swedish Embassy, Washington, D.C.*): We have also recognized the need to educate the worker, but comparatively more money is spent in Sweden for this purpose than is done here. Right now the Fund is in the process of trying to "internationalize" its information. They have a series of publications that go through the body, part by part, describing occupational hazards. The most important part of that series is available now in English.

The Fund is supported by industry. A fraction of a percentage of the employer tax goes to support the Fund, and the total amounts to several hundred million kronor per year, which provides quite a good platform for certain activities.

LINDA RUDOLPH (*California Health Department*): I want to comment on an initiative that we are currently working on in California. Following the Proposition 65 style, our initiative is actually a ballot initiative to restore the California Occupational Safety and Health Administration, which was dismantled by Governor Deukmejian in the summer of 1987. This model of community and worker education is a concept that we ought to look at more closely, because it is very interesting. The California Labor Federation has sponsored an initiative to reinstate CalOSHA onto the ballot for November 1988. It has spawned a tremendous outpouring of interest in occupational health and safety on the parts of organized labor, as well as a much broader constituency. Interest has been shown by such diverse parties as the California Medical Association and the California Trial Lawyers' Association. This initiative will create several months of tremendous publicity around occupational health; all of the environmental groups are involved, as are many of the public interest and voluntary groups such as the American Cancer Society and the American Lung Association. It is creating a tremendous opportunity for education for 10 percent of the citizens of the United States.

JOEL SHUFRO (*New York Committee for Occupational Safety and Health* [NYCOSH]): I would like to credit the importance of the study done by Drs. Landrigan and Markowitz and the other members of the Mount Sinai staff. Their study was pioneering in that it detailed the extent of occupational disease in New York State. But the New York State legislature has in its wisdom over the years commissioned hundreds of studies that have sat on the shelf and gathered dust. Consequently, the reason why we have a safety and health training program, a study of occupational disease, and the establishment of a clinic network in New York State is not because New York State legislators are particularly enlightened, but because we have an extremely active labor movement and an active COSH movement in the State. They put political pressure on the state legislators to adopt the recommendations made by people like Dr. Landrigan. Also I should note that it will not be studies that force the legislature to allocate funds for occupational clinics. It will be the force of the labor movement and the COSH groups throughout the state. I would plead with this august body that in your scientific deliberations here that you not omit consideration of the political process.

BINGHAM: In response to the various comments made about what California has done and New York has done and what has happened here and what has happened there: you all ratify my point that President Reagan was very successful—he has put all responsibility on the states. However, we have to have federal leadership on this issue; it cannot all come from the states. It is wonderful to have a laboratory in New York State, but what about the things that are not happening in South Carolina or in Ohio or in other states: mostly things are not happening. There are some isolated COSH groups and a clinic network here and there, but that is the best we can do. We need federal leadership, with some federal money going into grants like New Direction grants, and with some standards that require these initiatives throughout the United States.

Round Table Papers: 1. Risk Assessment and Regulation

Opening Statement

WILLIAM J. NICHOLSON

Division of Environmental & Occupational Medicine
The Mount Sinai School of Medicine
New York, New York 10029

In this round table session we are focusing on the role of risk assessment in the regulatory process. The next two papers are by investigators eminently qualified to discuss this issue. I will introduce the topic by following up on some of the remarks that Eula Bingham brought to our attention on the regulatory record of OSHA. She showed that in the history of OSHA, eighteen independent standards were issued, apart from the consensus standards that were initially adopted. Of those, about twelve involved chemicals for which a specific standard was established.

Prior to 1983, OSHA had begun regulatory action on approximately 100 agents, but had never completed action. OSHA sent the list of uncompleted standards to NIOSH, asking what their recommendation would be on these 100 agents. In 1984 NIOSH responded with reports stating that for 51 chemicals the current standard was not sufficiently protective and that rulemaking should proceed. So, three and a half years ago, there were 51 agents deemed to merit regulation. Of these 51 chemicals, criteria documents had been issued by NIOSH for 36, among which were 23 that had evidence of carcinogenicity. These 23 potentially and actually carcinogenic chemicals are listed in TABLE 1 along with the proposed standard for each.

Of the carcinogenic agents, there were fifteen for which a standard had been proposed 10 years previously. For one, the NIOSH-proposed standard was the same as the OSHA value; eight had a NIOSH-proposed standard 2 to 10 times lower; four had a standard 10 to 100 times lower; and 2 had a standard more than 100 times less than the current OSHA value. In sum, OSHA's lack of action in regulation is exposing numerous workers to agents that have evidence of carcinogenicity. This inaction is leading to increased mortality as the nonregulation continues. The total magnitude of that excess mortality for most of these agents is not yet assessed. It can, however, be assessed in a couple of instances where regulatory delay has been fairly extensive.

Let us consider the effect of delay in standard-setting with reference to standards recently promulgated, those for asbestos and benzene. In the case of asbestos, there was a proposed reduction in the existing standards of 2 fibers per milliliter in October 1975. At that time, OSHA suggested a standard of 0.5 and NIOSH a standard of 0.1 fibers per milliliter. Eventually, in June 1987, a standard of 0.2 was adopted. If a 0.2 fiber standard had been adopted in June 1977, there would now be 750 fewer deaths to be expected from exposure to asbestos in the workplace between June 1977 and June 1987.

A similar analysis for benzene from the period when the standard was first proposed in February 1978, until it was finally adopted in September 1987, leads to an estimate of 75 deaths which could have been prevented by more expedient standard-setting.

TABLE 1. A Comparison of Standards Recommended by NIOSH and Existing OSHA Standards for 23 Chemicals

Compound	NIOSH[a]	OSHA	Carcinogenicity Animals	Carcinogenicity Humans
Arsine	2 μg/m^3 C	200 μg/m^3 T	X	X
Beryllium	0.5 μg/m^3 C	2 μg/m^3 T	X	S
1,3-Butadiene	LTFL	1000 ppm T	X	
Cadmium	40 μg/m^3 T	100 μg/m^3 T	S	S
Carbon tetrachloride	2 ppm C	10 ppm T	X	S
Chromic acid	100 μg/m^3 C	100 μg/m^3 C	X	X
Chromium VI	1 μg/m^3 T	100 μg/m^3 C	X	X
Diazomethane	LTFL	0.2 ppm	X	
1,2-Dichloroethane	1 ppm T	50 ppm T	X	S
Dioxane	1 ppm C	100 ppm T	X	
Epichlorohydrin	0.5 ppm T	5 ppm T	X	S
Ethyl acrylate	LTFL	25 ppm T	X	
MOCA	3 μg/m^3	None	X	
Methyl iodide	NR	5 ppm T	X	
Nickel	15 μg/m^3 T	1 mg/m^3 T	X	
PCBs	1 μg/m^3 T	1 mg/m^3 T	X	S
1,1,2,2-Tetrachloroethane	50 ppm T	100 ppm T	X	
Tetrachloroethylene	1 ppm T	5 ppm T	X	
1,1,1-Trichloroethane	LTFL	350 ppm T	X	
1,1,2-Trichloroethane	LTFL	10 ppm T	S	
Trichloethylene	25 ppm T	100 ppm T	X	
Vinyl bromide	NR	5 ppm T	S	
Vinyl chloride	1 ppm C	1 ppm T	X	X

ABBREVIATIONS: C = ceiling; T = time-weighted average; X = evidence of carcinogenicity (IARC); S = sufficient evidence of carcinogenicity (IARC).

[a] Numerical value from Criteria Document for virtually all carcinogens; NIOSH now recommends that exposures be held to the "lowest technically feasible limit (LTFL)."

Risk assessment has served as a technique for delay in the regulatory process. That has been the case with respect to the benzene standard and was a major source of the delay in its final implementation.

A final comment I would like to make with respect to risk assessment is that it is an extremely useful tool, but a very crude tool. Very few published risk assessments present a measure of their accuracy. Usually their accuracy is extremely limited. In the case of asbestos, when a risk assessment was done determining the risk to workers per fiber exposure, the uncertainty around that risk estimate was found to be a factor of 10. In other words, the actual risk from asbestos exposure in an unstudied work circumstance could be 10 times greater or 1/10 as much as one would estimate from the best data available. Given such a background, arguments over a factor of 2, such as often occur in the regulatory process, are meaningless.

Outcome versus Process in Decision Making

NICHOLAS A. ASHFORD

Center for Technology, Policy, and Industrial Development
Massachusetts Institute of Technology
Cambridge, Massachusetts 02139

I would like to leave five thoughts with you in these few pages. First, I'd like to address the relationship between risk assessment and risk management, and ask whether you can separate the two. Then I'd like to examine whether one can separate facts from values. The paradigms of law and science are very different ways of looking at the world. An admonition Ralph Nader made in 1977 is very important here: "If scientists think lawyers present one-sided cases, they need to rediscover themselves." I think that's still good advice. Third, I'd like to ask questions about the decision-making process in the areas of environmental and occupational health. What is it that drives the way we make decisions about hazards, and whether to regulate and when? And finally, I want to make an important distinction between ensuring a fair *outcome*, i.e., a correct outcome of a decision, and achieving a fair *process*.

In his early days at the Environmental Protection Agency, William Ruckleshaus insisted that the way to separate risk assessment from risk management was to get the scientists to do the risk assessment and then hand the analysis over to the bureaucrats who would then make the decisions about whether to regulate or not.[1] However, even Bill Ruckleshaus has recanted[2] and said in effect "It's not that way, we don't know the science that well, I feel uncomfortable about what I recommended and I'm not sure the division can be made." And of course he's quite right, the division can rarely be made. In assessing risk, just think about the kinds of decisions you have to make. If the assessment is based on animal experiments or human epidemiology, you must make a choice of data sets: which data you are going to use, which studies you are going to examine, which dose-response curves you are going to use, which exposure data you are going to use. When you build uncertainties upon uncertainties, you realize, as Alice Whittemore has written very nicely,[3] your choices of models and data themselves reflect value judgments. The clear separation of risk assessment and risk management is understood to be very limited and not very helpful.

However, recognizing inherent values and then making a risk management decision involves more than simply doing a risk assessment. The crucial element here is to ask the following question: At what point in looking at a hazard do you spend money trying to refine the risk assessment? Where do you begin instead to look, for example, at the technological options, the substitutes, and new technology? Instead of spending money for a two-year animal feeding study to nail down the toxicologic parameters, it might be better to spend $300,000 in developing technological options to effect change. What you do about a risk could very well depend upon how you view the technological options. I would argue that you should start by doing a back-of-envelope risk assessment. Then you should see whether you really want a sophisticated risk assessment, a technological options assessment, or an economic assessment. It is important that we know the technological solutions to some degree of certainty, as well as the risk we are addressing.

Now with regard to the separation of facts and values, can you ever really do it? The central question is: At what level of certainty or strength of association for a risk assessment does the evidence become strong enough for you to do something about it? Three very different kinds of action are possible: (1) You can control the chemical. (2) You can notify those at risk. (At what level of strength of association or strength of evidence do you have to tell people that they're exposed to the hazard? That is a different question from determining the level of evidence required to control the hazard.) And (3) you can provide compensation. (Here there is yet another set of questions. At what level do you think the association is so strong that you want to compensate people for harm due to exposure to the chemical?) Now you might not think the evidence is strong enough to control a chemical, reflecting a kind of balancing in some environmental law, but fairness might dictate that you tell people there might be a risk. And if you don't think it is justifiable to control the chemical across the board, you still might want to compensate someone, perhaps through the Workers' Compensation system or the tort system. That is, you might decide not to impose all these costs on industry, but to pay anyone who might be a loser in the "risk lottery." And so what you do with the information reflects how you view the minimum evidence to trigger the action.

What happens when the uncertainty in risk is very large? As Bill Nicholson has indicated, sometimes it is not just a factor of ten, but a factor of 100 or 1000 (e.g., the case of vinyl chloride exposure at one part per million). How do you make a decision faced with uncertain costs and benefits? Analytically you are not balancing costs and benefits any more. What you are simply doing is valuing, as a decision maker, what kind of mistake you're willing to live with.[4] Do you want to "over-regulate" and impose larger economic burdens, living with the possibility that you need not have regulated? That is called a type 1 error in statistics. Or do you want to risk a type 2 error and fail to regulate and face the possible consequence later on that there are a lot more people who are sick than you counted on? The answer depends on the magnitude of the type 1 versus type 2 errors, and how you feel about that. There's a lot of talk these days about whether you should use worst-case estimates or most-likely estimates in risk assessment. The answer to this depends upon what you want to do. If you are dealing with a chemical for which there are very close substitutes, you want to ask how bad the health problem could be because it is easy to make the technical switchover. In the case of an essential chemical, like a radionuclide that is used in medical monitoring (or X rays used for medical diagnostics), it is hard to find a suitable substitute. And your decisions are then not based on a worst-case analysis. Instead, you're saying that this is an essential medical or industrial application and you then have to ask how bad a problem will most likely result. And so it is quite consistent from a values perspective to use a worst-case analysis in one case and a most-likely estimate in one another. In the former case, analysis should be focused on bounding the uncertainties of the risk estimates, that is, on identifying the set of not-clearly-incorrect estimates. In the latter case, analysis should be focused on improving the most-likely estimate.

Finally, let me say that *if*, in fact, we can look at the data and, by painfully teasing out what is there, we can decide about the science, then we can assist the decision makers in arriving at the correct outcome. We want to be correct about the risk assessment. However, if we don't have a ghost of an idea about how big the problem is, then the decision to regulate should not center ensuring that the *outcome* is correct; it should center upon ensuring that the *process* is correct.

Eula Bingham has touched on this point by suggesting that we might return to advisory committee deliberations, where representatives of a balanced set of interests—labor, the environmental community, and whoever is involved in the process—participates in the painful decision about what to do under a circumstance of uncertainty. We recommend this, not because the committee is going to decide that five parts per million or one part per million is where the level ought to be, but because somehow all parties have had part in a very difficult decision and at least the *process* is right. And I would submit that the very objectionable decisions are those in which the process has been violated and the decision has been disguised as a scientific question.

REFERENCES

1. RUCKELSHAUS, W. D. 1983. Science, risk, and public policy. Science **221:** 1026–1028.
2. RUCKELSHAUS, W. D. 1985. Risk, science, and democracy. Issues in Science and Technology **1**(3): 19–38.
3. WHITTEMORE, A. S. 1983. Facts and values in risk assessment in evironmental toxicologists. Risk Analysis **3:** 23–33.
4. ASHFORD, N. A. 1988. Science and values in the regulatory process. Statistical Science **3**(3): 377–383.

Risk Assessment and Occupational Health

Conceptual Problems

FRANK N. LAIRD

The Graduate School of International Studies
University of Denver
Denver, Colorado 80208-0280

Case studies can demonstrate *abuses* of risk assessment: suppressing information, ignoring data, or other forms of deception. When a clear abuse has been documented, it is easy to condemn it and point out how the risk assessment *should* have been done. However, abuses should not be dismissed as atypical aberrations. They may, in practice, be very hard to correct. It is worth asking why such abuses seem so prevalent.

Nonetheless, cases of clear abuse may leave unexamined some other conceptual issues. Even if it is done "right," is risk assessment a good tool for analyzing policies for occupational health and safety? This seemingly simple question contains profoundly difficult issues. Assume for a moment that we know what it means to do the assessment right, that is, in conformance with the best professional standards and with strict adherence to openness and honesty. How does risk assessment claim to be good for the policy process and what is problematic about that claim?

RISK ASSESSMENT: MAIN FEATURES

Risk assessment has been called "formalized common sense."[1] At first glance, the description seems apt. Different authors give slightly different descriptions of the process.[2-4] Nonetheless, all the descriptions include steps such as identifying hazards associated with some activity or policy, calculating their effects (usually on mortality and morbidity), estimating exposures to the hazards, and, finally, calculating the expected value of the harm actually entailed by the policy or activity in question.[1] The mathematical details may vary, but in general terms the final result is calculated by summing over all possible events the product of the probability of the event occurring and the consequences if it does occur.

This methodology is intuitively appealing. We would like the best possible information on the hazards workers face, the possible effects of those hazards, workers' exposure to them, and the total harm we expect to see as a result. Such information and analyses are important steps in protecting worker health. However, risk assessment also dictates the way we collect, structure, and use this information. Risk assessors make two additional claims about their technique. First, they argue that risk assessment should be done separately from risk management, that is, risk assessment should not determine policy choices, but rather should serve only as an objective input—one among several—to the policy process.[3,5] Second, the use of risk assessment to decision-makers is that it helps them understand the consequences of their choices, particularly the trade-offs that they must often make between levels of expenditure, for protection and lives lost. The argument implies that to confront such trade-offs explicitly is beneficial to the policy process.[3]

I will mention a few reasons why it may not be possible or desirable to keep risk assessment entirely separate from policy choices and to quantify explicitly all the trade-offs involved in different policy choices. My paper is synthetic, drawing on the work of scholars from a variety of fields, and is not comprehensive. It does suggest, however, that the choice of analytic framework for examining occupational health issues is a normative one, and that risk assessment, as it is conventionally described, may be the wrong choice.

PROBLEM FRAMING AND VARIABLE CHOICE

When doing risk assessment, there are many ways to frame the problem. No scientific criteria are available by which to attempt such framing. Thus, the choice of frame necessarily involves policy choices. The decision of how to do the risk assessment must be guided by choices about risk management. The processes are tightly linked.

Crouch and Wilson[3] illustrate this problem well. They present graphs of the trends in accidental deaths in the mining of coal. If the number of deaths per 10^6 tons of coal is measured, the trend from 1950–1970 is clearly down. However, if the number of deaths per 1,000 coal miners is measured, the trend is up. How should the problem be framed?

Crouch and Wilson (p. 14) state that risk assessment should not frame the problem. Rather, a "good" analyst should present both results to the decision-maker, and let him choose. However, that answer has several problems.

First, it assumes that the analyst thinks of all the different ways in which the data could be presented. Nothing exists in the methodology of risk assessment that insures or even suggests such completeness. Adherence to professional standards does not preclude mechanical, unimaginative, or pedestrian analyses.

Perhaps more importantly, the philosophic roots of risk assessment bias it in favor of aggregate, society-wide problem framing and away from concern with large risks for small numbers of people. One of the roots of risk assessment is cost/benefit analysis, which in turn has its roots in microeconomics. When cost/benefit analysis is applied to risks, it carries with it the assumption that the most desired outcome is the one that is most "efficient," that has the greatest net positive benefits, which usually means the greatest benefits in the aggregate sense.[6]

Such increasing efficiency, as in coal mining, may be purchased at the expense of a small number of people, that is, workers. The number of fatalities per million tons of coal dropped steadily from 1950–1970 (with the crucial exception of 1968) from 1.15 to 0.42.[7] However, mining was not getting safer. Miners were losing their jobs as new technology enabled mines to keep up production with fewer workers. The number of persons working daily fell from 483,000 in 1950 to 144,000 in 1970. Total coal production fluctuated during the same period, but increased somewhat, from 516 to 603 million tons.[8] Thus, hundreds of thousands of miners lost their jobs, and those who remained employed faced substantially increased risks, as the number of fatalities per thousand miners went from 1.33 in 1950 to 1.81 in 1970.[7] The distribution of risk in this industry raises important issues of social equity.

Crouch and Wilson[3] themselves subtly suggest that broad, aggregate variables are preferable to ones that reflect distributional issues. In discussing the two ways of framing coal miner death problems, they characterize them by noting that, "From a national point of view, given that a certain amount of coal has to be obtained, deaths per million tons of coal is the more appropriate measure of risk, whereas from a labor leader's point of view, deaths per thousand persons employed may be more relevant." (p. 13). Concern with aggregate measures is depicted corresponding to a broad public interest, whereas concern with the distribution of risk is seen as the pleading of a "special interest." Declaring distributional issues to be of secondary importance is a very powerful normative claim.

UNCERTAINTY AND THE BURDEN OF PROOF

In any risk assessment, there are always enormous uncertainties of a variety of types, such as the toxic effects of a substance, the patterns of exposure, and the dose-response relation. Judgment calls are always necessary to determine when to begin worrying about a potential hazard or when to declare some activity "safe." When for the purpose of regulation is a risk clearly considered significantly greater than zero? A methodology that stresses the use of expected values invites furious debate over the data and puts the burden of proof on those who claim that the risk is worth considering. Such a burden is greater than might be expected. It is often difficult, and always expensive, to prove that some substance or activity poses a significant risk to workers. For example, toxicologic data often come from animal experiments. Those experiments are costly, and their results can be disputed on numerous technical grounds, requiring more experiments and raising the cost of proof ever higher.

The burden of proof issue can be subtle in risk assessment. The methodology looks for hazard, not for safety. It does not "see" hazard unless empirical evidence of a statistically significant level of harm is actually in hand. These requirements clearly place the burden of proof on those at risk and have very clear implications for regulatory policy. Greenwood[9] found that industry's calls for "better scientific grounding" for regulation were often part of a deliberate strategy of deregulation. Whenever someone says that "There is no evidence that X is a risk," we should ask if there is any evidence that X is *not* a risk.

CONSENT AND CHOICE

Many people choose to engage in risky activities, such as skiing or hang gliding. However, when imposed risks are theoretically escapable, does choosing *not* to escape them imply consenting to accept the risk? If workers do not quit a job that they know entails risk, does that mean that they agree to accept those risks? Workers are not slaves. No one can force them to stay in a job. Does their freedom of choice mean that they have chosen their risk? Baier[10] gives a lengthy argument, based on moral theory, that such choice does *not* necessarily imply consent. There are several reasons, but the most salient is the distinction between work risks and leisure risks; taking a job is much more likely to involve economic compulsion or at least limited choices.

EXPLICIT VALUATION OF LIFE AND CALLOUSNESS

Assessing risks quantitatively, comparing them to benefits, and trying to maximize the benefits means, at least implicitly, attempting to monetize such things as injury, suffering, and death. Risk assessors argue, quite correctly, that we are not willing to spend an infinite amount of money to save lives, and that the amounts we do spend vary enormously by circumstance. However, is it wise to argue that we should state explicitly that we are willing to spend so much for a life, and no more? Bogen[11] has argued that such explicit statements can put us on a morally slippery slope, that talking about life in those terms can, over time, make us increasingly callous to life's value, and that the monetary value we affix to it will go down over time.

The refusal to monetize life does NOT mean that we impute an infinite monetary value to it. MacLean[12] argues that making life a *sacred* value has important ritual and symbolism connected with it. Those rituals and symbols contribute to the quality of life. Calculation that "deritualizes" the value of life may promote a cold attitude among people and exploitation of man by man.

Finally, it has been noted for years that many important risks and benefits have no market value and are very difficult to quantify, much less monetize. Hoos[13] has argued that emphasis on quantification will simply omit, or greatly downplay, factors that are difficult to quantify.

CONCLUSION

Much research and analysis on occupational health and safety remain to be done, and that work should be advanced as rapidly as possible. However, for the reasons just discussed, conventional methods of risk assessment as an analytic framework for that research pose serious problems for worker protection, even if the assessment is done right. The regulatory process must be made responsive to the issues discussed herein, such as the distribution of risk and the social effects of quantitative analysis.

REFERENCES

1. COVELLO, V. T. 1987. Decision analysis and risk management decision making: Issues and methods. Risk Analysis **7:** 131–140.
2. LOWRANCE, W. W. 1976. Of Acceptable Risk. William Kaufman, Inc. Los Altos, CA.
3. CROUCH, E. A. & R. WILSON. 1982. Risk/Benefit Analysis. Ballinger Publishing Co. Cambridge, MA.
4. ROWE, W. D. 1977. An Anatomy of Risk. John Wiley & Sons. New York, NY.
5. NATIONAL RESEARCH COUNCIL. 1983. Risk Assessment in the Federal Government: Managing the Process. National Academy Press. Washington, DC.
6. LEONARD, H. B. & R. J. ZECKHAUSER. 1986. Cost-benefit analysis applied to risks: Its philosophy and legitimacy. *In* Values at Risk. D. Maclean, ed.: 31–48. Rowman & Allanheld. Totowa, NJ.
7. U.S. BUREAU OF THE CENSUS. 1987. Statistical Abstract of the United States, 107th ed. USGPO. Washington, DC. See also 73rd to 106th editions.
8. PRESIDENT'S COMMISSION ON COAL. 1980. The American Coal Miner: A report on the Community and Living Conditions in the Coal Fields. U.S. Government Printing Office. Washington, DC.

9. GREENWOOD, T. 1984. Knowledge and Discretion in Regulation. Praeger. New York, NY.
10. BAIER, A. 1986. Poisoning the wells. *In* Values at Risk. D. Maclean, ed.: 49–74. Rowman & Allanheld, Totowa, NJ.
11. BOGEN, K. T. 1981. Quantitative risk-benefit analysis in regulatory decision-making: A fundamental problem and an alternate proposal. J. Health Politics, Policy, & Law **8:** 120–143.
12. MACLEAN, D. 1986. Social values and the distribution of risk. *In* Values at Risk. D. Maclean, ed.: 75–93. Rowman & Allanheld, Totowa, NJ.
13. HOOS, I. R. 1979. Societal aspects of technology assessment. Tech. Forecasting & Social Change **13:** 191–202.

Round Table 1: Discussion

SCOTT JACOBS (*Office of Information Regulatory Affairs at the Office of Management and Budget, Washington, D.C.*): I am not here to represent the OMB; I am here to learn how to do the job better. I want to engage in repartee with both of the previous speakers about the questions of cost-benefit, risk management, and risk assessment.

It is interesting to me, Dr. Ashford, that after saying that cost-benefit analysis was not legitimate, you engaged in it yourself in asking whether we should not apply a different standard for material for which there is an easy substitute. And you asked whether it was not different from having a diagnostic test, using X rays, for example, where the benefits might outweigh the risks. This gets to the core of the fundamental mistake that I believe both you and Dr. Laird made. The red herring you threw in consists of a kind of ledger with a series of costs and dollars on one side, and lives or health on the other. But cost-benefit analysis does not mean that; it means a trade-off process. The basic point of cost-benefit analysis is that a responsible decision maker looks at all of the implications of a decision, both positive and negative. Whether those sides are "monetized" or not is not important. In fact, you may or may not put a money value on either side. Both sides of the ledger contain monetary costs and benefits, and nonmonetary costs and benefits. All cost-benefit analysis, without this red herring about the value of life and health, is a technique that allows decision makers, properly and responsibly (particularly when they are making decisions that affect lives, as does safety and health regulation), to look at the full set of trade-offs in a decision. I must disagree with both of you, Drs. Ashford and Laird: it is so important to make that distinction between the trade-offs; it is so important to know the full consequence of a decision before you act. That is what cost-benefit analysis means as far as I am concerned and as far as I see it applied.

NICHOLAS ASHFORD (*Center for Policy Alternatives, M.I.T., Cambridge, Mass.*): Mr. Jacob's question needs to be heard and understood. Semantics and words are very important. First, I believe in trade-off analysis. I think I coined that term in Denver at an FDA conference about 8 years ago. Trade-off analysis is a technique in which you look at the full consequences of an act, as far as you know them, and then make a decision about how you are going to deal with those consequences. I think, though, that to call that activity cost-benefit analysis is neither within the practice of the profession nor helpful in terms of this political debate.

There is a real distinction between cost-benefit analysis and a rational process called trade-off analysis. Cost-benefit analysis consists simply of putting a money value on both the costs and the benefits and of looking for a net benefit of the result or a net benefit-to-cost ratio. In the examples I gave, I was not talking about evaluating cost and benefits; I was talking about evaluating the mistakes that you might make. My analysis was a "minimizing regret" type of analysis, to use a term from military analysis. You are seeking to minimize the chance of the maximum regret resulting from an event you want to avoid. Analytically, it is quite distinct from cost-benefit analysis.

In rejecting traditional cost-benefit analysis, I do not mean to reject rational trade-off processes. However, those are not the processes to which the OMB, OPP, EPA or OSHA have subscribed. There are lots of ways to perform trade-off and cost-benefit analysis. There are ways in which your values are very explicit, and ways in which they are hidden in the assumption, so there is no question about the fact that one makes value judgments in these decisions. Benefits can, for example, be discounted at 10 percent, the approach advocated in the OMB circular. It is important, therefore, that we articulate our values and not hide them behind some discount rate.

FRANK LAIRD (*University of Denver, Denver, Colo.*): I would also like to respond to a couple of points. First, the issue of whether or not you assign a money value to cost and benefits is important. The central point is that a cost-benefit analysis and a risk assessment, which is its child, imply more than a mere trade-off. For instance, several textbooks in the field, including Zeckhauser's and Meecham's, as well as the recent piece by Zeckhauser, talk about philosophical approaches; they all say very explicitly that a policymaker performing a cost-benefit analysis is not only just making lists and subtracting one from the other and computing ratios. Those pieces state quite clearly that buried inside those analyses are very clear assumptions about what is good policy. And according to those authors, a good policy is a microeconomically efficient policy. Indeed, those authors set forth a whole normative discussion as to why that is a good policy, an opinion which I think is particularly flawed.

Further, it is important to recognize that defenders of monetized cost-benefit analysis have learned to use two errors in logic in arguing with their opponents. The first claims that to deny cost-benefit analysis is to deny trade-offs, and the second says that to deny cost-benefit analysis is to insist upon zero risk, which is, of course, impossible. I have yet to read any serious scholar who argues for zero risk. There is no such thing as zero risk; everyone understands that. Moreover, trade-offs are something that all of us make in our lives every day; there is no reason to think that we can avoid them today. And there is no reason to think that we can avoid them in the workplace anymore than anywhere else. But the way in which you weigh those trade-offs makes a great deal of difference.

JACOBS: I understand that as an academician you want to be explicit about what terms mean. I would, however, refer you to guidance documents that have been prepared by the OMB describing the kind of analysis that is expected. I think that you will find that the OMB approach falls closer to the trade-off analysis you are talking about than to the kind of formal cost-benefit analysis that you mentioned earlier.

My second point is that finding a way of making decisions that are value-free, is a Sisyphean task—it cannot be done. In the public policy process, we are trying to arrive at a model that is better than the one used before; the process is always evolving and, we hope, improving.

I agree with your points about risk management and risk assessment, and I believe that the assumptions that go into the risk assessment have got to be public. But I do not agree that risk assessment and risk management are inexplicably intertwined; I think they can be separated by ensuring that the risk assessors are explicit about the assumptions they make and about their ranges of uncertainty, and that when they finish with their risk assessment, they do not end up with one definite number. They should come up with some estimate, an upper confidence interval limit, a maximum likelihood estimator, or a range of uncertainty. And that range of uncertainty is what the decision makers must use, after looking at the trade-offs involved, in making a risk management decision. Obviously, if in a trade-off you are talking about a range of uncertainty of 2000 times and the trade-offs are very small, you are far more willing to make that decision than you would be with a range of 2000 times but very large trade-offs. That is the kind of information which must be made public and which the risk assessors must give to the risk managers to enable them to make the correct and responsible decision.

WILLIAM NICHOLSON (*Mt. Sinai School of Medicine, New York, N.Y.*): I would note that in the occupational health standard setting, a cost-benefit analysis is not required. In fact, it is specifically precluded on the basis of the Supreme Court decision on the cotton dust standard. In the benzene decision, however, the Court ruled that, when possible, an estimate of the amount of harm that would exist at current standards and estimates of lives saved are required (i.e., a benefit calculation). The Court noted that such a calculation need not be balanced in any monetary way against lives.

BARBARA BERNY (*Washington, D.C.*): I want to say something about the distributive point. One of the critical issues in risk assessment and risk management is that they are not necessarily related. I participated in a study of methodologic problems in risk assessment. In the cases that we studied, it appeared that risk management decisions had a great deal more to do with politics, public pressure, and special interest groups than with risk assessment. I think that this distributive problem is particularly acute for several reasons. One is that the people making risk management decisions are invariably not among those people experiencing the effects of the decisions. This is a very critical problem that needs to be addressed systematically. Also, in terms of distributive effects, risk assessment analyses are inevitably made relative to some particular chemical or substance, but the analyses never deal with the fact that we are not really assessing the risk to rats, but rather to human beings who are exposed to numerous other risks. Generally speaking, the distribution of risks is not equal across society: there are people who tend to experience either a great deal of risk or very little risk; that is never taken into account in terms of the analyses.

LAIRD: The point that Ms. Berny has raised applies accurately to many fields, particularly to the siting of hazardous waste facilities. That is resulting in a crisis that now has government officials at the point of tearing out their hair, because people are getting very tired of not having their risks taken into account. As a result, there is a growing movement within the management community to take distribution into account and to make the process much more participatory. That is crucial also in the area of occupational risks.

HARRY TEITLEBAUM (*U.S. Environmental Protection Agency, Cincinnati, Ohio*): It has been a long time since I actually wrote a risk assessment directly aimed at a rule. The vast bulk of the risk assessment work we do at the EPA revolves around setting priorities for future work and most of that has to do with the factors Eula Bingham has spoken about: feasibility and identifiable populations. The point is that many of these important nonmonetary factors come into risk assessments at a very early stage.

The other point I want to make concerns the trade-off analysis that Scott Jacobs and Nick Ashford were talking about. When you look at the estimation of numbers in trade-off analysis, the vast bulk of the work is aimed at getting numbers that are useful in monetary analysis and that people are willing to use. The recent analysis of formaldehyde risks is an extremely good example of this point. An incredible debate developed about whether to use the maximum likelihood estimator or the upper 95 percent confidence limit to assess the risk from formaldehyde exposure. The reason for the debate is that there is an enormous difference between those two estimators if you are calculating cancer risks. The reason for this difference is that there are tremendous curvatures in the dose-response: at 2 parts per million, there are some adenomas and no carcinomas; at 5 parts per million, there are adenomas and carcinomas; at 15 parts per million, there are a lot of carcinomas. There is tremendous curvature in this dose-response curve, consisting of 3 points. However, you cannot determine the shape of a curve that is not a straight line by 3 points. It is clear that a rational decision maker would totally reject any kind of quantitative analysis based on the curve.

In summary, much of the reason for these interminable debates over the shape of a curve has to do with the ultimate primacy of the monetary analysis. We could talk all we want about the unimportance of monetary analysis, but the formaldehyde risk assessment has been hotly debated for four years over that one point, and I suspect it would not have been so debated had the financial stakes not been so high.

ASHFORD: I do not know how to respond directly except to say that the problem here is not that of the primacy of economic factors. The problem is a political unwillingness to make the Formaldehyde Institute angry. Had the EPA passed a regulation of formaldehyde—for example, a ban on the use of formaldehyde in permanent-press resins—an imperceptible increase in cost would have resulted for people who buy permanent press clothing. The only people whose ox would have been gored would have been the Formaldehyde Institute. The EPA did not have the moral fortitude to do the right thing. It is that simple.

ROBERT MCCUNNEY (*Cabot Corporation, Boston Mass.*): I practice occupational medicine in the Boston area. Dr. Laird and Dr. Ashford, you have both done a thorough and excellent job of pointing out some of the pitfalls involved in risk assessment. My concern with risk assessment is primarily in advising my patients, who may have been exposed to a carcinogen such as PCBs, asbestos or chlordane, and in trying to give them some perspective as to what risk these exposures may entail in terms of developing a serious illness later on in life. Surprisingly, more and more people are cognizant of the effects of latency. People without high school educations want to know whether or not exposure to certain materials will damage their liver later on. And while you both did an excellent job in pointing out the pitfalls of risk assessment, I am still left hanging as to what an effective approach to risk mangement is from both a policy and a clinical level. Clinicians must take the information that the regulatory bodies put together and try to relate it to the risk that their patient may have experienced. What, then, might constitute an effective approach to risk assessment in a clinical setting?

LAIRD: Dr. Ashford and I have talked about this issue from two different angles: substance regulation and political process. Dr. Ashford feels that the first thing you must do is to get involved in the decisions made by the people who are immediately affected by the risk.

MCCUNNEY: But that may not always be possible. As we have heard, the plethora of new substances that are introduced into commerce threatens to overwhelm such a process.

LAIRD: I am not suggesting that every single person who is exposed has to make a decision about every risk to which he or she is exposed: none of us could do that. But there must be better ways of insuring that those who are exposed to risks are included in decision making.

MCCUNNEY: Indeed; but unfortunately in many situations information is insufficient, and we are still left with what Dr. Ashford described as ultimately a value judgment. How then do we proceed?

NICHOLSON: Is there a clinician who wants to respond to that aspect?

JAMES KEOGH (*University of Maryland, Baltimore, Md.*): I sympathize with your situation, because it is shared by all of us who are seeing patients. The short answer is that there is no answer. The long answer is that in most circumstances patients are not actually asking us for a quantitative assessment of their risk, but are asking us for advice on what to do. Likewise, policy makers really do not care about the numerical outcome. They really want to know what to do. Just as the policy makers find those answers in the political exigencies of the moment, we have to find them for our patients and advise them about what to do in a practical circumstance, and to some extent reassure them. It is not our role to frighten people who are exposed and who ought to be concerned; it also involves giving them some direct advice about practical things that can be done in both the short and long run.

ASHFORD: I am of the opinion, and others may differ, that from an occupational perspective and maybe from an environmental perspective, there probably are not more than about 1000 to 1200 materials that are a problem. And if we could control about 1000 to 1200 materials, we would all be in a different business. It is nice to lobby around 50,000 existing chemicals, and 1000 new ones every year and to persuade Congress to give us Superfund money. Very frankly, however, I am concerned with only about 1000 substances. I think that they are within the grasp of being recognized and controlled, and their risks assessed.

I also believe that we should treat people as we would treat our own families. The advice to avoid the problem, if possible, should be given. Just think about the last 15 years. Almost every suspicion about a chemical's being harmful has been borne out. In fact, I do not know of a single suspicion that has not been later proved by finding an even greater risk than that which was anticipated, and I certainly know of none that was reversed. I know no substance for which the tip of the iceberg did not ultimately reveal the iceberg. Witness, for example, Dr. Selikoff's illustrations showing the signal-to-noise ratio for asbestos increase as the incidence of asbestos-related disease increases. We know that when we begin to think there is a problem, then there is a problem. And if we can get people to move and to put pressure on the authorities and on their employers and to make the judgments and trade-offs they can, and to get hazards out of the workplace, we are not being capricious. We do not manufacture problems; we are not chemophobic.

PHILIP LANDRIGAN (*Mt. Sinai School of Medicine, New York, N.Y.*): I would like to offer a further comment on Dr. McCunney's question because I think it is very important. The way a clinician deals with an individual patient requires a very different approach from that taken in confronting a recalcitrant regulatory agency. First you should assess the degree of risk, as Jim Keogh said, and grade your answer accordingly. Then you look for individual factors in the patient's own life which the patient may wish to modify if those influence his risk. For example, we reflexively tell persons exposed to asbestos to stop cigarette smoking. Then, over and above the prescription for individual action, I believe there is a real place in the practice of clinical occupational medicine for offering a prescription for social action. We must remind our patients that they are not just individuals, but also members of groups. We must remind them that as individuals in a workforce, they have co-workers; if they are members of a union, they have a union structure that they can mobilize; if they are in a workforce that does not have a union, there are other ways to mobilize action. It is important to remind folks that the clinical recourse is not the only recourse.

Round Table Papers: 2. Generic Standards—Prospects and Pitfalls

Opening Statement

BETRAM ROBERT COTTINE

Administrative Practice Manual
Bureau of National Affairs, Inc.
Washington, D.C.

In preparing for this panel, I viewed some of the *Annals of the New York Academy of Sciences* published 10 years ago to make some assessment of our governmental progress over the decade in preventing occupational disease. The framework for effective, preventive action was described by numerous participants, many of them here once again, including epidemiologists, physicians, scientists, the Assistant Secretary for Occupational Safety and Health, and the Director of NIOSH.

I had the honor of joining you then, and I welcome the honor of joining you again, and I trust that when we meet 10 years hence, I will be able to report more success in preventing occupational disease and a correspondingly diminished need for governmental reform.

In reviewing the real regulatory products of the past 10 years, and in paying particular attention to the hasty and ill-considered retreat of the past seven years, I felt a very definite sense of *déjà vu* as the problems and impediments of the first five years of OSHA surfaced again to disable governmental efforts to prevent occupational illnesses and injuries. As I reviewed the OMB's regulatory agenda from last October, I was impressed by how few regulatory accomplishments can be posted to OSHA's account. Moreover, I found that the promise of future action was unrealistic when measured both by the performance of these seven years and the realization that accomplishments on the regulatory front have not been a favored political achievement. But as I turned to the Administration's regulatory program, I discovered that the real impediment to effective governmental action to reduce occupational disease was none other than the Office of Management and Budget. The OMB has become the superregulatory agency of the United States; OSHA is simply the procedural device to implement the OMB's regulatory programs.

We need now to turn more specifically to the issues of generic standards. The next few panelists will outline their assessment of one of the potentially most powerful mechanisms to multiply the scarce resources of OSHA and to responsibly provide guidance to the private sector in its efforts to prevent occupational disease. The ensuing discussion will note the OMB's unwarranted interference with OSHA's regulatory actions and the essential reforms necessary to make generic rule-making possible.

Generic Standards: Prospects and Pitfalls

R. HAYS BELL

Health and Environment Laboratories
Eastman Kodak Company
Rochester, New York 14650

My definition of a generic standard is one that regulates similar situations or several chemical compounds through a single rule-making procedure. I will limit my presentation to a discussion of two types of generic standards.

First, I will discuss the pros and cons of a generic communications standard that serves as a guide for information sharing. The second part of this short presentation will be on the positive and negative aspects of a generic or chemical class standard.

We have a good example of a generic communications standard in the Occupational Safety and Health Administration's (OSHA) Hazard Communication Standard. Some of the advantages of a generic communications standard are: (1) flexibility; (2) opportunity for professional judgment; (3) a basis for consistency in evaluation; and (4) provisions for timely updating.

The OSHA Hazard Communication Standard permits flexibility in that it allows us to select a method for compliance that applies to a given situation. It allows for professional judgment, for example, in target organ labeling. There is consistency in the general guidelines for producing labels and Material Safety Data Sheets (MSDS). There are provisions for timely updating; complete rule-making is not required to revise a label or to make a change in an MSDS.

It is quite easy to list a number of advantages. Let us look at some of the disadvantages of a generic standard as they apply to the communications area.

One disadvantage is the potential for public confusion. This could happen through different interpretations of a data set that results in the selection of different labels for the same chemical by two or more companies.

Another disadvantage is the difficulty in enforcement. This is particularly true for those who choose to do the bare minimum to comply with a standard. Because of the flexibility that must be inherent in a generic standard, it is more difficult to document a violation.

I believe the advantages outweigh the disadvantages for a generic standard in the communications area.

In my second topic the pros and cons are not as easily defined. This is the area of a generic or chemical class standard in which multiple chemicals with similar structures, toxic endpoints, or physical properties can be regulated through a single rule. For discussion purposes, I found it easier to review the pros and cons together.

It can be argued that a generic standard allows for timely and cost-effective regulation of a large number of chemical compounds. On the surface this appears to be an advantage, but in practice it is difficult to get agreement on which chemicals are to be regulated or how they should be regulated. Such uncertainties can delay, rather than expedite, regulation.

The rule-making process for a risk manager is greatly simplified when a generic standard can be enacted. Establishing a standard is a process that consumes many agency resources, requires much legal input, and usually involves extensive public comment. It takes time. A generic standard in many cases is beneficial to the risk manager because it establishes one set of guidelines for multiple chemicals. In practice, however, it is possible for a generic standard to lead to overregulation. Generic standards tend to identify the chemicals to be regulated in general terms. For example, chemicals that may not show the toxicity characteristic of the class sometimes get included by virtue of the definition.

Another point I would like to make about generic chemical standards deals with basic toxicology. Sometimes the toxic properties of a molecule can change greatly with relatively small changes in structure. An example is provided by ethylene glycol ethers. 2-Methoxyethanol is widely recognized as a potent developmental toxicant in test animals. Adding one carbon to the methoxy chain to form 2-ethoxyethanol reduces the developmental toxicity about fivefold. Adding one more carbon to form 2-propoxyethanol apparently abolishes the prenatal toxicity. Thus, because general standards are based on toxicity, and the toxicity of chemicals can vary greatly with a small change in structure, it is important to define the class in terms of structure and toxicity, not structure alone.

A controversial subject is regulation of chemicals as carcinogens through the generic standard process. There are several classification criteria, guidelines, and models for estimating carcinogenic risk that appear to be leading us to a generic standard for carcinogens.

Our knowledge of the causation and mechanism of cancer induction has increased dramatically over the last few years. The more we know about the mechanism of and factors affecting the carcinogenicity of a specific chemical, the better we can assess the carcinogenic hazard of that agent to humans. Therefore, if there is to be a generic standard, it must be flexible so that it can be adapted as our understanding of cancer and risk assessment increases. For example, the role of oncogenes and the development of the two-stage theory of carcinogenesis, involving initiation and promotion, need to be considered in future risk assessments. In addition, we know from metabolic and pharmacokinetic studies that sometimes different species of animals, including humans, metabolize chemicals in unique pathways and at different rates.

Before leaving this subject, I would like to make several comments on the use of mathematical models for quantitative cancer risk assessment. Mathematical models have been used extensively in recent years in quantitative cancer risk assessment by regulatory agencies. Some of these models, however, do not take into account all of the underlying biology, nor can they make poor data good or compensate for a lack of data. In addition, some mathematical models oversimplify the scientific evaluation process and place undue weight on statistical procedures that use only part of the data. There is no alternative to the use of expert scientific judgment and consideration of all data in a weight-of-the-evidence evaluation of the carcinogenic potential of a chemical.

If there is to be a generic carcinogen standard, then I would like it to be: (1) flexible, to permit later inclusion of new scientific findings; (2) based on the weight-of-the-evidence approach; and (3) technology-driven, that is, with an incentive toward understanding the mechanism of action when a chemical is determined to be an animal carcinogen.

In summary, I have presented some thoughts on generic communication standards and generic chemical standards. I hope my comments will spur discussion and act as a general introduction to one point of view on generic standards.

ACKNOWLEDGEMENT

Thanks are given to William L. Hart, E. Scott Harter, and David P. Richardson for assistance in preparing these comments.

An Industrial Hygienist's Perspective On Generic Standards

JEFFREY S. LEE

*Rocky Mountain Center for Occupational
and Environmental Health, and
Department of Family & Preventive Medicine
University of Utah, School of Medicine
Salt Lake City, Utah 84112*

Although our past approach to standard-setting was appropriate for the time, history has taught us that the *framework* for standards is remarkably similar and that the 1990s warrant primary concentration on generic standards without abandoning a *mechanism* for supplementary substance-specific requirements where appropriate.

Pitfalls are undeniably associated with generic standards, but the advantages far outweigh the disadvantages. The precedents recently established by regulation, which I will briefly discuss, have created an opportune climate.

Of immediate and urgent importance is the need for a generic monitoring standard. Certainly the required elements of such a standard have become clear, and certainly it is defensible to support the right of workers who are significantly exposed to toxic materials to know what their exposure is.

Three historical endeavors come to mind when I think of generic standards: the joint OSHA/NIOSH Standards Completion Program, the OSHA Generic Carcinogen Policy, and the OSHA Hazard Communication Rule. The first two, although they failed, were probably ahead of their time and should be looked at again with today's hindsight. The Hazard Communication Rule set the stage for generic standards in the 1990s. I would like to discuss each of these briefly.

OSHA/NIOSH STANDARDS COMPLETION PROGRAM

In the mid-1970s, NIOSH and OSHA jointly undertook a massive multimillion dollar effort entitled the Standards Completion Program, intended to meet the mandate of the Occupational Safety and Health Act (Public Law 91–596, Sections 6 and 8) to provide requirements to protect employees beyond simply a Permissive Exposure Limit (PEL) when the potential for overexposure to chemical substances existed. The effort attempted to push through to promulgation expanded standards for groups of similar substances, but it was doomed to failure because the substance-specific approach hopelessly overloaded OSHA. The legacy of this effort was the logic used to formulate the expanded requirements. What we should consider for the 1990s is promulgation of a modern version of this logic as a complement to specific numbers.

By logic, I mean the decision process that systematically leads to a specific requirement. If the decision process can clearly be spelled out in regulations, or even not so clearly spelled out guidelines can be published, we will have achieved our objective.

The OSHA/NIOSH Standards Completion Program resulted in a comprehensive framework for standards—definitions, the concept of an action level, and all of the elements considered a part of expanded health standards that are promulgated today, including exposure monitoring, use of respirators and other personal protective equipment, sanitation, training, medical surveillance, record keeping, and use of nonmandatory appendices.

OSHA GENERIC CARCINOGEN POLICY

In the late 1970s an ambitious effort was undertaken by OSHA to develop a generic policy for carcinogens.[2] The effort captured the attention of all regulatory agencies as well as the broad public health community. A record 250,000 pages of extensive public hearings were produced. The effort, which remains perhaps the best example of an attempt to put into place a generic approach considering scientific uncertainty, unfortunately was never finalized. The policy prescribed the logic to be used to determine if a substance was to be considered a carcinogen, and the specific requirements to be contained in regulations for those substances meeting the criteria. It was reasoned that if agreement could be reached on the generic issues, they would not need to be reargued each time a substance was considered for regulation. The idea of reaching such agreement could be extended to the criteria for defining a "toxic" substance or a "significant exposure level."

OSHA HAZARD COMMUNICATION RULE

The OSHA Hazard Communication Rule (29CFR 1910.1200) broke significant new ground by requiring employers to identify and maintain a list of all "toxic materials" known to be present in their workplace and to inform workers of the hazards. The Rule defined what was meant by "toxic" (i.e., one positive study conducted in accordance with established scientific principles; oral $LD_{50} < 50$ mg/kg, rats; dermal $LD_{50} < 200$ mg/kg, rabbits; inhalation $LC_{50} < 200$ ppm or < 2 mg/liter, rats), but it did not specifically provide or reference any one listing or address what constituted a significant exposure level.

These attempts at generic standards lacked at least two fundamental concepts that should be considered in the future. First, there was no recognition of or requirement for a "qualified" or "competent" person with a mandated occupational safety and health responsibility to identify and quantify exposures and to develop a management plan for controlling exposures to toxic materials. Second, there was no recognition that employers who use toxic materials in significant quantities should have a basic occupational health program. I find it interesting that the precedents for these two missing regulatory ingredients can be found in recent EPA legislation.

THE ASBESTOS HAZARD EMERGENCY RESPONSE ACT (AHERA)

On October 22, 1986, President Reagan signed Public Law 99–519, the Asbestos Hazard Emergency Response Act of 1986 (AHERA).

AHERA amended the Toxic Substances Control Act (TSCA) to require the Environmental Protection Agency (EPA) to promulgate regulations requiring every school district to conduct inspections for asbestos-containing material in all school buildings, and to develop management plans and appropriate response actions, using accredited individuals, to deal with asbestos-containing materials in schools.

AHERA established a Model Accreditation Plan specifying in great detail the amount and content of training that individuals involved in asbestos abatement activities in schools must receive. Workers, contractors, supervisors, project designers, inspectors, and management planners all must be accredited for the type of work they perform. Further "awareness training" is required for all custodial and maintenance personnel with additional requirements for those who come in contact with asbestos-containing materials.

Using accredited individuals, school districts must inspect every school building for the presence of asbestos-containing material, must develop a management plan for each school building, must develop an ongoing operations and maintenance program for any school building where asbestos exists, and must reinspect buildings with asbestos at least every 3 years. Specific requirements are established for determining whether materials contain asbestos as well as for air sampling in an attempt to ensure that air levels are not increased as a result of abatement actions.

There are lessons to be learned from the AHERA legislation. Although it currently applies only to public and private schools, kindergarten through grade 12, legislation has already been introduced that extends it to all public buildings. The next logical step is to look beyond asbestos to all toxic materials.

Fundamental to taking this next step and to developing generic standards in general is the well-recognized and controversial need to define what is meant by "toxic" and "significant exposure." I simply propose that on a regular basis NIOSH publish a listing of recognized safe exposure levels. I call your attention to Section 20(a)(6) of the OSHA Act (Public Law 91–596) which mandated NIOSH . . . "to publish . . . at least annually a list of all known toxic substances by generic family or other useful grouping, and the concentrations at which such toxicity is known to occur." NIOSH has addressed this mandate by publishing the Registry of Toxic Effects of Chemical Substances (RTECS), which identifies those compounds having recognized safe exposure levels. What is needed is merely a sublisting of RTECs, which would become a standard guidance document for employers. I define "recognized" as referring to established organizations, principally OSHA, NIOSH, and ACGIH, who establish or recommend exposure limits.

I further propose that "significant exposure" be defined as exposure in excess of one half the *lowest* recognized safe exposure level that occurs either under normal conditions or in a forseeable emergency. These levels could be referred to as action levels. The idea of action level triggering monitoring, medical and employee information, and training requirements is not new, having originated as previously mentioned in the Standards Completion Program and having become an expected ingredient of modern standards.

I next propose that generic standards of the 1990s require the use of "competent" persons. OSHA, in its new Asbestos Construction Standard (29 CFR 1926.58, effective July 21, 1986), for the first time in its history, introduced the requirement for a competent person, defining him or her as "one who is capable of identifying existing asbestos in the workplace and who has the authority to take prompt corrective action to eliminate [asbestos]." The duties of the competent person [were defined to] "include at least the following: establishing the negative-pressure enclosure, ensuring its integrity, and controlling entry to and exit from the enclosure; supervising any employee exposure monitoring required by the standards; ensuring that all employees working within such an enclosure wear the appropriate personal protective equipment, are trained in the use of appropriate methods of exposure control, and the use of hygiene facilities and decontamination procedures specified in the standard; and ensuring that engineering controls in use are in proper operating condition and are functioning properly (p. 22756)." The standard further explains that "the competent person will generally be a Certified Industrial Hygienist, an industrial hygienist with training and experience in the handling of asbestos, or a person who has such training and experience as a result of on-the-job training and experience (p. 22780)." . . . "The competent person shall be trained in all aspects of asbestos . . . abatement, the contents of [the] standard, the identification of asbestos . . . and their removal procedures, and other practices for reducing the hazard, such training shall be obtained in a comprehensive course, such as a course conducted by an EPA Asbestos Training Center, or an equivalent course (p. 22757)."

RECOMMENDATIONS

If the definition of toxic substance and significant exposure, and the need for a competent person defined to be an industrial hygienist are accepted, I can conclude with a recommended generic standard involving six elements, which for political expediency, may be considered independently. These six elements are: (1) initial determination; (2) employee-exposure monitoring; (3) medical surveillance; (4) sanitation; (5) training and education; and (6) the management plan.

Initial Determination

I am convinced that many, if not most, overexposures to toxic materials that are occurring in the workplace are unrecognized by employers and employees. Each employer should be required to conduct an initial inspection of his or her workplace, using a competent person, to determine if exposures in excess of action levels are present. This initial determination may not require air sampling, but it may be based on objective data supported in writing by a competent person. The only burden on employers at this point, beyond that already required by the Hazard Communication Rule, would be to assess the potential for exposure in excess of action levels. If employees are likely to be exposed in excess of action levels, then the remaining five "preventive health" elements would be required.

Employee-Exposure Monitoring

When exposures are in excess of action levels, periodic monitoring by competent persons "at such frequency and pattern to represent with reasonable accuracy the levels of exposure of employees" should be required. In no case should sampling intervals be greater than 6 months. If periodic monitoring reveals that exposures are below action levels, the employer should be allowed to discontinue monitoring until there is reason to suspect that exposures may be increased above action levels as with a change in production, process, control equipment, personnel, or work practice.

The requirements for an initial determination with subsequent employee-exposure monitoring, when warranted, could be combined into a generic monitoring standard. Such a standard, in my opinion, is long overdue and urgently needed.

Medical Surveillance

Medical examinations should be made available at no charge to employees exposed in excess of action levels. The current proposed high-risk occupational disease and prevention legislation provides for medical examinations of high-risk employees. However, periodic medical examinations should be routine for all workers exposed to significant levels of toxic materials. Examinations could be performed by a physician's assistant, nurse practitioner, or other health professional, acting under the direction of a physician, to reduce the burden on existing medical facilities.

Sanitation

Laundering of contaminated employee work clothing should be required when a toxic material may cause acute or chronic illness due to resulting exposure if the employee wears the contaminated clothing home. The definition of toxic could be the same as that used in the Hazard Communication Rule.

Employees exposed to toxic materials should be provided showers.

Training and Education

Employees should be informed of the nature and possible effects that could result from overexposure to toxic materials consistent with the OSHA Hazard Communication Rule.

Management Plan

Employers should be required to develop and maintain a management plan for controlling exposures to toxic materials in their workplace. One essential element of such a plan should be the long recognized principle that engineering controls should be implemented wherever and whenever feasible to reduce employee exposure, before reliance on respiratory protection is permitted.

I propose that employers who have exposures in excess of recognized safe exposure levels, but not in excess of PELs (accepting that a PEL may not exist), should not be *required* to take corrective action to reduce exposure unless they are in excess of established PELs. The conservative tendency, however, would be to control exposures below recognized safe exposure levels, to avoid liability, and even further below action levels, to avoid the requirements of the generic standard discussed earlier. We all know that the fear of liability often forces compliance with recommended levels and accepted state-of-the-art good work practices.

Accreditation of Competent Persons

NIOSH could establish minimal criteria for competent persons. As a minimum, these persons should be trained industrial hygienists. Perhaps multiple levels of accreditation should be considered, with larger programs required to be under the supervision of a board-certified industrial hygienist. Smaller employers would not require these individuals on a full-time basis, but they could contract for their services from consulting firms. NIOSH could approve training programs and serve a quality control function.

Implementation

It could be argued effectively that this proposal would overwhelm our current resources in occupational health, particularly industrial hygiene. It would seem reasonable to provide a phase-in plan, requiring initial compliance of larger employers with timetables for smaller employers.

CONCLUSIONS

Regulatory activity in the 1990s should first reassess, refocus, and broaden current approaches by defining what is meant by significant exposure. Once this is accomplished, a generic standard (or standards) should be proposed that relies on a competent person and that involves the requirements for the following:

1. Initial inspection of all workplaces to determine the presence of toxic materials consistent with the requirements of the OSHA Hazard Communication Rule and further the potential for significant exposure;

2. Periodic exposure monitoring of workers in excess of action levels (i.e., one-half the recognized safe exposure levels);

3. Medical surveillance for all employees exposed significantly (i.e., in excess of action levels) to toxic substances;

4. Sanitation, including laundering of contaminated work clothing and providing show facilities;

5. Training and education, on a regular basis, of all employees who are significantly exposed; and

6. A management plan for controlling exposures to toxic materials, incorporating the basic requirement that engineering controls must be implemented, in preference to personal protective equipment, wherever feasible to reduce exposure.

It is neither unreasonable nor indefensible to require that employers who have employees exposed to recognized toxic materials identify that exposure, quantify it, provide basic medical surveillance to ensure workers are protected, and to inform workers of the nature and magnitude of their exposures. It could be conceded that a requirement to control levels below Permissible Exposure Levels, which have been carefully evaluated and considered as part of a formal extensive rule-making procedure, may place an unjustified burden on employers and put organizations who recommend safe exposure levels in an inappropriate regulatory position. Thus, required Permissible Exposure Levels could continue to be promulgated, but far more expediently. The time is opportune to move forward to promulgate generic standards to achieve these objectives.

SUMMARY

OSHA and EPA regulations promulgated to date contain the necessary framework to consider generic standards in the 1990s. Missing in OSHA standards has been the requirement for a competent person to define and manage an occupational health program and the requirement for all employers who have toxic materials with significant exposures to have a basic occupational health program. Certainly we have evolved to a point where every worker significantly exposed to toxic materials has a right to know what that exposure is.

Fundamental to generic standards is the need to define what is meant by toxic substance and significant exposure level. It is suggested that NIOSH maintain a list of recognized safe exposure levels that have been recommended by credible organizations including NIOSH.

It is suggested that action levels be defined as one-half the lowest recognized safe exposure level. It is proposed that all employers be required to conduct an initial inspection of their workplace, using competent persons, to determine if exposures exceed action levels. This is only one step beyond the requirements of the OSHA Hazard Communication Rule which requires that employers identify and maintain a list of all hazardous materials known to be present in the workplace and to inform workers of the hazards.

If exposure levels are found in excess of action levels, then the basic elements of current standards would be required, including regular employee-exposure monitoring, medical surveillance, sanitation, training and education, and a management plan.

REFERENCES

1. LYNCH, J. R., N. A. LEIDEL, R. A. NELSON, & R. F. BOGGS. 1978. The Standards Completion Program, Draft Technical Standards Analysis and Decision Logics, USDHEW, PHS, CDC, NIOSH, NTIS Pub. No. PB-282-989.
2. Occupational Safety and Health Administration (OSHA); Oct. 4, 1977. Identification, Classification and Regulation of Toxic Substances Posing a Potential Carcinogenic Risk. Federal Register Part VI 54148. Jan. 22, 1980; Identification, Classification and Regulation of Potential Occupational Carcinogens. Federal Register Part VII 5001.
3. MCGARITY, T. 1979. Substantive and procedural discretion in administrative resolution of science policy questions: Regulating Carcinogens in EPA & OSHA. Georgetown Law J. **729:** 733-749.
4. RUTTENBERG, R. & E. BINGHAM. 1981. A comprehensive occupational carcinogen policy as a framework for regulatory activity. Ann. N.Y. Acad. Sci. **363:** 13.

Occupational Safety and Health Standards

RICHARD A. LEMEN, LAWRENCE F. MAZZUCKELLI,
RICHARD W. NIEMEIER, AND HEINZ W. AHLERS

National Institute for Occupational Safety and Health
U.S. Department of Health and Human Services
Cincinnati, Ohio 45226

The Occupational Safety and Health Act[1] is the product of years of human experience with industrial environments. Unfortunately, the American work force had to endure a series of particularly shocking tragedies that eventually led Congress to take steps to "assure so far as possible every working man and woman in the nation safe and healthful working conditions."

What has been the history of standards development in the United States? In 1877, Massachusetts passed the first occupational safety law, and in 1893 legislation was passed by the U.S. Congress regulating railroad safety.[2] Between 1920 and 1948 all of the States had passed worker compensation laws; Mississippi was the last.[3] According to Gersuny,[3] most of these laws emphasized safety-related problems and had the support of conservative economic groups. The purpose of these workers' compensation laws was to undercut unionists and other advocates of adversary posture in labor-management relations.

The first air-quality standards or guidelines were published in 1912 by Rudolf Kobert[4] titled, "The Smallest Amounts of Noxious Industrial Gases Which Are Toxic and the Amounts Which May Perhaps Be Endured." This list included 20 compounds such as HCl, chlorine, bromine, and ammonia. Other lists followed, and most were based on least-detectable odor or least amount required to cause irritation. In 1921 the Bureau of Mines published the first federal technical paper with limits for 33 compounds.[5] The first list to consider not only acute effects, but also effects from prolonged exposure was that of Henderson and Haggard[6] in 1927. The U.S. Public Health Service issued a manual listing recommended values based on its collective experience in 1943. In 1946 the American Conference of Governmental Industrial Hygienists (ACGIH) published its list for 140 substances.[7] Others, such as Cook[8] in 1945 and Smyth[9] in 1956, also published suggested limits on expanded lists. Smyth's list contained 240 substances. This trend of publishing exposure limits continues to the present time.

There are several federal laws that have affected the standards-setting process. The first was the limited legislation concerning coal mine and railroad safety enacted in the 1880s.[2] The next significant law addressing workplace safety in the United States was the National Labor Relations Act, commonly known as the Wagner Act of 1935,[10] legitimizing unionization and collective bargaining. The Walsh-Healy Public Contracts Act of 1936[11] provided federal jurisdiction in areas of regulation of working hours and also standards concerning safety and health, but it was limited to only those with government contracts of $10,000 or more. The Labor Management Relations Act of 1947 provided that the employee might quit work in good faith because of "abnormally dangerous conditions," without it being considered a strike.[12]

The Metal and Nonmetallic Mine Safety Act of 1966[13] followed by the federal Coal Mine Health and Safety Act of 1969[14] marked the beginning of the federal government's effort to provide a safe workplace through specific and detailed regulations.

As recently as 20 years ago, the American workforce still faced the risk of job-related death and injury. At hearings before the Senate Subcommittee on Labor of the Committee on Labor and Public Welfare in 1966, Secretary of Labor Willard Wirtz provided the following testimony:

> Mr. Chairman, and members of the Committee, while we sit here talking, from now until noon, seventeen American men and women will be killed on their jobs.
>
> Every minute we talk, 18 to 20 people will be hurt severely enough to have to leave their jobs—some of them never to work again.
>
> In the time these two sentences have taken, another 20 people—one every second—have been injured on the job—less seriously, but in most cases needlessly.
>
> Today's industrial casualty list—like yesterday's—and tomorrow's—and every working day's week after month after year— will be 55 dead, 8,500 disabled, over 27,200 hurt.
>
> The figures for the year will be 14,000 to 15,000 dead, over 2 million disabled, over 7 million hurt.

The testimony given by Secretary Wirtz and others clearly described the magnitude of the problem.

Data published by the Office of Technology Assessment (OTA) of the U.S. Congress in 1985[15] concluded that between 1979 and 1983 at least 4,650 and as many as 12,200 workers died as a result of occupational injuries each year. The total number of occupational deaths each year will obviously be greater than this, if one includes delayed deaths due to exposure to chemicals and physical agents such as asbestos, coal dust, and benzene. The point is obvious. In 1966, Secretary Wirtz estimated the annual occupational death toll to be about 14,000. In 1985 the U.S. Congress estimated the annual occupational death toll to be about 12,000. The similarity between these two figures tells you how far we have progressed, at least in absolute numbers.

When Congress passed the Occupational Safety and Health Act in 1970,[16] its members realized that until the Occupational Safety and Health Administration (OSHA) could implement the rule-making procedures established in the Act, there must be a set of workplace health standards that OSHA could implement. The solution that Congress arrived at was to allow OSHA to adopt existing guidelines for workplace exposure limits as OSHA standards for airborne contaminants. At the time the largest collection of such guidelines was the list of Threshold Limit Values (TLVs) published by the ACGIH. Additional standards were adopted from consensus standards produced by the American Standards Association, now called The American National Standards Institute, and the National Fire Protection Association. Thus, OSHA began its existence with exposure standards for about 400 substances of industrial importance. They are contained in the Z-Tables of the current Code of Federal Regulations.[17] In Section 6(b) of the Occupational Safety and Health Act[1] it is made clear that Congress intended that OSHA should promulgate new standards to update those on the Z-Tables using information supplied to them by the National Institute for Occupational Safety and Health (NIOSH) or other interested parties. The process established by Congress required that new OSHA standards be established following public scrutiny and discussion of the most current data. Congress also directed NIOSH to provide OSHA with data necessary to promulgate new standards.

Since passage of the Occupational Safety and Health Act of 1970, NIOSH has supplied OSHA with recommended standards for about 125 individual chemical substances. And since passage of the Act, OSHA has promulgated new standards for about 26 chemical substances.

At the current rate of promulgation (about 1.5 standards a year), about 270 years will be needed to establish new standards for the 400 substances in the OSHA Z-Tables. On the basis of the history of the first 15 years of NIOSH, it will take about 50 years to produce recommended standards for the remainder of the substances in the Z-Tables.

OSHA is currently considering a proposal to update and expand the Z-Table containing those old start-up standards. This is a laudable idea, because the old table contains standards based on 1968 or earlier data; however, it can entail a number of problems. One major problem lies with the depth and reliability of documentation in the various data sources OSHA has to draw upon. If, for example, OSHA were to again use the ACGIH TLVs as their basic resource instead of NIOSH recommended standards, they would not be following the mandates of the OSHAct. NIOSH recommended exposure limits[1] are intended to present: ". . . criteria dealing with toxic materials and harmful physical agents and substances which will describe exposure levels that are safe for various periods of employment, including but not limited to the exposure levels at which no employee will suffer impaired health or functional capacities or diminished life expectancy as a result of his work experience." The ACGIH TLVs, however, are intended as guidelines for health professionals to use in establishing protective procedures and are threshold limit values which: ". . . refer to airborne concentrations of substances and represent conditions under which it is believed that *nearly all workers* may be repeatedly exposed day after day without adverse effect."[18] ACGIH TLVs are not intended to be used as exposure limits according to ACGIH's testimony at the October 1987 OSHA hearings on the proposed rule for hazardous waste site workers.

In one analysis of 12 chemicals found on the top 100 National Priority List for hazardous waste cleanup sites, three—lead, benzene, and arsenic—already have permissible exposure limits (PELs) established by OSHA through the public rule-making process. For these three chemicals, the current ACGIH TLVs are 3–20 times higher than the OSHA PELs. Analysis of six of the other nine chemicals revealed some interesting findings.

The TLV documentation for trichloroethylene stated that "A TLV of 50 ppm, as a time weighted average, is recommended to control subjective complaints such as headache, fatigue and irritability. A STEL of 200 ppm is recommended to protect against incoordination and other beginning anesthetic effects from trichloroethylene. These levels provide a wide margin of safety in preventing liver injury."[18]

In this same documentation, the ACGIH cited three studies in which neurotoxic effects were reported at concentrations that ranged from 1–335 ppm and became particularly noticeable at concentrations of about 40 ppm. This same recommendation also cited a National Cancer Institute bioassay[19] that demonstrated hepatocellular carcinoma in mice.

In a NIOSH evaluation of these same data,[20] it was concluded that the reports of neurotoxicity and carcinogenicity were sufficient to warrant a reduction of the PEL to 25 ppm as an 8-hour time-weighted average (TWA). NIOSH also noted that this is a concentration that can be attained through the use of existing engineering controls.

The 1986 TLV for chloroform[18] states: "In view of recent reports on carcinogenicity and embryotoxicity of chloroform, the Committee recommendation for a TLV is 10 ppm, as a TWA, and classification as an Industrial Substance Suspect of Carcinogenic Potential for Man (A2). A concentration of 10 ppm is one-fifth the concentration at which organ injury was observed and one-half the concentration which would be derived comparing the toxicity of other organic solvents." NIOSH in 1976 lowered their recommended exposure limits to 2 ppm because of the suspected carcinogenic potential of chloroform.[21]

The ACGIH have two TLVs for polychlorinated biphenyls (PCBs) based on their chlorine content.[18] For those compounds containing 42% chlorine, the TLV is 1 mg/cm as an 8-hour TWA with a STEL of 2 mg/cm. Those PCBs having 54% chlorine have a TLV of 0.5 mg/cm as an 8-hour TWA with a short-term exposure limit (STEL) of 1 mg/cm. The most recent study cited in this 1986 documentation was published in 1977. The documentation carries no mention of carcinogenicity but does carry a statement of intent to delete the STEL.

In response to data on the carcinogenicity of the PCBs, NIOSH in 1977 recommended an exposure limit of 0.001 mg/cm of air[22] (the minimum reliably quantifiable concentration using the recommended sampling and analytic methods). These recommendations should be considered in the context of the EPA ban on the use of PCBs as a dielectric in transformers and capacitors, and the fact that PCBs are the only substances specifically mentioned in the Toxic Substances Control Act.[23]

The most recent data cited by the ACGIH in support of its TLV for 1,1,2,2-tetrachloroethane were published in 1972. The ACGIH[18] states that there are no data on carcinogenicity, mutagenicity, or teratogenicity in either animals or humans.

In 1978 NIOSH[24] recommended that tetrachloroethane be controlled to the lowest feasible concentration because of its carcinogenicity and its effects on the liver, gastrointestinal tract, and nervous system. The International Agency for Research on Cancer (IARC) listed it as a suspect animal carcinogen in 1979.[25]

The ACGIH also cites[18] data from Schmidt, indicating pathologic changes in rats at 2 ppm, and data from Navrotsky, indicating hematologic changes in rabbits at 1.5 ppm, before concluding that 1 ppm is safe for human exposure.

The most current information cited by the ACGIH in their 1986 documentation for cadmium was published in 1977.[18] Although they cited the 1976 NIOSH criteria document on cadmium in which NIOSH concluded that the available information was insufficient evidence of cadmium's carcinogenicity, the ACGIH did not acknowledge information published in 1979, 1980, 1982, and 1983 or the *revised* NIOSH policy in 1984 that described cadmium's carcinogenicity, and recommended that exposures be reduced to the lowest feasible level.[26] It should also be noted that IARC[27] recognizes cadmium as a carcinogen. All of these reports noted associations between cadmium exposure and carcinogenicity in both animals and humans.

The literature on chromium and its compounds is not clear, particularly that on chromium VI compounds, some of which are water soluble and some of which are not.

NIOSH recommends 0.001 mg/m^3 for carcinogenic Cr VI and 0.025 mg/m^3 for other chromium VI compounds.[28] The latter includes a 15-minute ceiling of 0.05 mg/m^3. NIOSH has a separate recommendation for chromic acid of 0.025 mg/m^3 as a TWA and 0.05 mg/m^3 as a 15-minute ceiling. It is important to note that the ACGIH recommendation for Cr VI compounds, 0.05 mg/m^3, cites data from Mancuso and Hueper estimating that workers who developed lung cancer were exposed to Cr VI concentrations as low as 0.01 mg/m^3, a concentration one fifth of the recommended TLV.[18]

For toluene,[29] phenol,[30] and xylene,[31] both NIOSH and the ACGIH[18] essentially agree on similar exposure limits.

SUMMARY AND CONCLUSION

If we are to approach developing a safe and healthful workplace in a more timely fashion, a more generic approach must be considered and applied instead of developing recommendations and standards simply on a substance-by-substance basis, an approach that has been the most prominent. Some examples in which developing generic standards may be appropriate are: cholinesterase-inhibiting substances, neurotoxic agents, reproductive hazards, cold environments, and vibration syndrome, to name but a few.

It is important to recognize that developing standards based on individual substances often does not allow for the role of synergism, a reaction that has had little study, but it is important in controlling occupational disease and injury.

These concerns can be addressed in several ways. One is to look at processes or conditions found in the workplace; for example, coke oven emissions that OSHA has promulgated into a standard[32] and, as NIOSH has done in their recommendations to OSHA for foundries,[33] coal tar products,[34] the manufacture of paint and allied coatings,[35] field sanitation,[36] hazardous waste management,[37] hot environments,[38] and confined spaces.[39] Another is to address groups of similar substances such as NIOSH has done with alkanes,[40] benzidine-based dyes,[41] diisocyanates,[42] dinitrotoluenes,[43] and glycol ethers.[44] A third comprehensive approach is to look at general categories of hazards, such as the generic carcinogen policy,[45] and the hazard communication rule.[46]

Finally, risk must be considered in the development of any standard. Nelson Rockefeller once said in relation to an incidence involving a radiation hazard that, "you can't have a riskless society." I would amend this to say that you cannot have a reckless society either. Safety and health regulations are essential and must be designed, promulgated, and then enforced so that a reckless society is avoided or controlled, with a riskless society being the ultimate aim.

[**Note added in proof:** OSHA published a time rule on air contaminants on January 19, 1989 in the Federal Register (**54**(12): 2329–2984) updating the OSHA PELs.]

REFERENCES

1. Occupational Safety and Health Act of 1970, 29 USC 651, *et seq*. Public Law 91–596.
2. Safety Appliance Acts, Act of March 2, 1893; 45 USC 1, *et seq*. 127 Stat 53., and Employers Liability Act, Act of April 22, 1908; 45 USC 51, 35 Stat 65.
3. GERSUNY, C. 1981. Work Hazards and Industrial Conflict. University Press of New England. Hanover, NH.
4. SCHRENK, H. H. 1947. Interpretation of Permissible Limits. Am. Indust. Hyg. Assoc. Q. **8:** 55–60.
5. FIELDNER, A. C., S. H. KATZ & S. P. KINNEY. 1921. Gas masks for gases met in fighting fires. Bureau of Mines and Tech. Paper **248:** 56.
6. HENDERSON, Y. & H. HAGGARD. 1927. Noxious Gases and the Principles Influencing Their Action. New York. (Cited in Schrenk[4].)
7. ACGIH. 1946. Threshold Limit Values for 1946. American Conference of Governmental Industrial Hygienists. Cincinnati, Ohio.
8. COOK, W. A. 1945. Maximum allowable concentrations of industrial atmospheric contaminants. Indust. Med. **14:** 936–946.
9. SMYTH, H. F. 1956. Improved communication-hygiene standards for daily inhalation. Indust. Hyg. Q. **17:** 129–185.
10. Wagner Act of June 5, 1935 and Labor Management Relations Act of 1947; 29 USC 151, *et. seq*.

11. Walsh-Healy Act, Act of June 30, 1936; 41 USC 35, 49 Stat 2036.
12. Labor Management Relations Act of 1947; 29 USC 143, 61 Stat 162.
13. Metal and Metallic Mine Safety Act of 1966; Public Law 89–577.
14. Federal Coal Mine Safety and Health Act of 1969; 29 USC 801, *et seq*. Public Law 91–173.
15. OFFICE OF TECHNOLOGY ASSESSMENT. 1985. Preventing Illness and Injury in the Workplace. U.S. Congress, Office of Technology Assessment, OTA-H-256. Washington, DC.
16. MINTZ, B. W. 1984. OSHA: History, Law and Policy. The Bureau of National Affairs, Inc. Washington, DC.
17. Code of Federal Regulations. 1987. 29 CFR 1910.1000, Air Contaminants.
18. ACGIH. 1986. Documentation of the Threshold Limit Values and Biological Exposure Indices, 5th ed. American Conference of Governmental Industrial Hygienists. Cincinnati, Ohio.
19. National Cancer Institute: Carcinogenesis Bioassay of Trichloroethylene. 1976. National Cancer Institute Technical Report Series No. 2, DHEW Pub. No. (NIH) 76-802. Washington, DC.
20. PAGE, N. & J. ARTHUR. 1978. Special Occupational Hazard Review of Trichloroethylene. DHEW (NIOSH) Pub. No. 78–130.
21. 1975. NIOSH Criteria for a Recommended Standard . . . Occupational Exposure to Chloroform. DHHS (NIOSH) Pub. No. 75–114.
22. 1977. NIOSH Criteria for a Recommended Standard . . . Occupational Exposure to Polychlorinated Biphenyls. DHHS (NIOSH) Pub. No. 77–225.
23. Toxic Substances Control Act, Public Law 94–469.
24. 1978. NIOSH Criteria for a Recommended Standard . . . Occupational Exposure to 1,1,2,2-tetrachloroethane. DHHS (NIOSH) Pub. No. 77–121.
25. WORLD HEALTH ORGANIZATION 1979. IARC Monographs on the Evaluation of the Carcinogenic Risk of Chemicals to Humans. Some Halogenated Hydrocarbons, Vol. 20. 1,1,2,2-tetrachloroethane, p. 477.
26. 1984. NIOSH Current Intelligence Bulletin 42: Cadmium (Cd). DHHS (NIOSH) Pub. No. 84–116.
27. WORLD HEALTH ORGANIZATION 1979. IARC Monographs on the Evaluation of the Carcinogenic Risk of Chemicals to Humans. IARC Monographs, Suppl. 1.
28. 1975. NIOSH Critera for a Recommended Standard: Occupational Exposure to Chromium (VI). DHHS (NIOSH) Pub. No. 76–129.
29. 1973. NIOSH Criteria for a Recommended Standard . . . Occupational Exposure to Toluene. DHHS (NIOSH) Pub. No. 73–11023.
30. 1976. NIOSH Criteria for a Recommended Standard . . . Occupational Exposure to Phenol. DHHS (NIOSH) Pub. No. 76–196.
31. 1975. NIOSH Criteria for a Recommended Standard . . . Occupational Exposure to Xylene. DHHS (NIOSH) Pub. No. 75–168.
32. 1987. Code of Federal Regulations. 29 CFR 1910.1029, Coke Oven Emissions.
33. 1985. NIOSH Recommendations for Control of Occupational Safety and Health Hazards . . . Foundries. DHHS (NIOSH) Pub. No. 85–116.
34. 1978. NIOSH Criteria for a Recommended Standard for Occupational Exposure to . . . Coal Tar Products. DHHS (NIOSH) Pub. No. 78–107.
35. 1984. NIOSH Recommendations for Control of Occupational Safety and Health Hazards . . . Manufacture of Paint and Allied Coating Products. DHHS (NIOSH) Pub. No. 84–115.
36. 1984. NIOSH Testimony to U.S. Department of Labor, Occupational Safety and Health Administration Proposed Rule: Field Sanitation Docket No. H-308.
37. 1987. NIOSH Testimony to U.S. Department of Labor, Occupational Safety and Health Administration Proposed Rule: Hazardous Waste Sites. Docket No. S–760A.
38. 1986. NIOSH Criteria for a Recommended Standard . . . Occupational Exposure to Hot Environments (Revised Criteria). DHHS (NIOSH) Pub. No. 86–113.
39. 1979. NIOSH Criteria for a Recommended Standard . . . Working in Confined Space. DHHS (NIOSH) Pub. No. 80–106.
40. 1977. NIOSH Criteria for a Recommended Standard . . . Occupational Exposure to Alkanes (C5-C8). DHHS (NIOSH) Pub. No. 77–151.

41. 1980. NIOSH Special Occupational Hazard Review for Benzidine-Based Dyes. DHHS (NIOSH) Pub. No. 80–107.
42. 1979. NIOSH Criteria for a Recommended Standard . . . Occupational Exposure to Diisocyanates. DHHS (NIOSH) Pub. No. 78–125.
43. 1985. NIOSH Current Intelligence Bulletin 44: Dinitrotoluenes (DNT). DHHS (NIOSH) Pub. No. 85–109.
44. 1983. NIOSH Current Intelligence Bulletin 39: Glycol Ethers, 2-methoxyethanol and 2-ethoxyethanol. DHHS (NIOSH) Pub. No. 83–112.
45. 1987. Code of Federal Regulations. 29 CFR 1990, *et seq.*, Identification, Classifications, and Regulation of Potential Occupational Carcinogens.
46. 1987. Code of Federal Regulations. 29 CFR 1910.1200. Hazard Communications.

Round Table 2: Discussion

EILEEN TARLAU (*New Jersey Department of Health, Trenton, N.J.*): I am an industrial hygienist. I would like to point out that we have, in the general duty clause of OSHA, the most generic of all standards. The creative use of this OSHA general duty clause could transform OSHA. However, the biggest obstacle to creatively using the clause for chemical hazards is the presence in OSHA standards of the permissible exposure limits in Tables Z1, Z2, and Z3. I propose that an easily achievable goal would be to get rid of the PELs as a first move in a new OSHA. That action would enable OSHA inspectors to completely change the way they do business. Right now OSHA inspectors spend their time going around taking samples, 95% of which show that employers are in compliance with the PELs. Freed from that bias, OSHA inspectors could go into workplaces and look for sick people and hazardous practices. They could creatively invoke the general duty clause, which could also be used for other hazards, such as repetitive trauma, in addition to chemical hazards. I would like to point out, also, that the Standards Completion project only solidifies the impediment that the PELs provide to cleaning up the workplaces.

R. HAYS BELL (*Eastman Kodak Company, Rochester, N.Y.*): I certainly concur that the general duty clause could be a fine example of a generic standard, but it would be very difficult to eliminate the PELs and to depend then on the general duty clause to substantiate violations; it would take too much time in the courts and tie up resources.

BERTRAM COTTINE (*Bureau of National Affairs, Washington, D.C.*): While you may view the general duty clause creatively, regrettably, none of my colleagues or their successors on the Commission have a very creative view of its legislative purpose. After having seen more than 60 cases involving the general duty clause come before the Commission, they indicated two things to me. First, the cases involved a tremendous investment of the technical and scientific resources of OSHA; and, second, they created factual questions that were almost impossible to resolve in an adjudicatory setting. As a result, one could hardly find unanimity, and rarely majority views, on the general duty clause. This is a very serious practical impediment. So, while I believe the general duty clause is an important component of the statute, I would agree with Dr. Bell that proceeding under that provision might not be the best investment of the Agency's resources.

JORDAN BARAB (*American Federation of State, County and Municipal Employees, Washington, D.C.*): We have been discussing the mistakes that OSHA has made during the last 18 years in terms of not having enough generic standards; in addition we should also be talking about correcting those mistakes and looking ahead and not making the same mistakes again.

In particular, I want to mention the area of infectious diseases. OSHA has been petitioned and is now embarking on regulating certain infectious diseases, focusing mainly on AIDS and hepatitis B. OSHA is starting off here with an Advanced Notice of Proposed Rule Making for blood-borne infectious diseases alone, completely leaving out the rest of the infectious diseases that workers encounter. We petitioned OSHA more than a year ago to regulate not only bloodborne, but also *all* infectious diseases in a generic standard. However, OSHA is not responding. We are finding this particularly frustrating because exposures to several diseases often occur together. For example, in connection with AIDS, we find a direct connection between the increase in AIDS and the increase in the rate of tuberculosis. Assuming that a standard goes into effect for bloodborne diseases, we would have a paradoxical situation where workers would be trained to take precautions for hepatitis B and for AIDS but not for tuberculosis. This seems like a foolish mistake on the part of OSHA.

MITCHELL ZAVON (*Agatha Corporation, Cincinnati, Ohio*): The Occupational Safety and Health Act states that the employer shall provide a safe and healthful workplace. I have always been mystified as to how OSHA can indicate that the workplace is safe and healthful when the employer is not required to properly characterize the workplace. I would suggest for your consideration that whether or not generic standards are proposed, OSHA should propose over the next 25 years a mandatory schedule of characterizations of workplaces throughout the nation; it would take a week to figure out such a schedule. All places of employment would be required to characterize the workplace so that OSHA inspectors could determine from the data available whether or not a particular workplace is safe and healthful. And if a workplace has not been characterized properly and thoroughly, it would automatically not be considered safe and healthful. I know of very few firms that have ever done a proper industrial hygiene survey of their plants. A wall-to-wall industrial hygiene study of the workplace will often show all sorts of things that might be suspect, but whose effect is not known at this time. And often, certainly in chemical plants, this finding will alert management to the fact that they are wasting a product, or wasting intermediates, or that they do not know what the reaction really is. Such surveys can have a very salutary effect on our competitiveness as an industrial society by making us more interested in what is really happening within the plant while at the same time contributing to a database that will make it easier and more feasible to create a healthy working environment.

JEFFREY LEE (*University of Utah, Salt Lake City, Utah*): I agree, but I am struggling with the question of whether an employer or workplace that was completely free of any significant hazard should be excluded from inspection. Therefore, I suggested that when the potential existed for excess exposure, an excess of one-half of the recognized safe exposure levels be set.

DOROTHY WIGMORE (*Manitoba Federation of Labor, Occupational Health Center, Winnipeg, Manitoba*): In my former role as a hygienist with the Manitoba government, I was principally responsible for the initial drafting of a regulation for the Province that sounds very much like your proposal for a generic approach to an occupational hygiene program in workplaces. I am pleased to say that five and a half years later, the Cabinet passed a regulation in two parts, and that this regulation will be taking effect in Manitoba in October 1988. It basically involves a combination of the hazard communication regulation which has been implemented on a national level in Canada, and the requirements for the evaluation and the control measures that you discussed. Also, as part of this regulation, there is a requirement for the development of occupational exposure limits for any substance to which workers are exposed. These regulations can be based either on TLVs properly used and/or other information. There will be lowest detectable levels set for more than 130 substances that are considered to be carcinogens, mutagens, respiratory sensitizers, or reproductive toxins based on certain criteria that have been developed at the national level under the hazard communication scheme.

A lot of the material currently discussed is of great interest to me because I have been involved with these issues in the last few years. These regulations are not perfect by any means, but one of the elements that has helped them along is an advisory committee. In our case, the committee consisted of labor and management representatives who then worked with persons in the government to draft acceptable regulations. Although a technically qualified individual is defined in these regulations, it must be recognized that they are few in number. Thus, the role of workers is very important, because they are very able to do such tasks as taking inventories or conducting effective occupational hygiene surveys, once they are trained. Training is another very important component that the labor movement has been pressing for and one on which the labor movement in Canada has a good record.

JAMES CONE (*The Northern California Occupational Health Center, San Francisco, Calif.*): The issues addressed here have touched on many of our concerns, although one that has not been—and that lies within the artificial barrier between occupational and environmental health—is building-associated illness, a syndrome afflicting large numbers. Many of the problems that I have to deal with would not be addressed by new PELs. As far as I know, there are no buildings where anything approaching even 10% of a PEL has ever been measured, except in a rare circumstance. This issue would also not be addressed by generic medical surveillance programs, because the action limit would never be reached. The issue of the building syndrome raises the question of why an artificial separation exists between occupational and environmental health. Why is there a double standard in the field? Clearly, buildings should be looked at as a kind of an environmental arena where we need to look at performance standards in terms of ventilation. Building owners must be made to maintain their buildings in a way that provides for a healthy and safe working environment. If we begin to look at regulations in that area, putting the onus on the persons who designed these buildings inadequately, we would begin to see some progress in prevention.

LEE: Dr. Cone, your public radio broadcast on the "tight building syndrome" in Florida was well received in Salt Lake City. I agree with you that we are moving toward a basic occupational health program again, one requirement of which could be a generic standard approach. Once that is in place, the program could address the tight building syndrome as well as other problems.

I am currently the past chair of the American Conference of Governmental Industrial Hygienists, the ACGIH. And, although I am not here representing the ACGIH, I think it is appropriate that I comment on Dr. Lemen's presentation with regard to Threshold Limit Values or TLVs. TLVs have never been intended to be adopted into legislation; that was clearly the view of the ACGIH and has remained its view throughout the years. Furthermore, the ACGIH and its TLV Committee recognize that many TLVs are inadequate and suffer from lack of information. They really reflect a rather herculean effort by a volunteer group with fairly minimum resources, and they have offered very useful guidance to professionals. On a substance-by-substance approach, I am sure you can find many inadequate TLV documentations with very out-of-date references. However, to balance that impression, I would urge you to look at how many TLVs there are for which there are no NIOSH standards or recommendations and no PELs.

RICHARD LEMEN (*NIOSH, Cincinnati, Ohio*): Thank you, Dr. Lee—you have corroborated my position. I hope that the ACGIH will make all of this information on the shortcomings of the TLVs immediately known to OSHA, so that OSHA does not make the mistake that I am afraid they are about to make of adopting TLVs wholesale in lieu of proper standards. Also, given the acknowledged lack of documentation for most TLVs, I am not so sure that using the ACGIH's threshold limit values can be expected to provide adequate protection.

In summary, I think it would be a very serious error to adopt any of the TLVs as standards without looking at them extremely carefully.

Special Address

SCOTT LILLY[a]

*House of Representatives
Rayburn House Office Building
Washington, D.C. 20515*

I first met Dr. Selikoff 14 years ago this spring when Congressman Obey sent me to New York to a conference to hear about a chemical called vinyl chloride and what it was doing to workers in Louisville. After I got the call from him to make this presentation, I reflected on how much things have changed since then. I remember how in 1974 the business community was trying to gut OSHA. We thought that was a problem. Now, though, we wish that they were sufficiently concerned that they would feel that they *needed* to gut OSHA!

The other thing that has changed in the last couple of years is the American economy. In 1974, we had a view of the United States as the sole producer in the world; in many ways that was true at the time. We saw corporate profits as having risen steadily for nearly 30 years. At that time, we saw family incomes having gone up by 4 and 5% steadily year after year, and hourly wages rising year after year. In 1974 things looked a lot different that they do today. Half of American families have less in real income today than they did in 1973. As a result of these changes, when you think today about occupational health and you think about what people are willing to give up to make sure that their workplace is clean and healthful, you have to also take account of the magnitude of the economic downturn.

A country that went from the end of the Second World War through the 1950s and '60s and saw spectacular increases in income had one view of what the economy could stand and what we could do in terms of cleaning up the workplace. They also had an idea of what corporations ought to be willing to sacrifice to make sure that everyone was in a job that was not going to shorten his or her life or worsen health. Most families have had a hard time just trying to maintain their financial position, wondering about what happened to the dream they once had of having more in their life than their parents had. That change dramatically affects expectations in terms of controls and regulation of the workplace.

The idea that we had, which was never written into the original Occupational Safety and Health Act, was that no one should give up any aspect of his or her health as a result of a job. That concept is far more elusive today than it was at the time we put it into the law. Thus, the question now is whether the changes affect the importance of the work of those in occupational health. My answer is that the good work of such persons is, in fact, *more* important; the cost that today's economy extracts from health and well-being has to be measured even more carefully, because the economic demands are greater. That means that we need to know more about the processes that result in the loss of one's health and well-being, and we need strong advocates for workers' health to make sure that the cost is put on the line and that people understand it and balance it every day; otherwise they will pay an unwise price for a short-term return.

[a] Mr. Lilly is the Chief Aide to Congressman David Obey of Wisconsin.

DISCUSSION OF THE PAPER

QUESTION: With regard to your point about disposable family income, I would note that at the APHA meeting in New Orleans, Professor Vincent Navarro of Johns Hopkins University reported that the average American family had lost 20% of its disposable family income in real dollar terms since the 1970s. Do you have any actual figures on that?

LILLY: There are a number of different figures and there are different ways that you can look at them. It depends on the year that you pick and on the kinds of families that you look at. But the median family income is about 6% lower in 1986 than it was in 1973. It is lower than it was in 1978; it basically flattened from '73 to '78; it dropped down during the recession in 1981, and it has never gotten back up to where it was. The disturbing aspect about that is that most families have had to send more workers into the workforce simply to keep that loss from being much greater than it would have been. For two-earner families or for two-parent families, the loss in income would have been more than twice what it would have been had not both parents gone into the workforce. And, of course, there are a lot of intangible costs associated with having two parents in the workforce. Families are worse off, but how much worse off depends on how you put the statistics together. That fact has a lot to do with the way people think about the demands they want to put on employers to provide health and safety at work.

QUESTION: Despite the economic realities you are alluding to and the clearly antiregulatory posture of the current administration, the polls certainly indicate that there is continued interest in improving the general environment as well as the work environment. From your perspectives in the Congress, is that view representative of reality and, if so, how are members responding to these issues?

LILLY: My general reaction is that the members of Congress react more strongly in terms of environmental issues than occupational issues because persons who are interested in the broader environmental issues tend to be more politically and socially influential. The environment inside the workplace is a less sensitive issue to most members and is not being translated politically right now, but the opportunity to do so is there. Enough interest about health issues in the workplace exists among workers and the general public so that members of Congress who want to address these issues would get a good response. But I do not think that many of them have decided that these are issues they want to support or for which they want to work very hard.

QUESTION: What are the specific problems that occur with our current decrease in family income? What are the results of having both people in a family work? Would you address these questions on a microeconomic and on a global or macroeconomic scale?

LILLY: We see that families are making a lot of adjustments to try to compensate for this economic change. First, many families do not really realize that they are living on less. They are not paid in real dollars; their check comes in nominal dollars, and thus it appears to be a lot more than what it was 10 years ago. They do not understand what the adjustment for inflation has done to the paycheck. So they tend to think that they ought to be able to live better than their parents, when in fact that is not really the case. So, to compensate, more members of the family go into the workforce. They save quite a lot less, and they stretch in a lot of places we do not recognize. People think of yuppies as eating out all the time, drinking chablis and eating brie, but the fact is that young families today spend about the same as families did 10 years ago on restaurants, even though more of them work and food preparation is more of a problem. They are stretched to the limit in terms of time; they spend less time with their children and more money on day care; they contribute considerably less to charity; and they save much less.

QUESTION: What bad things are happening?

LILLY: The situation is bad in terms of home ownership, it is bad in terms of people having less time to spend with their children, which I think is disinvesting in the next generation. It is bad in terms of family savings because people are not saving in their middle years, which is when they should be saving, years in which Americans have always put away substantial savings to meet needs later in life, such as ill health or childrens' education or the additional costs of retirement. So currently middle-aged people are not able to prepare for the future.

QUESTION: Has the current state of the labor organizations in this country reached a level where Congress no longer feels it has to listen to them?

LILLY: No. Labor continues to be the major source of funding for Democratic members of Congress and a major source of volunteer workers in elections. Members of labor unions represent a large number of voters. The problem lies in determining the agenda of those voters; what are they interested in? The fact that these persons are members of a labor union does not change their perspective that much. They are facing the same pressures and constraints that all Americans are facing and they are concerned about their jobs, about wage increases, and about a lot of the more fundamental economic issues. Unfortunately, most workers have never been as sensitive to their own health questions as they should be.

PART III. RIGHT TO KNOW AND DISEASE PREVENTION

The Right to Know in the Workplace

The Moral Dimension

J. DONALD MILLAR

*National Institute for Occupational Safety and Health
Centers for Disease Control
Atlanta, Georgia 30333*

It is significant that this workshop is taking place during the week of our national celebration of the life of Dr. Martin Luther King, Jr. It reminds us of the clear awareness that the American Civil Rights Movement had for the specific concerns of workers. Indeed, the part of the struggle that cost Dr. King his life was the attempt to secure economic justice for garbage workers in Memphis.

The timing also was excellent in that it permitted me the opportunity to hear late last week a splendid talk by Congressman John Lewis of Atlanta, a remarkable man who embodies the history of the Civil Rights Movement. The son of an Alabama sharecropper, he marched shoulder to shoulder with Dr. King. He faced the dogs, the firehoses, the jails—he was one of the frontline soldiers. He went on to earn two academic degrees and an honorary degree from Princeton. He is now a member of the U.S. House of Representatives.

Hearing Congressman Lewis reminded my wife Joan and me that part of my decision in 1961 to join the U.S. Public Health Service and seek assignment at the Centers for Disease Control in Atlanta was our mutual desire to return south and be active participants in nonviolent change. Joan especially has reason for pride. In the mid-60s while I was fighting smallpox in various places around the world, she worked with John Lewis' Student Nonviolent Coordinating Committee in voter registration in Georgia. Congressman Lewis talked about that. He noted that in 1964 in the states of the old Confederacy, there were less than 100 elected black officials. Today, there are more than 5,000!

Significantly, Congressman Lewis tied the victories of those days to very contemporary problems. Because of those struggles, he said "We have come a distance as a people, and as a nation. We are now free to ask other questions, such as: What's in the water I drink? What's in the air I breathe?," or I might add, "What's in the place where I work?"

He reminds me, by both his words and his life, that progress *does* occur in this country—productive change *does* happen. I remember the promise in Psalms 9:18, "For the needy shall not always be forgotten: the expectation of the poor shall not perish forever."

BACKGROUND

But you asked me here to speak on the "right to know." This most challenging subject has been under increasing public scrutiny for several years. Underlying the debate are widely divergent views, strongly defended by responsible people, all of whom consider themselves well informed and concerned about the health and safety of workers. Because the issue is both very broad and very complex, it is well to start with some definitions.

Just what is a right? The Random House Dictionary[1] says a right is "a just claim whether legal, prescriptive, or moral." Now one can see that there is ambiguity here. The definition raises almost as many questions as it answers. Today, when I speak of the right to know, I will be talking about the "just claim" of workers to have knowledge of the risks they face in their workplace. In general, rights are always seen as *relational*, that is, they are correlated with *obligations*. In other words, if I have a right to something, then somebody has an obligation or duty to grant it to me. Here again, in this discussion, my use of right to know should generally be understood to incorporate the correlative "duty to inform."

I have chosen to focus my remarks on the *moral* dimension of right to know. I have done this for two reasons: (1) I believe there are important moral issues associated with the right to know in the workplace that should be discussed. (2) I find myself typically prone to make snap judgments about moral issues without going through the disciplined dissection that characterizes the work of professional philosophers. To do so is a dangerous practice; I would never make such snap judgments in my own field, epidemiology, and I want to learn to avoid such abuses in the philosopher's field.

I have no personal professional credentials as a philosopher. However, I have a good friend, Dr. Robert F. Almeder, who is Professor of Philosophy at Georgia State University and who is also a national figure in biomedical and business ethics. We have collaborated on several endeavors in the past, including most recently a National Conference on Moral Issues in the Use of Quantitative Risk Assessment. That meeting was cosponsored by the National Science Foundation, Georgia State University, and NIOSH. Out of it came a book edited by Professor Almeder and his associate, James M. Humber. The book is entitled, "Quantitative Risk Assessment, Biomedical Ethics Reviews, 1986" (Humana Press, Clifton, NJ, 1987).

With your invitation I went to Dr. Almeder and asked for his advice and help. What he presented is the result of our collaboration. If there is erudition in what I say, it is his; if there is confusion and befuddlement, it is very likely to be mine!

Although not really a definition, perhaps the most useful depiction I have seen of rights is that by David Lyons in his book of that name.[2] He describes rights as "centers of controversy." This rings true to our national experience; since our origins as a nation, much of our national consciousness has focused on rights. Moreover, as David T. Ozar notes,[3] "rights talk," such as we are doing here, "is in the western world . . . one of the most common ways of formulating moral issues. For this reason, it is important to understand rights talk and to see how it can be used to explain the moral components of the situation we face in our lives" (pages 3–4).

THE NATURE OF MORAL RIGHTS

Explaining the nature of a moral right is more than even a professional philosopher could handle adequately in the time allotted to me. Hundreds of books and treatises have been and are being written on the nature of moral rights. There are very different and mutually exclusive views on the nature of moral rights and no lack of profoundly thoughtful people who are willing to define what they regard as the *correct view* about morality. However, the sad truth is that there is no consensus, either public or academic, on just what a moral right is. Accordingly, when it comes to the nature of moral rights, anyone taking a clear and dogmatic stand is like the proverbial "fool rushing in where angels fear to tread." It seems that the best one can do is to adopt a particular view that one finds congenial and then "sallie forth to do battle." Even so, refusal to honestly and energetically confront the issue of human moral rights seems a reprehensible abandonment of our human responsibility. In short, "woe to those who seek to understand human moral rights, and woe to those who don't."

In spite of these woes, I will rush in and outline a major obstacle I see facing us in the construction of a problem-free public policy on the right to know in the workplace. This obstacle is a philosophic one. Therefore, in this discussion I hope you will tolerate my using distinctions and concepts that moral philosophers consider commonplace, but that others, including me, may find unfamiliar and hard to follow. I will, it is hoped, end up with some practical observations on how to reduce the obstacle.

TWO BASIC VIEWS ON MORAL RIGHTS: CONSEQUENTIALIST AND NONCONSEQUENTIALIST

There are two basic and mutually exclusive views about the nature of human rights. The first is the consequentialist theory of rights, and the second is the nonconsequentialist theory of rights. Under the first theory, consequentialists say that a right exists if recognition of the right would produce the best outcome for all those affected by the exercise of that right. As the name implies, the consequentialist says we must look at the consequence of exercising the right, and if the consequence promotes the best outcome, given all the available alternatives, then the right exists. For example, consider the question, "Is there a right to life?" For the consequentialist it is a matter of determining the consequences of letting people kill without a very good reason. As these consequences clearly would not produce the best general outcome for all those affected by the behavior, the consequentialist asserts that there *is* a right to life for everybody—by this he or she means only that nobody ought to take anybody else's life without a very good reason.[4]

Conversely, the nonconsequentialist says that rights can and do exist even if recognition of them does *not* produce the best general outcome. The nonconsequentialist holds that even if killing one innocent person would save the lives of a thousand other innocent people who would otherwise surely die, it is still wrong to kill that one innocent person. Thus, the nonconsequentialist says there are certain things one should *never* do (or should *always* do), no matter what the consequences. The famous German philosopher Immanuel Kant argued that no matter what the consequences, one should *never* lie, steal, or murder.[5]

Perhaps the best way to depict the differences between these two theories on the nature of rights is to cite a hypothetical example that moral philosophers frequently use when contending over the nature of morality, the famous "Commandant Example."[6] Suppose you are an occupant of a POW camp, and the commandant (who is reliable but insane) approaches you and says, "Either kill one of the innocent babies in this camp, or I will kill 5,000 innocent inmates." Assuming you cannot kill the commandant, what would be the morally correct course of action? If you choose to kill the innocent baby to save the lives of a much larger number of innocent persons, then you have opted for the consequentialist theory of rights, namely, that the baby does not have the right to life, because recognition of such a right would result in 5,000 deaths which does not produce the best general outcome. Conversely, if you refuse to kill the innocent baby, you have opted for the nonconsequentialist view that no matter what the circumstances, it is never morally permissible to kill an innocent person.

Consequentialists attack nonconsequentialists on the grounds that anybody who would not kill an innocent baby to save 5,000 innocent people is more like a moral fanatic than a responsible agent acting on moral principle. After all, they say, anybody who would not be willing to kill an innocent baby to save the world is surely morally blind! Nonconsequentialists, however, stand in amazement over what they consider the total moral blindness of anybody who would kill an innocent baby even to save a larger number.[7] The consequentialist who sees morality as a matter of the greatest good for the greatest number regards the nonconsequentialist as morally blind; the nonconsequentialist who sees morality as a matter of doing certain good things no matter what the consequences, equally sees the consequentialist as morally blind. An important point is that no matter which position you choose, there does not seem to be any decision procedure for effectively resolving the dispute over which view of moral rights is the correct one. Those of us who must make public policy from such opposing viewpoints see no good way to resolve the dilemma in terms of an agreeable principle.

What then are we to do? Should we ignore the philosophers and make decisions on some other, nonmoral basis? Is there a means by which we can resolve these conflicts?

A CASE IN POINT

Lest you think this is so much intellectual esoterica, I offer you a very real and very personal experience with just exactly this type of moral dilemma. In late 1981, early in my tenure as Director of NIOSH, I took on the question of what NIOSH should do about workers whose records had been analyzed in retrospective cohort mortality studies, leading to the finding of a risk of some sort for the cohorts involved. Given that NIOSH generally publishes its findings in scientific literature and the like, should the individuals in these cohorts be individually notified of the observed risks or not?

I posed this question to (1) the Office of General Counsel of the Public Health Service, and (2) the CDC Ethics Committee. Here are the responses. From the lawyers of the Office of General Counsel I got a lengthy discussion of pertinent case and common law leading to the following general summary: "NIOSH *has no legal duty to advise* individual workers. . . ." Moreover, in a follow-up note, we were warned that should NIOSH decide to undertake individual notification anyway, NIOSH would incur certain legal liabilities as a consequence. In other words, not only had we no legal duty to inform, but also we might enhance our likelihood of legal trouble if we did.

The CDC Ethics Committee, in its draft report, advised the following: "NIOSH does have a general responsibility to ensure that workers have knowledge of their exposure to hazardous materials. The general responsibility *should be interpreted as a moral duty to inform.* . . ."

In short, the well-meaning counsel I got on the question consisted of two opinions that are 180 degrees apart! What to do next was not so esoteric an issue!

IN DEFENSE OF THE CONSEQUENTIALIST

When we specifically turn to the debate about the right to know in the workplace, we recognize immediately the two distinct views on the nature of moral rights. On the one hand, there are clearly nonconsequentialists who insist that no matter what the consequences of informing workers about possible risks in the workplace, workers have an absolute right to that information as an extension of their right to autonomy and even of their right to life.[8] On the other hand, there are also consequentialists who insist that failure to look at the consequences of notifying workers is unjustifiable moral fanaticism. The problem for those of us who fashion public policy is to struggle with the moral question of whether or not the right to know in a particular case is a valid right only if informing workers causes less human harm than not informing them. We can imagine instances in which more harm would be created by revealing information than by withholding it.[9] In fact, some aspects of the present public reaction to information on AIDS suggest this. After all, the Surgeon General has publicly said, "Most of the people who are scared to death of AIDS couldn't catch it if they tried!"[10] Obviously, circumstances in which untoward results of notification outweigh benefits are expected to be exceptional, but because such exceptions are conceivable, we should be willing to examine the consequences of dispensing information about risks in the workplace. Those who object to such a policy from the basis of the nonconsequentialist theory of moral rights must recognize that their position is no more morally privileged than is that of the consequentialists.

The nonconsequentialist often overlooks the crucial fact that this society has already opted very strongly for the consequentialist view on the moral right to life. Certainly as a nation, we grant that human life is sacred and that everyone has a fundamental right to life. However, we do not hesitate to endorse an institution that conscripts and kills large numbers of innocent persons in the interest of preventing predictable deaths of even larger numbers of innocents. I refer, of course, to the institution of war. If having a right to life meant that a life would never be taken no matter what the consequences, then war would never be morally acceptable to us. The fundamental reality is that this society is unwilling to live with the principle that a human life should never be taken, no matter what the consequences. One may ask then, why should we act differently when it comes to the moral right to know, especially if the moral right to know is construed as an extension of the moral right to life itself?

Whether we talk about war or capital punishment, we as a society endorse the view that the right to life means only that one must have a *very good reason* for taking another person's life, and that the only "very good reason" may well be the anticipated greater harm (in terms of lives lost) that would result from *not* taking that person's life. Is there reason to adopt a different general attitude when it comes to the moral right to know?

IN DEFENSE OF THE NONCONSEQUENTIALIST

Although it makes sense to examine the consequences of informing workers in order to determine if there is a moral right to know, the concern behind the nonconsequentialist posture should not be dismissed too easily. After all, as we have already noted, the Kantian view that morality has nothing to do with the consequences has commanded the respect of serious and profound thinkers. But where are the nonconsequentialists "coming from" on the moral right to know in the workplace?

First, there is a long-standing and deeply felt suspicion that some corporations are more than willing to be indifferent to the safety and health of workers if the costs of compassion are sufficiently burdensome to the shareholder. Nobody denies that these abuses have occurred. Unless a good watchdog is in place, such abuses also are likely to occur in the future. To some extent this concern may be addressed by the effect of strict liability law and its capacity to engender real fear in the hearts of those who might otherwise be tempted to play loose with the health and safety of workers. Of itself, however, liability law works only *after* harm (including loss of life) has occurred. Although it may allay some of the moral concerns of nonconsequentialists, liability law is certainly no substitute for a mechanism that would *prevent* harm.

Secondly, what often bothers the nonconsequentialist is the ominous prospect of measuring the life of the worker in purely economic terms. Some people erroneously believe that such estimates are a legitimate part of cost-benefit analyses as associated with workplace protections. Certainly, however, the responsible consequentialist does not endorse measuring the sanctity of human life purely in terms of dollars. Neither does the responsible consequentialist imply that any worker should be exposed to risks simply as a cost of doing business.

The core concern of the nonconsequentialist perhaps could best be dispelled by adopting the same strategy toward the moral right to know that we, as a nation, adopt toward the moral right to life, namely, that a person has a right to life only if nobody can take his or her life without *a very good reason*. Those who would take it must assume the burden of proof and demonstrate that compelling reason. Similarly, those who would withhold from workers the information on occupational risks would need to assume the burden of proof and demonstrate the presence of a similarly compelling reason. Indeed, such a reason may be "compelling" only if informing the worker is demonstrably more likely to involve loss of life, than is not informing. This kind of strategy, assuming we can suitably implement it, should allow us to alleviate the root concerns of the nonconsequentialist, without having to abandon the consequentialist view of the moral right to know in the workplace.

PHILOSOPHICAL CONCLUSION

Many other problems exist in implementing a broadly agreeable public policy on the right to know in the workplace. There are questions involved in the determination of risks as well as the quantitative degree of risk that must be present before a worker's right to know is materially affected. Also, I have said nothing as yet about legal rights. I have sought only to confront what I see as the major obstacle posed by the nonconsequentialist's view that no matter what the consequences, no worker should ever be exposed to any risk in the workplace without his enlightened and informed consent.

In sum, I have urged that the moral right to know in the workplace is best construed as the consequentialist construes it. This implies that the worker has a *prima facie* moral right to know about any reasonably harmful condition or substance in his or her workplace; this amounts to saying that nobody can morally withhold that information without a very compelling reason. Those who would withhold such information must bear the burden of proof and demonstrate the compelling reason. By extrapolation from the moral right to life, the "compelling" reason would probably have to be that there is more likely to be a greater loss of life by informing workers than by not informing them. It seems to me that such a circumstance is highly unlikely to occur in reality.

NOW, WHAT ABOUT THE "REAL WORLD?"

So much for philosophical theories. Is any of this relevant in a practical sense? You bet it is. Decisions to inform or not to inform are very important in the prevention of work-related diseases and injuries. As Dr. Lorin Kerr expressed to me just last week, "No law alone can protect the worker. There never will be enough inspectors to insure protection. Therefore, what the worker *knows* is crucial to protection."

Having been very much a part of the debate concerning the right to know, I believe that participants in the debate are all genuinely concerned about finding practical ways to protect workers. The debate has revolved around how best to do that. No one seriously suggests that workers should not have information about the risks that they face. The storms of debate have swirled around ways to provide the needed information while neither sacrificing ongoing prevention activities nor provoking problems that would leave workers worse off than they were.

The concern to notify workers of their risks is not new and some of these concerns have been addressed in law. The Occupational Safety and Health Act (PL 91–596, Dec. 29, 1970) is rife with references to a legislative imperative to inform workers. Some examples follow.

1. As regards employers, Section 5 of the Act, known as the "General Duty Clause" reads, "each employer . . . . (2) shall comply with occupational safety and health standards promulgated under this Act." Turning to Section 6(b)(7), where such standards are described, one finds the requirement that "any standard promulgated under this Subsection shall prescribe the use of labels or appropriate forms of warning as are necessary to assure that employees are apprised of all risks to which they are exposed. . . ." Hence employers are charged to comply with standards, and standards are mandated to include information on risks.

2. Section 8(c)(3) is even more explicit in charging that: "Each employer shall promptly notify any employee who has been or is being exposed to toxic materials or harmful physical agents in concentrations or at levels which exceed those prescribed by applicable occupational safety and health standards promulgated under Section 6."

3. Section 13(c) mandates that whenever an OSHA inspector finds "eminent dangers" in "any place of employment, he shall inform the affected employees and employers of the danger. . . ."

4. Section 17(i) prescribes penalties such that "any employer who violates any of the posting requirements as prescribed under provisions of this Act, shall be assessed a civil penalty of up to $1,000.00 for each violation."

5. Section 20, which deals with research, provides in Part (d) that "information obtained by the Secretary, and the Secretary of Health, Education, and Welfare, under this Section, shall be disseminated by the Secretary to employers and employees and organizations thereof."

6. In Section 12(g) even the Occupational Safety and Health Review Commission is mandated to inform, by a provision that "every official act of the Commission shall be entered of record, and its hearings and records shall be open to the public."

I conclude from all this that, conflicting ethical theories aside, the framers of the Occupational Safety and Health Act clearly wanted workers informed of their risks. Viewed in this light, the worker notification efforts of NIOSH, the recently expanded OSHA Hazard Communication Standard, and all the legislation currently being considered by the Congress in this area represent predictable further steps toward fulfilling a dream first elaborated in the Occupational Safety and Health Act.

SUMMARY

The makers of public policy cannot avoid the deep and often strident public controversy over the nature and scope of basic moral rights. There are persuasive defenders on both sides of the issue. Forging public policy in the absence of a broad public consensus is nothing more than the arbitrary imposition by government of some preferred, but not necessarily privileged, moral view. It hardly seems the legitimate role of a democratic government, even in the name of moral leadership, to so impose views that are deeply controversial and not capable of broad-based support by the population at large. It is better by far, for reasons of stable public policy, that we seek the painful path of building a general public consensus among the well-informed and well-meaning citizenry. If no such consensus can be achieved, then the law will, as a matter of necessity, settle the issue in the interest of the efficient discharge of general social functions . . . and that is really not a particularly unfortunate outcome.

NOTES AND REFERENCES

1. Random House Dictionary of the English Language, 2nd Ed., 1987. Unabridged. :1656. Random House. New York.
2. Rights. Wadsworth Publishing Co. Inc. Belmont, California, p. 1.
3. WERHANE, P. H., A. R. GINI & D. T. OZAR, eds. 1986. Philosophical Issues in Human Rights. Random House. New York.
4. For a general discussion of consequentialist and nonconsequentialist theories of ethics, see: FRANKENNA, W. 1982. Ethics. :15–45. Prentice Hall. Englewood, NJ. See Also: LYONS D. 1979. Human rights and the general welfare. In Rights. D. Lyons, Ed. :187ff. Wadsworth Publishing Co. and WILLIAMS, B. 1976. Utilitarianism For and Against. Cambridge University Press. Cambridge, England.
5. For a general discussion of Kant's views see FRANKENNA, W. 1982. Ethics. :25–29, Prentice-Hall, and Kant, I. 1959. The Foundation of the Metaphysics of Morals, Liberal Arts Press, New York. See also, as an example of the nonconsequentialist position, ANSCOMBE, G. E. M. 1958. Modern Philosophy :7. Philosophy.
6. WILLIAMS, B. & J. J. C. SMART. 1976. Utilitarianism For and Against, Cambridge University Press. Cambridge, England. (The example was initially offered by B. Williams.)
7. ANSCOMBE, G. E. M. 1958. Modern moral philosophy. Philosophy :7. See also GEWIRTH, A. 1979. Moral Philosophy. University of Chicago Press. Chicago, IL.
8. FADEN, R. R. & BEAUCHAMP, T. L. 1982. The right to know in the workplace. Canad. J. Phil. 8(suppl.): 199 ff.

9. FADEN, R. & BEAUCHAMP, T. 1982. The right to know in the workplace. Canad. J. Phil. 8: 197–200. The point Faden and Beauchamp make is that one sometimes has a responsibility to beneficence that may well conflict with the worker's right to autonomy. In which case, depending on the circumstances, we may withhold information for reasons of beneficence.
10. Opening General Session, Annual Meeting of the Association of Military Surgeons of the United States. Las Vegas, Nevada, Nov. 9, 1987.

DISCUSSION OF THE PAPER

PAUL BRANDT-RAUF (*Columbia University, New York, N.Y.*): This dichotomy between consequentialists and nonconsequentialists has troubled me for many years, particularly as applied to occupational health. At least on a theoretical basis, the conclusion I have reached is that ethical reality probably mirrors physical reality. Let me explain that statement. Particle physics has no trouble dealing with two mutually exclusive, simultaneous, differing realities. Taking the electron beam as an example, a physicist can tell you whether it is acting as a waveform or a particle form, but it cannot be both at the same time. I suggest that ethical reality reflects that. Furthermore, I suspect that there is some superethical reality that we cannot approach on a rational basis; that is the underlying problem between the two camps who logically address this dichotomy. There is a consequentialist side and a nonconsequentialist side, and they exist simultaneously; they are mutually exclusive, but they are both right.

The trick in practical reality is to be able to approach problems from both points of view in an intellectually sound way. When training professionals in the field, we should be teaching them more about these different approaches, so that when faced with ethical problems they will be able to make a sound judgment and then reach a conclusion.

PETER BARTH (*University of Connecticut, Storrs, Connecticut*): I appreciate your approach to this issue, but I would like to suggest that you might also want to address the question of legal rights as you consider these questions.

States have given workers rights to compensation for conditions that may be the consequence of occupational exposures; those rights have now existed for 60, 70, and in some cases 75 years. It seems to me, however, that those rights are very hollow in a job where workers are not informed as to the kinds of substances or the kinds of hazards to which they have been exposed. Without such information, workers may not even recognize that their diseases are occupationally derived and that they have a right to present themselves for compensation before the various state bodies.

Given the problem of long latency, it is not enough to wait for the illness to develop, to wait for the worker to bring this illness to a compensation arena, and then to raise the question of whether or not there was an exposure. We may after all be talking about businesses that no longer exist, processes that are no longer being used, and issues of proof that are very difficult. As to the question of right to know, it seems, therefore, that we ought to examine it in the context of the rights that workers were given 60, 70, or 80 years ago when the compensation system was first put into place.

J. DONALD MILLAR: I agree that there certainly are such things as hollow rights. Faden and Beauchamp make this point in their landmark summary of the issue, *The Right To Know In The Workplace*. They say that to make the right to know truly meaningful and functional in the context of the workplace, other worker rights must also be secured. They point out six different rights that are assured by the Occupational Safety and Health Act which are peripheral and supportive to the right to know. They are: (1) the right to complain to OSHA about perceived safety and health problems; (2) the right to accompany OSHA officials during plant inspections; (3) the right to contest the reasonableness of OSHA-proposed abatement periods; (4) the right to participate in relevant adjudicatory proceedings; (5) the right to request a NIOSH health hazard evaluation; and (6) the right to employee training and education funded by OSHA.

Clearly the question of support for right to know is important. I believe that the only really satisfying way to deal with this problem is through the establishment and recognition of legal rights. At least in that process, we have to reach a societal consensus in order to get a bill passed and implemented. There is the added advantage that a great deal more can be done about implementation and enforcement if a law is in place, than if simply a moral principle is cited.

M. A. EL BATAWI (*World Health Organization, Geneva, Switzerland*): I greatly enjoyed your talk, Dr. Millar, and the philosophical discussion associated with it. Nowadays, however, it has become a fashion throughout the world not only that workers should know, but also that workers should participate in discussions on occupational health problems. By their participation they should know a number of the things that you have just listed including exposure limits, early manifestations of disease, how to save a life in an emergency, and how to be self-sufficient in taking care and doing self-care for health. This notion in this country has extended to programs for health promotion, which are intended to educate workers to follow a lifestyle that would prevent aggravation or causation of diseases.

MILLAR: The idea of worker participation in the decisions and programs that affect workers' health is a fundamental operating principle that we have always cherished in NIOSH. For example, in formulating our policy recommendations, whether they be recommended standards or other policy statements, we have insisted for many years that there be tripartite review of these policies and decisions. Furthermore, we are very reluctant to make decisions or to enunciate policies unless there has been thorough participation in that process by labor, management, and government.

DAVID WEGMAN (*University of Lowell, Lowell, Mass.*): I took substantial comfort from your discussion of consequentialist versus nonconsequentialist theories of rights, because the right to know is a right that needs to be accepted by either theory. I cannot imagine a way that it could be denied. What interests me is the next step to which you referred, namely, the cost of implementing the Right-to-Know bill and the consequences of using dollars for this purpose. It reminded me of yesterday's discussion on risk assessment and cost-benefit analysis. It troubled me, not in terms of what you said, but in terms of planning for the future. We seem too willing to try to reduce risk assessment to cost-benefit analysis. A consequence of this approach is that considerations of cost too often dominate the debate. However, it is equally, if not more important in public debate to consider the issue of risk. We must move away from cost-benefit analysis and back to informed judgment in order to decide what is a risk and to know when and whom to notify.

MILLAR: Dr. Wegman and others working with the NIOSH Board of Scientific Counselors have produced a very helpful document, *Guideline for Worker Notification*. It spells out the concerns that Dr. Wegman has discussed and offers recommendations for dealing with the identification and assessment of risks. Moreover, it considers what levels of risk warrant notification. These are very important, indeed crucial, issues for implementation.

Round Table Papers: 3. High-Risk Worker Notification and The Prevention of Occupational Disease

High-Risk Worker Notification
A Necessary Public Health Program

JAMES M. MELIUS
*New York State Department of Health
Albany, New York 12237*

This roundtable will address three different perspectives on the high-risk worker-notification legislation currently before Congress. Mr. Martin Connor from General Electric will provide a business perspective on the legislation. Dr. Alan Engelberg from the American Medical Association will present a medical care perspective. Finally, Dr. Knut Ringen from the Workplace Health Fund will describe his experience in conducting worker-notification projects. These three perspectives will provide a sound basis for understanding why worker-notification programs are needed and how thousands of workers and former workers might benefit from these programs.

Our usual efforts at primary prevention of occupational health problems often fail. Sometimes this failure is due to our ignorance of the health consequences of exposure to specific toxic substances. By the time we understand the potential health effects of these substances, many persons have been exposed in the workplace and, as a result, are at increased risk of developing adverse health effects from these exposures. Often, our efforts at primary prevention fail for other reasons. Lax enforcement efforts, inadequate standards, and poor dissemination of information on the toxicity of the substances are some of the factors that may allow workers to be exposed to these substances for many years without adequate control and hence place these workers at increased risk of subsequent disease. These failures of primary prevention, for whatever reason, provoke the need to develop worker-notification programs to attempt to provide later assistance and preventive steps for these workers.

The legislation for high-risk worker notification provides a sound public health approach to this problem. Notification efforts will be targeted at those who will most benefit from this type of program. They will be determined by an expert review board who will select specific groups for notification based on credible scientific evidence of their potential health risk and the potential benefit of the notification program for these groups. After selection of the groups to be notified, the National Institute for Occupational Safety and Health will have the responsibility for identifying, locating, and notifying the subjects. This notification process is similar to procedures used for some epidemiologic studies and provides a very feasible method for such notification.

Once a subject has been notified, he or she may require medical screening, counseling, and other assistance. The guidance for this aspect of worker notification will be provided by university centers with occupational and environmental medicine programs and by other groups with this expertise. However, much of the burden for medical screening and counseling will be placed on primary care physicians. Although this part of the program will require a focused effort to ensure that these physicians have sufficient knowledge to adequately provide this screening, it also will provide an important opportunity for bridging the gap between occupational health and the medical care system. Occupational health must become more integrated with the provision of primary medical care if prevention of occupational diseases is to be achieved. Educating primary medical care providers on the appropriate follow-up of notified workers not only will directly benefit the workers but will also begin to involve primary care providers in the recognition, screening, and prevention of occupational diseases.

In summary, high-risk worker notification is an important and feasible public health program. Thousands of current and former workers may be assisted by this effort, and some of the adverse consequences of our failure to properly control workplace exposures may be prevented.

The Politics of the Worker-Notification Bill

MARTIN F. CONNOR
Public Affairs Counsel
General Electric Company
1331 Pennsylvania Avenue, N.W.
Washington, D.C. 20004

Let me confess at the start, for it is undoubtedly the reason I have been invited to make this presentation, that General Electric is one of the few companies that is working for enactment of the High-Risk Disease Notification Bill of 1987. We are in the company of IBM, Digital Equipment, Crum & Forster Insurance Co., the Chemical Manufacturer's Association, and the National Paint and Coating Association. The rest of the business world is opposing enactment of this legislation. You will recognize that a company does not casually break ranks with most of industry. We decided about a year ago, however, that that is exactly what we would do. Let me briefly review the process we went through within General Electric and then make some comments on the politics of the worker-notification bills.

THE WORKER-NOTIFICATION BILL

In summary, S.79, which has been reported out of committee and is ready for floor action, and H.R.162, which has passed the House, have three basic components. They would (1) establish a Risk Assessment Board in the Department of Health and Human Services that would *identify* employee populations at high risk of occupational disease, (2) require that the Secretary *notify* members of identified populations, and (3) require employers to *monitor* the health of notified employees when the exposure occurred in the course of their current employment. The key words are "identify," "notify," and "monitor." The intent of the bill is to permit early medical intervention. As we at GE reviewed the bills, we agreed that they would fill a gap in our nation's effort to provide for the health and safety of its working people. We agreed that legislation promoting medical intervention between the time of workplace exposure and the occurrence of occupational disease might save thousands of lives and billions of dollars in health-care costs.

Conversely, we had serious problems with the bills as drafted. We therefore went to Senator Metzenbaum and Congressman Gaydos and asked them, among other things, (1) to redefine the factors to be used in identifying populations at risk in order to assure that Board determinations would be scientifically sound, (2) to permit judicial review of Board actions to assure that they would be supported by substantial evidence, (3) to establish a process of independent physician review of employee requests to be transferred to less hazardous jobs, as permitted by the bills, and (4) to prohibit use of Board findings or other actions taken under the Act, as a basis for, or as evidence in support of, a workers' compensation or tort claim. These changes, and many others, were agreed to and are reflected in S.79 as reported out of committee and H.R.162 as enacted by the House. I should add that we were joined in these and subsequent requests by the Industrial Unions Department of the AFL-CIO, which has had a consistently open mind as we have continued to suggest improvements in the bills.

INDUSTRY OPPOSITION

The interesting question, I suppose, is why most of industry opposes these bills, as indeed they do most bitterly. Their coalition, in its printed handouts, regularly raises four objections. I suppose it is safe to assume they are the points made face-to-face to Congressional members and staffs. The bill, it is said, will: (1) create a new and unnecessary bureaucracy; (2) mandate employee benefits; (3) require transfer from hazardous jobs to less hazardous jobs at no loss of pay; and (4) trigger thousands of multimillion dollar lawsuits.

What these four objections come down to is a claim that costs will greatly outweigh benefits. It is never put that way, however, because opponents of the bills, for some odd reason, never discuss their benefits. In any event, our view is that while ignoring the substantial benefits of the bill, they are grossly overstating its costs. There will be no new bureaucracy; transfers will be permitted only when there are objective grounds for fearing impairment of employee health; total annual cost of the monitoring program will be well under $100 million per year.

FEAR OF A LITIGATION EXPLOSION

The principal ground on which the bill is opposed is the last one just mentioned: that it will produce a flood of workers' compensation claims and lawsuits that would not have been brought were it not for this legislation. Let me say, first, that I am not sure that is true. Notwithstanding statements to the contrary by opponents of the bill, it did not happen in two of the NIOSH pilot notification projects on which this legislation is based. It did happen in the Augusta, Georgia, pilot project, but the circumstances were very unusual. In that project, involving an employee population exposed to a potent bladder carcinogen, betanaphthylamine (BNA), 47 of 696 respondents were found to have bladder cancer or suggestive symptoms of bladder cancer; 171 of the 696 (25%) filed suit against their employer. The parties settled 120 of the claims for about $500,000. The Georgia Supreme Court later affirmed dismissal of the rest on the ground that workers' compensation was the employees' exclusive remedy.

The claim is made that the Augusta pilot project is typical of what will occur in implementing these bills. I submit that there is no reason to think this. BNA has been a suspected carcinogen since 1895 and a known carcinogen since the 1930s. I understand that it was banned in Great Britain and Switzerland in the 1950s. The Augusta company was the only American company producing and using BNA. The detected health effects (6.8% of screened employees with bladder cancer or "suggestive characteristics" of bladder cancer) were extreme. The Senate Labor Committee report on S.79 understates the case when it suggests that the number of claims filed in Augusta "may be attributable to certain unusual aspects of that situation"!

There were, however, two other pilot projects to which I already referred. The first, in 1978, involved a population of 854 glass and insulating-materials workers in Port Allegany, Pennsylvania. The second, in 1980, involved 12,000 employees represented by the Pattern Makers League of North America. The diseases involved were, respectively, lung cancer and colon and rectal cancer. It has been reported that few, if any, personal injury claims were filed that would not have been filed except for those notification programs. Don't these give us a better basis for prediction than does the Augusta pilot project? I would suggest that they well might.

But if I am wrong, then what? There is a very basic fact that is ignored in most discussions of this issue: any new claims either will be meritorious or will not be meritorious. If they are not meritorious, the flood will turn into a droplet because, all rumors to the contrary notwithstanding, lawyers do not find it worthwhile to bring frivolous lawsuits. If they are meritorious, what is the problem? I am appalled by an argument that we should not tell workers that they are at exceptionally high risk of occupational disease because they might thereby be alerted to the fact that they have, or may someday have, legitimate claims for compensation. If we are concerned that today's workers' compensation systems and tort systems do not adequately discriminate between meritorious and nonmeritorious claims or that the amounts of compensation payable to holders of meritorious claims are inequitable, then that is ground for reforming these systems, not for opposing the worker-notification bill.

It seems to me, in any case, that the House and the Senate Labor Committee have done what they reasonably could do to meet these concerns. Both the House and the Senate bills provide that no state or federal claim for compensation may be based on an action taken by the Risk Assessment Board, by NIOSH, or by an employer pursuant to the Act. This substantive rule is then reinforced with a rule of evidence: no evidence of actions taken by the Board, by NIOSH, by the employer, or by others pursuant to the Act is to be admissible. Thus, to turn specifically to the most frequently expressed concern, claims seeking compensation for stress, fear of disease, or other emotional harm arising from the notification process itself would be barred. Anything more than that would be full-blown tort reform, which is not what these bills are about.

What I am suggesting is that, to the extent that explicit reasons are given for opposition to the bills, they have to do with compensation for occupational disease, not with the subjects directly addressed by the bills. I too am concerned with the adequacy and efficiency of our system for compensating victims of occupational disease. These systems cry out to heaven for reform. That is not, however, a reason to oppose the worker-notification bills.

THE LARGER POLITICAL CONTEXT

Although these are the reasons given for opposition to the worker-notification bills, they do not fully explain the violence of industry opposition to the bills. As anyone familiar with the public-policy process would expect, the debate over these bills is inevitably caught up in a larger clash between interest groups. Industry tends to view the worker-notification bills not on their merits but simply as one of many items on the ambitious agenda of the AFL-CIO. The worker-notification bills must be opposed, on this view, because to do otherwise would be to risk defeat on such unrelated issues as plant closings, parental leave, and mandated benefits. I can attest to the truth of this proposition from personal experience. The strongest criticism of our decision to support the worker-notification bills has been on this ground.

I make this point because it is so seldom said that it is often overlooked. What I am suggessting is that those who support the worker-notification bills are implicitly dissenting from the current majority opinion of what public-policy processes are about. We are dissenting from the very fashionable view that if industry strenuously pursues *its* selfish interests and workers strenuously pursue *their* selfish interests, the Invisible Hand made famous by Adam Smith will guide us to the common good. To put it affirmatively, we at General Electric are suggesting that it is appropriate for industry to examine issues one at a time and to take a stand for what it believes to be in the public interest, even if the AFL-CIO supports it!

The High-Risk Disease Notification and Prevention Program

Role of Personal Physicians

ALAN L. ENGELBERG[a]

Department of Public Health
American Medical Association
Chicago, Illinois 60610

This presentation focuses on the implications of the High-Risk Disease Notification and Prevention bills (S.79 and H.R.162) for personal physicians and how these implications may affect the preventive focus of the bills. Three topics will be discussed: (1) the personal physicians' role in the notification program; (2) payment for medical services; and (3) training for nonoccupational physicians. Most activists who labor for or against the passage of these bills work full-time in the occupational health arena, and see these bills as they would affect employees, businesses, and academic institutions. Some sections of the bills mention specifically the "employee's personal physician," yet most "personal physicians" are not occupational medicine physicians. As we are all painfully aware, with the lack of time in medical school curricula (an average of 4 hours in 4 years), most medical students and physicians barely realize that the specialty of occupational medicine exists, that people can become diseased because of exposures at work, and that physicians and other health and safety professionals can prevent disease and injury at work and even enhance the health of workers. Despite this general lack of knowledge, the American Medical Association (AMA), which represents the broad base of "personal physicians" in the United States, has long supported occupational safety and health legislation, especially since the late 1960s, when the great concerns about worker safety culminated in the passage of the Occupational Safety and Health Act of 1970. The AMA's position on the high-risk disease notification and prevention bills follows this trend: early on, the AMA's Council on Legislation supported the concept of notifying employees at high risk for developing occupational disease; however, the Council was troubled by many specific provisions of the bills, partly because it was not sure how these bills would affect "personal physicians" and their relations with their employee-patients.

Now that the two bills are nearly identical, their objectives and implications are clearer. Section 9 of S.79 describes the medical monitoring procedures, and paragraphs (c)(1) and (c)(2) of this section mention specifically the roles of the employee's personal physician. Paragraph (c)(1) states that the employee's physician may "medically determine that an employee who is a member of a population at risk shows evidence of the development of the disease described in the notice or other symptoms or conditions increasing the likelihood of incidence of such disease." This language is far superior to the language in previous versions of the bill by relating directly to what physicians normally do: physicians determine whether or not diseases are present or if in a particular individual a heightened

---

[a] Present address: Monsanto, 800 N. Lindbergh Blvd., St. Louis, Missouri 63167.

likelihood of disease is present (even though in the case of occupational diseases most employees' personal physicians may be a little out of their territory). Previous versions of the bill gave the employee's physician the power to authorize removal of the patient from the job. This power to effect a job action should never rest with a personal physician; rather, it is vested in an employer, a regulatory administrator, or a court, and perhaps the employee. I refer to this past language to state what I believe are the proper and improper roles of personal physicians in the high-risk notification process, so that the proper role is not altered when regulations are drawn up to implement the bills.

Alternative bills have been introduced, whose sponsors argued (speciously) that S.79 and H.R.162 are not designed with prevention in mind. Medical monitoring is a form of secondary prevention rather than primary prevention; nonetheless, the medical monitoring provisions constitute prevention. But this does raise a dilemma when it comes to payment for medical monitoring services. There are three groups of employees who are covered by these bills. First are the employees whose high risk resulted from exposures while employed by their present employer. For them, the employers must pay for medical monitoring. Second are the employees whose high risk resulted from exposures while employed by past employers. H.R.162 mentions this group and provides for a cost-sharing mechanism between the present employer and the notified employee. Third are the retirees; neither bill mentions them, which implies that the retirees would have to pay for their own medical monitoring services. Thus, two of the three groups of employees would have to pay for all or part of the medical monitoring services. As we all know, many persons in the United States are medically underinsured or uninsured. It is not hard to imagine that a large number of present and past employees who would be notified under the program would also be counted among the legions of uninsured or underinsured and therefore would have to pay out-of-pocket. Even those who have "adequate" medical insurance may face a problem, and herein lies the dilemma. Those of us in prevention know that medical monitoring constitutes prevention. So do third-party payers, who generally do not cover clinical preventive services. By calling the disease notification program "preventive," we may be limiting its effectiveness.

Finally, there is the issue of training. The bills would establish centers of excellence in occupational health whose functions would be to perform medical monitoring and train others to do the same. The notification letter itself will mention the name of the nearest center of excellence, and perhaps those who live nearby would benefit from the center's expertise. However, the number of notified workers who use these centers would be vanishingly small, indeed. Most notified employees would not live close to these centers, and they and those who live close more than likely would favor visits to their personal physicians rather than to faceless academic institutions. An example of this was recently highlighted in *Medical Benefits*,[1] which reported that employers were facing difficulty in getting their retirees to use either health maintenance organizations (HMOs) or preferred provider organizations (PPOs) as a way of cutting down health care coverage costs; the retirees wanted to remain under the care of the personal physicians with whom they had built up trusting relationships. The entire medical monitoring process, and hence the preventive nature of the notification program, may fall apart unless the many physicians who are untrained in occupational medicine learn enough about occupational medicine to function appropriately under the notification program. These physicians will no doubt follow suggested monitoring protocols, but they will certainly fall short of providing adequate counseling that must accompany physical examinations and laboratory procedures. Unless physicians understand the need for lifetime, periodic follow-up on a 6-month or yearly basis, they may not instruct their patients to return.

As with most bills, Congress will appropriate insufficient funds to implement the program the bills envision. Most of the funding should go to strengthen the program where it is to have the greatest effect—at the level of the individual employee. Those who allocate the resources should understand that the training of personal physicians in all aspects of high-risk notification and medical monitoring should be given high priority. The effectiveness of the program should not end at the physician's office door.

REFERENCE

1. GIESEL, J. Doctor loyalty deters retirees from use of HMOs. Business Insurance December 21, 1987. Reported *In* Med. Benefits, January 15, 1988 :3–4.

The Case for Worker Notification

KNUT RINGEN[a]

Workplace Health Fund
Washington, D.C. 20006

In the late summer of 1981 the national news media reported a story that was referred to in the most extreme form by the tabloid *Weekly World News* as "Cancergate."[1] The federal government, notably the National Institute for Occupational Safety and Health (NIOSH), had conducted studies on large groups of workers in which serious disease risks had been found. The problem was that the government had not informed the subjects in those studies of their adverse health risks.

Although these issues had been debated in policy terms for a half decade before 1981,[2] they became known widely when the Workers' Institute for Safety and Health (WISH) and NIOSH launched three intervention projects to demonstrate the feasibility of notifying and offering medical and related assistance to members of occupational high-risk groups. Those projects were conducted between 1980 and 1983. Since then, legislation has been introduced in Congress. The High Risk Occupational Disease Notification and Prevention Bill was passed by the House of Representatives on October 15, 1987, but was withdrawn after a lengthy filibuster in the Senate. The legislation was reintroduced in the 101st Congress in 1989. This legislation has been opposed strongly by the executive branch of the federal government. Since 1983, no new efforts have been made to notify occupational high-risk groups. Within the U.S. Public Health Service these efforts have been neglected with vigor.[3]

DEMONSTRATION PROJECTS

The three demonstration intervention projects conducted are summarized comparatively in TABLE 1. These projects have been discussed in detail elsewhere.[4] Their key characteristics are as follows:

Augusta Chemical Company. The first notification involved predominantly black male workers who between the 1940s and 1972 were exposed to betanaphthylamine at the Augusta Chemical Company, Augusta, Georgia. These workers were unskilled, received relatively low pay, and were not unionized. Extraordinary efforts went into the identification and location of the workers, including the use of commercial personal tracing firms.[5] TABLE 2 summarizes the results of this effort. Of the workers who were alive and could be located, over 90% of those living within the Augusta area participated in the medical program, and the majority of those workers who had dispersed to all parts of the country participated as well.

---

[a] Present address: Laborers' National Health and Safety Fund, 905 16th Street, N. W., Washington, D.C. 20006.

TABLE 1. Comparative Characteristics of the Cohorts Notified in Demonstration Projects

Cohort	Location	Size/Race/Sex	Type of Work	Comparative Characteristics of Cohorts					
				Carcinogen	Target Cancer	Average Period of Exposure	Latency Period	Relative Risk	Medical Intervention Potential
Augusta Chemical Workers	Augusta, GA	1,150/70% black/male	Unskilled Industrial Nonunion Low pay	Beta-naphthyl-amine	Bladder	1949–1974	18.6 yr	4–111	Good
Pattern makers	Nationwide	10,000 current, 2,000 former/all white/male	Skilled Industrial Craft Union High pay	Undetermined	Colon-rectal	Unknown	Unknown	2	Good
Flint Glass Workers	Port Allegany, PA	1,200/all white/male	Unskilled Industrial Union Medium pay	Asbestos	Lung	1964–1972	20 yr	10–53	Poor

TABLE 2. Augusta Project Notification and Participation Rates

Total no. in cohort	1,385		
No. assumed deceased before notification	272 (20%)		
No. with no address available	19 (1%)		
No. lost to follow-up[a]	245 (18%)		
No. assumed alive and notified	849 (61%)		
Geographic Distribution	In Area	Out of Area	Total
No. assumed to be notified	611	238	849
No. participating (% of those notified)	566 (93%)	138 (77%)	749 (88%)

[a] Notification letters returned as undeliverable.

Pattern Makers League of North America. In 1980, three independent epidemiologic studies were published that indicated that pattern and model makers may have a double risk of colon and rectal cancer.[6-8] These workers are almost entirely white men who are skilled, well-paid, and belong to a craft union. This cohort consisted of 10,000 current and 2,000 retired members of the Pattern Makers League of North America (PML). The PML represents members employed in 700 workplaces in 27 states and several Canadian provinces.

Port Allegany Asbestos Health Program. Approximately 1,200 workers, who are members of the Flint Glass Workers' Union in Port Allegany, Pennsylvania, have been determined to be at high risk of developing cancer associated with workplace exposure to asbestos at a glass and insulation products plant. In 1981, after lengthy discussions involving the Pittsburg Corning Corporation and the union, a nonprofit community program was set up with representations from the union, management, community groups, and medical providers, to provide notification, medical examinations, outreach, counseling, and education.[9] Because of the possibility of secondary exposure of family members to asbestos, the program has been extended to include workers' families.

These projects differ in major respects and provide a good cross-section of the medical, social, and political nature of the notification problem. The Augusta project was conducted in a situation of great social tension arising from ignorance, discrimination, and a history of neglect towards a serious health problem on the part of all responsible institutions.[10] The project employed a combination of "top-down" action on the part of a government agency (NIOSH) and grass-roots organizing of the afflicted workers and their social networks on the community level. This project was selected for inclusion as a pilot study because of the serious health risk to workers and because it represented a "worst case" scenario.

The Pattern Makers project represented a union-initiated response that was immediate once a problem became known. Although hesitancy about the program was expressed both by union representatives and by employers in some cases, on the whole its implementation was smooth. To some extent, this undoubtedly reflected that by 1980 our society had come a long way in recognizing the need to address occupational hazards with some degree of vigor and urgency. The Pattern

Makers project is unique in that it is the first multicenter intervention program in occupational medicine in the United States, and a great deal of valuable clinical research on early detection of colorectal cancer has been gained from it.[11]

The Port Allegany Asbestos Health Program celebrated its fifth anniversary last year and is an ongoing community health program. Although its genesis was a lengthy struggle between labor and management, once established this program became known as a "model of community cooperation" on a serious health problem.[12]

These projects demonstrated that notification and intervention programs for workers at high risk of occupational diseases can be conducted feasibly within the structures of community health and labor management relations in the United States. They also demonstrated that many different approaches can be used to achieve these ends. Consequently, policies directed at worker-notification and intervention should be flexible and build on the structures that already are in place.

OBJECTIONS TO WORKER-NOTIFICATION

In the course of hearings and debate on this issue within the U.S. Congress and the private sector, a number of objections to worker-notification and intervention programs have been raised. These objections, which can be found in the minority views in the House *Report*,[13] Senate *Report*,[14] as well as the debate on the floor of the House of Representatives,[15] are summarized under five headings which will be addressed:

1. There are no medical benefits for notified workers.
2. The legislation is a duplication of existing OSHA activities.
3. The legislation is too costly.
4. Notification promotes litigation.
5. Notification is damaging to workers.

No Medical Benefits

Too often the current bill in Congress has been thought of as a cancer bill, and lung cancer has been raised as a case in point to illustrate that medically nothing is gained by intervening. Apart from this damaging assessment of U.S. medicine in general and the 12% of the Gross National Product currently expended on medical care, the argument is tendentious and wrong in many respects as follows:

The legislation covers all occupational diseases, some with excellent survival potential and some with poor survival potential.

It is a utilitarian error to argue that medical benefits are the essential justification for this bill. The real justification resides in fundamental ethical and moral principles grounded in democracy: the right to self-determination, as reaffirmed in the Nuremburg code on medical research and the Helsinki declaration on informed consent, the precedent of notification in other areas of public health, such as victims of childhood thyroid irradiation therapy, and the principle of not withholding health information laid down after the Tuskegee syphilis natural experiments.[16]

This argument neglects the medical experience that even after exposure to lung insults such as asbestos, much can be done to reduce mortality from superimposed respiratory infections.[17] Additionally, on January 13, 1988, a professional consensus meeting at NIOSH concluded that intervention through early detection is valuable in lung cancer. This determination is being reaffirmed by officials of the National Cancer Institute.[18]

Bill Duplicates Existing OSHA Activities

It has been claimed that occupational high-risk notification and intervention is a duplication of activities carried out by the U.S. Department of Labor Occupational Safety and Health Administration (OSHA) under existing health standards and the Hazard Communications Standard. The deficiencies of this position were discussed extensively by Dr. Philip Landrigan, Professor of Pediatrics and Community Medicine, Mt. Sinai School of Medicine, New York, on February 24, 1987, and Dr. John Finklea, Professor of Preventive Medicine, University of Alabama, on May 15, 1986, in testimony before the Subcommittee on Labor of the Senate Committee on Labor and Human Resources. They have pointed out three areas not currently covered that would be covered by the new legislation:

Past exposures. In a dynamic economy many of the occupational diseases detected will relate to past exposures, given the long latency periods that may separate exposure from its clinical manifestation.

Former workers. Similarly, most workers will change occupations or places of work during their lifetimes.

Family members. Occupational household contact disease is not covered in any current programs despite the increasing recognition of this problem.

Legislation is Too Costly

Cost estimates as high as $53 billion have been attributed to this legislation. Debate on the floor of the House of Representatives suggested that it would threaten the economic competitiveness of the United States in world trade and have global economic consequences. These are gross overstatements. The fact is that the costs are already incurred, as is evident in the following simple calculation:

Assume the U.S. Department of Labor's estimate from 1980 that there are 1.88 million disabled workers in the United States.[19]

Although it is difficult to estimate the economic cost of occupational disability,[20] assume that the estimate of average costs from Johnson and Heler's study of 515 asbestos disability cases is representative of all occupational disability cases. They estimated a total cost to the worker and his or her family of $475,000 and of an additional $95,000 to society.[21] This means a total cost per case to the victim and society in excess of $500,000.

If both of these assumptions are correct, the total cost of occupational disability in the United States at present is approximately *one trillion dollars*.

The issue then is not the cost associated with notification and intervention, but rather who should pay these costs. Workers and their families are currently paying the bill. Not only that, but since these costs are being carried by the workers as individuals, these workers are paying a premium arising from the lack of an organized program of intervention. Consider the following estimates for the Pattern Makers program:

Cost of developing the program is $120,000, or $10 per worker for each of the 12,000 persons covered.

Cost of medical examination, including detailed occupational and medical history, physical examination, lung function testing and chest x-rays, urinalysis and blood work, stool hemoccult, and flexible sigmoidoscopic examination to 68 cm. The cost negotiated for this medical testing program ranged from $130 to $240 per worker examined, depending on location, number of workers involved, and the like. These low costs were obtained because they were negotiated for an organized group program. If these workers had arranged individually to obtain this same battery of exams and tests, the cost would easily have exceeded $1,000.

Another way of looking at this legislation, then, from a societal point of view, is that it would save significant amounts of money. An approach to calculating this has been developed by Ruttenberg and Powers.[22]

The Legislation is Litigious

It has been argued repeatedly that this legislation will open the floodgates for tort suits brought by workers against third parties and employers. Surprisingly, much of the hysteria about litigation has been caused by the U.S. Department of Justice, arguing that the U.S. Treasury may be vulnerable to a run against it by aggrieved workers who have been notified. This argument is disturbing for two reasons. First, the U.S. Constitution set up the Judiciary as a third branch of government to protect minorities against the excesses of majorities and to allow aggrieved individuals to seek redress. In this case, the government would effectively deny workers this constitutional right by withholding from them the information about their risk. Second, much of the concern about litigation has been expressed by referring to the demonstration projects presented here. The record from these three projects with regard to litigation is as follows:

In Augusta, 171 suits totaling $300 million in claims were filed. Of these, 120 were settled out of court for an estimated total of $500,000. The remaining suits were thrown out of court on statute of limitations grounds. Thus, for the 1,000 eligible, living workers in this group, the average recoupment through the courts was about $500. That is hardly a windfall.

In Port Allegany, only two suits are known to have been filed since September 1981, when the asbestos health program was started. Both of these cases were mesotheliomas.[23]

Among pattern makers, not a single suit is thought to have been pursued.

We have long held the position that tort litigation is a poor way to resolve social problems on a large scale and that a national system of prompt and equitable compensation for occupational diseases is needed.[24] These projects suggest that litigation does not arise from the act of notifying workers, but rather from the failure to have notified them in the first place. Furthermore, the litigation is substantially a response to the lack of an organized system to deal with the special needs of workers at high risk.

Notification is Damaging to Workers

The final and most patronizing objection to worker notification is that workers cannot deal with this type of information. It is true that, in the short run, the act of notifying a high-risk cohort may create discriminatory responses against the workers, especially in employment and financial dealings. Instances of this were reported in the Augusta project. More dramatic, but similar, actions were experienced recently by HIV-positive individuals, much as lepers were treated in the past. Yet, based on carefully conducted psychosocial studies of the cohort in Augusta, no adverse affects were evident.[25]

This finding, which scientists were able to discern using sophisticated psychometric scales, was summed up by a woman in her late forties—the spouse of one of the Augusta chemical workers—who said one night during a community meeting in response to a question about whether the notification program was beneficial, "When you live from day to day, from hand to mouth, this is just one more in a series of life crises. We are just glad someone was willing to help us with one of them."

CONCLUSION

In the convoluted debate over the need for a national system of notification and intervention for workers with a high risk of disease it is easy to lose a sense of perspective, particularly when confronted with doomsday predictions on the grand scale that opponents of such a system present. Yet, tear away the fluff, and the issues present themselves clearly:

> A large number of workers are known to be at high risk of disease because of past or present exposure to serious health hazards on the job. These individuals are identifiable and have rights as members of a democratic society to be informed about their risk.

> The projects reported on herein demonstrate that notification and intervention can be provided feasibly within the structures of community health and labor management relations at minimum cost.

> The suggestion that an organized program of notification and intervention is litigious simply is not supported by the facts as presented by these demonstration projects. Workers do not sue because of organized programs to address their needs; they sue as a measure of last resort in the absence of such programs.

> The suggestion that an organized program of notification and intervention is economically not viable ignores the reality that the costs of occupational disability and premature death today are borne by the victims and society in the amount of approximately one trillion dollars. These costs are excessive in the

absence of an organized system because of the vast inefficiencies incurred by dealing with each case individually.

The High Risk Occupational Disease Notification and Intervention Act is an important step towards creating a national system for dealing with this problem. The legislation is not perfect, but then neither is our society. It is a start. It will give workers at risk a means to aid them in protecting their lives.

SUMMARY

There is currently a heated debate about whether the U.S. Congress should enact the High Risk Occupational Disease Notification and Prevention Act. This Act would set up an orderly system for identifying, notifying, and assisting workers at high risk of occupational disease. Significant underpinning for this legislation comes from three pilot projects conducted by the National Institute for Occupational Safety and Health and the Workers' Institute for Safety and Health. These projects demonstrate that notification and intervention for occupational high-risk groups can be implemented feasibly within the existing structures of community health and labor management relations. These projects also suggest that, contrary to the views of opponents of current legislation, it is the absence of systematic programs that leads to massive litigation and high costs. At present, these costs are borne by workers and society.

ACKNOWLEDGMENTS

This work was conducted collaboratively with Paul Schulte, Ph.D., of NIOSH, and Sandra Tillett and Kenneth Miller, M.D., at the Workers' Institute for Safety and Health. We are indebted to two preceding generations of intellect and action on this problem: Irving J. Selikoff, M.D., Professor Emeritus, Mount Sinai School of Medicine, New York, and Sheldon W. Samuels, Director of Health, Safety and the Environment, Industrial Union Department, AFL-CIO.

REFERENCES

1. "CANCER SCANDAL." 1981. Weekly World News **2**: 1.
2. GUMBERT, D. 1977. Workers right to know. The Wall Street Journal, July 1.
3. BAYER, R. 1987. Notifying workers at risk: The politics of the right to know. Am J. Public Health **76**: 1352–1356.
4. TILLETT, S., K. RINGEN, P. SCHULTE, K. MILLER, & S. W. SAMUELS. 1986. Interventions in high-risk occupational cohorts: A cross-sectional demonstration project. J. Occup. Med. **28**: 719–727.
5. SCHULTE, P. A., K. RINGEN, et al. 1985. Notification of a cohort of workers at risk of bladder cancer. J. Occup. Med. **27**: 19–28.
6. SWANSON, G. M. & S. H. BELLE. 1982. Cancer morbidity and workers in the U.S. automotive industry. J. Occup. Med. **24**: 315–319.
7. SCHOTTENFELD, D. et al. 1980. Study of cancer mortality and incidence of wood shop workers of the General Motors Corporation. Memorial Sloan Kettering Cancer Center, New York; April 18.
8. ROBINSON, C. et al. 1980. Pattern and model makers proportionate mortality 1972–78. Am. J. Ind. Med. **1**: 159–165.

9. HOLSTEIN, E. C., K. W. DEUSCHLE, S. BOSH, et al. 1984. Port Allegany Asbestos Health Program: A community response to a public health problem. Pub. Health Rep. **99**: 193–199.
10. OMANG, J. 1981. Augusta: Case study of difficulties of telling workers of old job perils. The Washington Post, September 3, A2.
11. BANG, K. M., S. TILLETT, S. K. HOAR, et al. 1986. Sensitivity of fecal hemoccult testing and flexible sigmoidoscopy for colorectal cancer screening. J. Occup. Med. **28**: 709–713.
12. DAILY, J. E. 1981. A neighborly way to fight asbestosis. Business Week, September 7: 24B-C.
13. U.S. CONGRESS, HOUSE OF REPRESENTATIVES. 1987. Report on the High Risk Occupational Disease Notification and Prevention Act of 1987 [to accompany H.R.162]. 100th Congress, 1st Session, Report 100–194, June 26.
14. U.S. Congress, Senate. 1987. Report on the High Risk Occupational Disease Notification and Intervention Act. 100th Congress, 1st Session, Report 100–166, September 23.
15. U.S. Congress. 1987. Congressional Record. **133**(160): H 8615-H 8671; **133**(161): H 8692-H 8712.
16. SCHULTE, P. A. & K. RINGEN. 1984. Notification of workers at high risk: An emerging public health problem. Am. J. Public Health **74**: 485–491.
17. SELIKOFF, I. J., Professor Emeritus, Mount Sinai School of Medicine, New York. 1987. Letter to the Committee on Labor and Human Resources, U.S. Senate.
18. SMART, C., Chief, Early Detection Branch, Division of Cancer Prevention and Control, National Cancer Institute. 1988. Personal communication, February 3.
19. Assistant Secretary for Policy, Evaluation and Research. 1981. An Interim Report to Congress on Occupational Diseases. Washington, DC: U.S. Department of Labor.
20. JOHNSON, W. G., Professor of Economics, Syracuse University. 1987. Letter to the Subcommittee on Labor, U.S. Senate. Senate Report 100–166 on the High Risk Occupational Disease Notification and Prevention Act, September 23.
21. JOHNSON, W. G., & E. HELER. 1983. The costs of asbestos-associated disease and death. Milbank Memorial Fund Q. **61**: 210.
22. RUTTENBERG, R. & M. POWERS. 1986. The economics of notification and medical screening for high risk workers. J. Occup. Med. **28**: 996–1005.
23. COHEN, G., Attorney, Bredhof and Kaiser, Washington DC, and a Plaintiff's Lawyer for the Port Allegany Population. 1988. Personal communication, February 19.
24. RINGEN, K. & W. J. SMITH. 1983. Occupational diseases and equity issues. Va. Natural Resources Law J. **2**: 213–231.
25. HORNSBY, J. L., J. T. SAPPINGTON, P. MONGAN, et al. 1985. Risk for bladder cancer: Psychological impact of notification. JAMA **253**: 1899–1902.

Round Table 3: Discussion

LAURA FLEMING (*Yale University, New Haven, Conn.*): Approximately half the patients I see in our occupational health clinic at Yale are minority workers, Spanish- or non-English-speaking, transients, with no insurance, with no union, and often without visas. How will this bill, which I support, take care of these people?

ALAN ENGELBERG (*American Medical Association, Chicago, Ill.*): It will not take care of them.

KNUT RINGEN (*Workplace Health Fund, Washington, D.C.*): This bill will not do anything specifically for those workers, unless they are covered in some study that becomes part of the notification program of the government.

FLEMING: I am concerned that those are the people who had the worst exposures and are probably at highest risk.

RICHARD RABIN (*Massachusetts Division of Occupational Hygiene, Boston, Mass.*): It is important to recognize that the right to know, whether it is called notification or hazard communication, is only a first step towards workers' right to act. Knowing that a worker risks getting a disease, or that he is being exposed to a hazardous substance is of only minimal use unless he has the right, both legal and contractually guaranteed to actually limit exposure in the workplace and to control what goes on there.

LINDA RUDOLPH (*California Department of Health Services, Berkeley, Calif.*): I would like to hear comments on the role of the occupational health researcher in notification, in terms of his responsibility to notify the cohorts on which he does research, other people at risk, and the appropriate public health agencies of his research findings.

RINGEN: There has been a lot of discussion, particularly in the Society of Epidemiological Research, about the role of investigators. Is their purpose to study the world or to change the world? That is a discussion that has been going on in epidemiology for 100 years. It is my feeling that an epidemiologist who undertakes a study of a population has a responsibility beyond that which is implied in publishing an article in a journal. He has a responsibility to the workers, to their representatives, and to the public health community to see that there is follow-up for that population. Just as any clinician who examines a worker has the responsibility to see that something detected on a screening examination should be followed-up properly.

RUDOLPH: Is there a concomitant responsibility of the researcher to adequately notify a study group before a study about the implications of either a positive or a negative result?

RINGEN: Probably, yes.

PHILIP J. LANDRIGAN (*Mount Sinai School of Medicine, New York, N.Y.*): An approach to achieving that goal is to hold an open tripartite meeting at the beginning of the study in which the goals, the aims, and the possible outcomes are explained; I have been involved in studies at the National Institute for Occupational Safety and Health (NIOSH) and at Mount Sinai School of Medicine where that has been done with satisfactory results.

JAMES M. MELIUS (*New York State Department of Health, Albany, N.Y.*): We also need to make funding agencies more keenly aware of that responsibility.

FRANKLIN E. MIRER (*United Automobile, Aerospace, and Agricultural Implement Workers' Union, Detroit, Michigan*): My comment concerns the implementation of this bill. Should it pass, let us not forget that it was initiated over concern

ROUND TABLE 3: DISCUSSION

for informing the populations who were in particular studies undertaken by NIOSH and the National Cancer Institute (NCI). To illustrate this, several years ago, looking through the *Journal of the National Cancer Institute*, we saw an article about a mortality study performed in a large automotive foundry in the Midwest by the National Cancer Institute. We figured that this plant had to be one of ours, but we did not know which one. After considerable looking and one false start, we eventually found the plant. Management told us that they were aware that somebody had turned over records to NCI about 10 or 15 years before. However, the published report was the first word they too had had of the results of the investigation.

We are now doing a considerable amount of joint research in the auto industry, and one of the principal issues we must resolve is how to notify people of the results when they come in. It would be very helpful to researchers, management, and the unions, if one of the first stages of the rule-making under this law were to establish the criteria and the nature of the information to be released to subjects of cohort studies when these studies are completed.

RINGEN: I would like to comment on that point. I believe that Dr. Paul Schulte of NIOSH has developed a protocol for notification that covers all of the issues you have raised. It would be nice if his protocol were made more public than it is at present.

Worker-Notification Activities at the National Institute for Occupational Safety and Health

Past and Present

EDWARD L. BAKER,[a] PAUL A. SCHULTE,[b]
AND JEAN G. FRENCH[a]

National Institute for Occupational Safety and Health, CDC
[a]*Atlanta, Georgia 30333, and*
[b]*Cincinnati, Ohio 45213*

It is the right of workers to know the agents to which they are exposed in the workplace and the potential consequences of such exposures. Yet, workers have labored for years without being informed of their workplace exposures. Only recently has public attention been drawn to this important issue.

Worker notification has two components: informing presently employed workers of their current exposures and informing workers, both presently employed and no longer employed, of their past exposures and risk. The first component can be achieved by a multiplicity of actions on the part of the employer, the manufacturer, and governmental agencies and permits the worker to participate in responsible action to prevent or minimize his exposures. The second component, notification after the fact of exposure, which may permit the worker to initiate secondary preventive action, is heavily influenced by social, economic, ethical, and scientific considerations.

I would like to share with you NIOSH activities, both past and present, in the area of worker notification.

NIOSH has been extensively engaged in informing present workers of their current exposures and potential subsequent effects throughout its existence. As part of the more than 500 health hazard evaluations performed by NIOSH each year, reports are sent to the requester, the company, employee representatives, union headquarters, the Department of Labor, appropriate state representatives, and local agencies. Furthermore, the report is posted at the worksite for 30 days or sent individually to all affected employees.

Whenever we perform a medical test on workers, we send the results of the test to the individual, and to the health care provider, if designated by the individual. By similar means, we report widely the findings of industrial hygiene surveys and cross-sectional medical studies. Moreover, all of our field and laboratory findings are reported extensively in the scientific literature.

NIOSH involvement in notifying workers of past exposures relates primarily to informing surviving cohort members of the findings of retrospective cohort studies conducted by NIOSH. This involvement stems from a 1977 Senate Subcommittee Hearing during which the directors of NIOSH and the National Cancer Institute (NCI) were asked why the government failed to individually notify the subjects of retrospective cohort studies of their potential risks. As part of that hearing the NIOSH Director and members of his staff prepared a paper entitled, "The Right to Know," which outlined practical problems and policy issues arising from notifying workers of their past exposure to hazardous chemical and physical agents in the workplace.[1] The following issues were identified:

Uncertainties relating to individual risk: A retrospective cohort mortality study involves identifying a cohort of workers, following that cohort, and evaluating the mortality experience within the cohort by comparing what you would expect to find with what is observed. A measure of that comparison is the Standardized Mortality Ratio. This type of study is typically a records search with no direct contact of living members of the cohort. Epidemiologic information is group specific and does not directly assess the experience of an individual within the group. If the total cohort is found to be at risk, then individuals in the group are presumed to be at varying levels of individual risk depending on the extent of their individual exposure and other causal factors.

Need for adequate follow-up: In some cases, notification could be detrimental to the individual if provision has not been made for counseling, medical follow-up, and treatment, if appropriate. A necessary part of worker notification and counseling is the provision for access to medical expertise whereby the workers, their physicians, and others may obtain additional information on the significance of follow-up procedures.

Subsequent to 1977, NIOSH had embarked on various projects aimed at evaluating the problems of notification and identifying possible solutions.

In 1979, NIOSH completed a small pilot study of individual worker notification of a selected group of 55 terminated workers whose medical records had been submitted to NIOSH pursuant to the provisions of the Occupational Safety and Health Act and the Occupational Safety and Health Administration's regulations on 13 carcinogens (29 CFR part 1910.10). The workers were sent letters that told of possible exposure to a carcinogen. No medical surveillance or follow-up was planned. Forty-nine percent of those who presumably received a letter responded by asking NIOSH to send medical information to their physician. However, on the basis of a telephone survey, none were known to have contacted their physician. It was established that the cost of this notification alone was about $150 per worker notified.

In 1980, a major pilot study was begun (1) to evaluate the problems inherent in notifying individual workers of their potential health risks, and (2) to identify criteria and develop a conceptual model for subsequent notification efforts. The pilot project examined the problems resulting from the individual notification of members of a cohort of workers in Augusta, Georgia, who manufactured textile dyes and had exposure to aromatic amines, most notably 2-naphthylamine and benzidine.

The cohort studied involved 1,385 plant workers employed between 1940 and 1972. In tracing the cohort, it was found that individuals were dispersed over 30 states; however, most of them still remained within the Southeast. Despite the best efforts in locating members of the cohort, 22% were not located. Tracing mechanisms included the Social Security Administration, Internal Revenue Service, State Bureaus of Motor Vehicles, and some credit tracing organizations. From a vital status follow-up of the cohort, it was assumed that 1,094 were still alive, and 798 of these were in and around the Augusta area. A screening program of these 1,094 individuals was conducted with a 77% participation rate. Special methods were employed to screen individuals living outside a 50-mile radius of the Augusta area.[2]

Of the 1,385 people, 14 were identified as having bladder cancer.[3] Four of the cancers were identified from death certificates. Seven patients were under treatment by community urologists, and three were identified in the first phase of the screening program. Since that time, two others have been identified. The cohort had an approximate fourfold risk of bladder cancer, but some of the subsets had a much greater risk—the highest being among black workers with over 10 years of employment. These individuals had a 111-fold risk.[3]

The pilot project in Augusta confirmed many of the issues and concerns raised in the 1977 "Right to Know" paper that individual worker notification is not just a simple process of sending a letter to a former worker about some employment experience.[4] It requires initiating a large, diverse, complex process in which a variety of information is involved. Some of the information needed includes: personnel records; epidemiologic findings; information to locate the cohort; appropriate information about the cohorts to develop the method and message to be sent to them; information regarding the substance or substances to which the cohort is exposed; and information, not only for the workers, but also for their physicians. Notified workers also have concerns about: medical surveillance, particularly medical screening; obtaining the appropriate information to relay to their personal physicians; counseling needs, both psychologic and legal; and financial concerns.[4] In the Augusta experience, some of the workers would not participate in the screening program for fear that detected health problems would be too costly for them. Some of these people need various kinds of support (such as economic, psychologic, or legal) to help them cope with their risk status.

Following the Augusta Pilot Project, a decision logic outlining the criteria that could be used as a basis for worker notification was developed by NIOSH staff. After review by the NIOSH Board of Scientific Counselors, the decision logic was revised and renamed, "Guidelines for Notification of Individual Workers,"[5] and contained the following recommendations:

These guidelines are meant to be flexible and applied on a case-by-case basis. They are not to supplant scientific interpretation and judgment. The cohort studies under consideration are complex and we consider it inappropriate to apply simple, rigid rules to complex studies.

A. Determine that the study is appropriately designed and analyzed.

The study needs to be carefully reviewed in the context of questions such as:

1. Was an appropriate hypothesis formulated for the study?

2. Was the study population appropriate and of sufficient size to address this hypothesis?

3. Is there adequate documentation of cohort selection? Could this selection be biased?

4. Was there adequate follow-up of the cohort?

5. Were the causes of death adequately documented particularly for diagnoses where death certificate data needs confirmation?

6. Were appropriate statistical methods used to analyze the collected data?

7. Are the risk estimates from the study reliable? The determination will include confirmation of the definition of the study groups and the confidence in the study results.

All of these factors (and others) need to be reviewed in determining whether the study is appropriately designed and analyzed.

B. Consider whether the findings are consistent with those of other studies.

The study results then should be reviewed to determine whether other information supports the conclusion of the study. This other information may come from animal studies, other human health studies, accepted mechanisms of action and metabolism to substances having similar activities. Findings consistent with such information would be likely candidates for notification. A finding not supported by other studies would need greater evidence of elevated risk to be considered for individual notification.

C. Establish whether the survivors are or are not at risk.

Another important aspect of a notification decision is a determination that the survivors are still at risk from their previous exposure. Often the lack of information will make this difficult to determine, and the cohort will have to be assumed to still be at risk. However, in some instances, a change in production process control or a substitution in the process may place a subpopulation of the cohort survivors at much less risk than cohort members who worked prior to the change. Such factors must be very carefully evaluated before deciding *not* to notify on this basis.

Another consideration relates to the selection of only certain cohort groups for notification. In some cohort studies it may be possible to identify a portion of the cohort who are at increased risk as compared to others in the study. This selection will usually be based on work in certain areas of the plant with unique or much greater exposure to the toxic substance. This differential notification will be very carefully reviewed prior to leaving certain cohort members out of the notification process.

D. Determine that the cohort has not been previously notified.

The review of each cohort study must also address whether the cohort has already been notified. The nature of the previous notification effort, the information included in that notification, and its timing would need also to be assessed. This may have been done through special screening programs at the plant or other efforts. If over 75% of the group has already been notified, no further notification is proposed. As with other criteria, this cutoff must be judged with flexibility.

E. Notification Options

The following options are sufficient but not necessary criteria to trigger notification actions. Other factors to be considered include the potential for medical intervention or other steps that would alter the individual risk. Also, it is important to reduce false-negative and false-positive notifications.

1. If the attributable risk[a] is less than 25% (or the SMR[b] is less than 133), and the absolute risk[c] is less than 10^{-5}, then:

  a. Employers and union representatives for the same type of industries

---

[a] As used here, attributable risk (AR) is synonymous with the terms attributable risk (exposed) or attributable fraction (exposed) as defined by J. M. Last in *A Dictionary of Epidemiology*, p. 7. The definition as adapted to mortality studies is as follows: In a situation in which exposure to a given factor is believed to cause a given outcome, the attributable risk among the exposed is the proportion of the outcome among those exposed to the factor that can be attributed to the exposure factor. In these guidelines, it will be expressed as a percent. It is computed as: AR = (SMR−100) / SMR. For example, if the SMR for a specific disease is 133, the AR would be (133−100) / 133 = 0.25 or 25%. If information on other risk factors was available, appropriate adjustments in attributable risk could be made. However, this other information is usually not available.

[b] The Standardized Mortality Ratio (SMR) is the ratio of the number of deaths observed in the study population to the number of deaths expected if it had the same rate structure as had the standard population. An SMR that is greater than 100 indicates an excess of observed deaths in a study population.

[c] As used here, absolute risk represents the actual risk in a population, that is, the probability of cause-specific deaths occurring within the lifetime of the population. Absolute risk is expressed here in a shorthand form according to orders of magnitude. For example, an absolute risk of less than 10^{-5} means that the risk of dying of a given disease in a population during its lifetime is less than 1 in 100,000.

should be notified of the results through a general notification effort.

b. The cohort should be notified through information on the study being provided to the involved company and union officials and, where possible, posting of the report in the involved locations.

2. If the attributable risk is between 25 and 50% (or the SMR is between 133 and 200) and the absolute risk is between 10^{-3} and 10^{-5}, then:

a. Notify the involved industry and unions as outlined in E.1. above.

b. NIOSH Alert: Through appropriate mechanisms such as a Hazard Alert, NIOSH should take active steps to notify the industry and workforce of the hazard.

c. Notify the local newspapers and media in the areas where the cohort is located of the findings of the study and the implication of these findings for the study participants.

d. Notify the appropriate public health agencies.

3. If the attributable risk is greater than or equal to 50% (or the SMR is greater than 200) and the absolute risk is greater than 10^{-3}, then individual worker notification will include:

a. Efforts to locate individual members of the cohort.

b. Individual letters of notification to the cohort participants, informing them of their assumed increased risk.

c. Notification of noncohort workers, which will be the same as E.1 and E.2.

d. Appropriate provision for workers to contact NIOSH personnel to obtain further information.

When considering this option and when individual worker notification takes place under E.2., the provisions for support services in connection with notification must be thoroughly evaluated before proceeding.

Note: The three options do not cover all possible combinations of absolute and attributable risk. When studies have risk combinations that do not meet the options as described, great care should be taken to ensure that the appropriate worker notification option is applied.

F. Other recommendations

In considering the foregoing guidelines, again flexibility and case-by-case decision-making are to be used. Additional considerations that the Director of NIOSH should use for the individual decisions include:

1. When considering the SMR, the comparable population should be reviewed carefully. National statistics may not always be appropriate.

2. Attributable risk, as defined, should be given greater weight than should the other criteria.

3. The setting of a limiting statistical p value is probably not appropriate for this use.

4. Adjustment for simultaneous inference should be used cautiously and only if the unadjusted estimates of probability are also presented.

5. Individual worker notification as described in E.3. would be used if worker notification as described in E.2. is not possible, because the plant is closed and the cohort is geographically dispersed or if selected groups within the cohort have a much higher risk.

6. Decisions regarding individual worker notification, after the guidelines have been applied by NIOSH to their studies, should be audited by an external peer review group.

7. After implementation the notification effort should be evaluated for effectiveness. Early efforts should be fully evaluated, with periodic evaluations

thereafter. There should be a behavioral scientist on the evaluation team. The primary questions to be answered are:

   a. Were the individual workers notified?, and
   b. What happened after notification?

8. Systems should be in place to deal with health inquiries stimulated by worker notification and to provide health care as may be appropriate.

9. There should be a disproportionate use of resources for those subjects of cohorts at greater risk.

Thus far the guidelines have been applied to four NIOSH retrospective cohort studies. The following example illustrates the notification decision derived from the application of the guidelines to one of the NIOSH retrospective cohort studies[6]:

In the early 1970s, NIOSH researchers evaluated the health effects of occupational exposure to vinyl chloride in a cohort of 1,294 workers at four polymerization plants. Analysis of 136 deaths showed statistically significant SMRs of 149 for all malignant neoplasms and 1,155 for biliary and liver cancer. For workers with more than 15 years since onset of exposure, statistically significant SMRs of 184 occurred for all malignant neoplasms, 498 for brain and CNS cancer, and 194 for respiratory system cancer. Eleven of 14 biliary and liver cancers were angiosarcomas.

In 1987 the study results were subject to detailed analysis which yielded the following conclusions:

   A. The study is appropriately designed and analyzed.
   B. The findings are consistent with other studies.
   C. The cohort has not been extensively notified.
   D. The SMR for liver cancer is considerably in excess of 300, the attributable risk percentage is greater than 50, and the absolute risk is in the order of 10^{-3}; therefore, individual worker notification of this cohort would be warranted. Also found in excess and thus eligible for notification, although of lower priority, were cancers of the brain and respiratory system.

CONCLUSION

With the beginning of fiscal year 1990, NIOSH will apply these guidelines to all current and newly planned studies. With the assistance of the NIOSH Board of Scientific Counselors, we are using the guidelines to assess the backlog of approximately 90 studies to determine which ones should result in notification and the type of notification to be done.

NIOSH is firmly committed to the concept of worker notification. The institutional strengths and the consolidation of creditability that has occurred in NIOSH over the past 15 years place it in a unique position to enter the 1990s—an era in which notification and surveillance will be of particular importance to the field of occupational health. The challenges will be substantial, but the rewards for the health and safety of U.S. workers will be proportionately great.

REFERENCES

1. The Right to Know: Practical Problems and Policy Issues Arising from Exposures to Hazardous Chemical and Physical Agents in the Workplace. Prepared by the National Institute for Occupational Safety and Health, Centers for Disease Control, July 1977.

2. SCHULTE, P. A., K. RINGEN, W. GULLEN *et al.* 1985. Notification of a cohort of workers at risk of bladder cancer. J. Occup. Med. **27**: 19–28.
3. SCHULTE, P. A., K. RINGEN, G. HEMSTREET *et al.* 1985. Risk assessment of a cohort exposed to aromatic amines: Initial results. J. Occup. Med. **27**: 115–121.
4. SCHULTE, P. A. 1985. The epidemiologic basis for notification of subjects of cohort studies. Am. J. Epidemiol. **121**: 351–361.
5. Report of the subcommittee on individual worker notification. NIOSH Board of Scientific Counselors, February 15, 1986.
6. WAXWEILER, R. J. *et al.* 1976. Neoplastic risk among workers exposed to vinyl chloride. Ann. N.Y. Acad. Sci. **271**: 40–48.

Round Table Papers: 4. The Consequences of High-Risk Worker Notification

The High-Risk Occupational Disease Notification and Prevention Act

From Primary to Secondary Prevention—From Paternalism to Autonomy

PAUL W. BRANDT-RAUF[a] AND
SHERRY I. BRANDT-RAUF[b]

[a]*Department of Occupational Medicine
Columbia University
New York, New York 10032*

[b]*Center for the Study of Society and Medicine
Columbia University
New York, New York 10032*

The High-Risk Occupational Disease Notification and Prevention Bill of 1987 (H.R.162[1] and S.79[2]) has been characterized as an effort to rectify the deficiencies of prior legislation in the area, the Occupational Safety and Health Act (OSHAct[3]). The OSHAct, passed in 1970, represented an attempt to cure the problem of widespread occupational injury and disease through primary prevention. The primary preventive approach involved the setting of safety standards and exposure limits for hazardous substances, both of which employers had to meet or risk the imposition of a fine. This approach left little opportunity for worker participation or decision making. Because the OSHAct reflected an assumption that workplace health risk could be eliminated, it made no provision for informing workers of any such risks. And because it was, and remains, prescriptive in the first instance, it left no sphere for workers to decide to encounter known occupational health risks. As such, it might be described as representing a paternalistic approach to the problem of worker health.

The OSHAct has clearly failed in its mission of maximizing the safety of the American workplace. Its effectiveness has been hampered by inadequate funding and manpower, lengthy and cumbersome judicial challenges, and changes in the political climate. Rep. Joseph M. Gaydos (D.-Pa.), the original sponsor of the new bill, has stated that Congress hoped the OSHAct ". . . would substantially reduce the number of deaths and injuries arising from occupational accidents and diseases. Unfortunately, it hasn't worked out that way. Each year, 100,000 American workers die from occupationally related diseases. Another 400,000 become disabled."[4] Rep. Gaydos believes that H.R.162 "will take a giant step toward solving this serious national occupational health problem."[4]

Although the new law, which recently passed the House of Representatives, follows in the footsteps of the OSHAct, it represents a major policy shift along two dimensions. The basic mechanism of H.R.162 is one of identifying occupational health risks and then notifying the workers who are at risk. On the basis of the information provided them, workers can then decide on an appropriate course of action for detection and, if necessary, treatment for the disease in question.

This represents a secondary, or even tertiary, attempt at preventing disease, in that rather than simply eliminating the source of the risk, it depends on future action, such as union negotiations or government regulation, to eliminate it. In addition, although the decision as to which workers merit notification is still essentially paternalistic, the decision to apply the information in pursuit of the goal of prevention would become an exercise in individual choice. Thus, the proposed legislation, rather than simply following the approach of its predecessor, actually represents a dramatic shift in both philosophy and underlying public health policy.

The philosophical shift is neither unprecedented nor without justification. A consumer-oriented approach rooted in autonomy considerations and free choice has become predominant in other areas of health care decision making, in particular in relations between doctors and patients. Other pieces of federal legislation reflect the rights of other groups to different types of information.[5,6] Such an approach may be justified on pragmatic grounds as well. A paternalistic approach requires the expenditure of considerable resources in money and manpower. Employer compliance must be verified by inspection, and noncompliance penalties must be assessed through often lengthy administrative and judicial proceedings. The OSHAct failed in its goal, in part, because it never commanded the kinds of resources that might actually have made it work. In fact, the new legislation may continue in that tradition by diverting some of the already scarce resources we devote to occupational health away from enforcement of the OSHAct.

The shift from primary to secondary preventive strategies can also be justified on several grounds. For example, outlawing the sale of tobacco products would be a primary approach to the prevention of lung cancer. Its opponents might suggest that similar primary strategies failed to stop alcohol abuse during Prohibition and that secondary strategies make practical sense while better preserving the rights of the individual.

Despite the fact that these changes, from paternalism to autonomy and from primary prevention to secondary, can be justified theoretically does not mean that they make the best sense as applied to worker health. These changes require further examination and thought as to their immediate and long-range implications for the likelihood of the bill's achieving its goals.

In fact, the goals of the new bill are not entirely clear. In its findings section, H.R.162 states that "workers have a basic and fundamental right to know they have been and are being exposed to an occupational hazard and are at risk of contracting an occupational disease."[1] But the bill goes beyond this in intent. It seeks not only to inform workers but also to eradicate or at least reduce the incidence of occupational disease. Although these goals do not necessarily conflict, the goal selected as primary will color the approach in areas of ambiguity.

H.R.162 is geared primarily toward situations in which a disease process is clearly understood: a hazardous substance induces a physiologic change in an employee that increases that employee's risk of disease. Problems of interpretation will most likely arise in cases in which the process diverges from this prototypical one. Several examples of such areas include the treatment of subclinical pathophysiologic changes, in which the relation between the change and the risk of disease is not well understood; the definition of hazardous exposures, in which that relation is understood but the agent may not fall within the purview of the bill; and the management of paraoccupational exposures, in which the employee is exposed but someone else may be at risk for disease.

First, the language of the bill requires that workers be notified of risks of "occupationally induced disease,"[1,2] which the Senate version defines as "acute or chronic health affects."[2] Physiologic alterations that correlate with future disease outcomes clearly fall into this category. But in some instances, biochemical or molecular biologic abnormalities occur at a significantly increased rate in certain worker populations exposed to toxic materials, abnormalties that have not yet been clearly linked to ultimate morbidity. For example, consider the case of new markers for monitoring potential occupational cancer risk such as urinary mutagenicity, sister chromatid exchanges, chromosomal aberrations, micronuclei, DNA adducts, and oncogene proteins. These markers, which occur at increased frequency in mutagen-exposed populations, are suspected of contributing to the evolution of malignant disease.[7] Should workers in these groups be informed of these changes before an association is conclusively established? On the one hand, if the guiding purpose of the bill is to satisfy the workers' right to know, one would err on the side of informing them, even in the absence of meaningful counseling or prognosis. On the other hand, if the predominant goal is disease prevention, we may refrain from informing workers of subclinical changes.

A second difficulty concerns establishing which exposures trigger notification. The bill requires that employees be informed that they are at risk because of a "hazardous occupational exposure."[1] It defines the latter as including "any harmful chemical, physical, or biological agent found in the workplace,"[1] and S.79 adds the phrase "generated or integral to the work process and found in the workplace."[2] Such language is reminiscent of workers' compensation statutes, most of which define compensable occupational injuries and diseases as those "arising out of and in the course of . . . employment."[8] As we have indicated elsewhere, such language may logically be extended to cover many nontraditional occupational hazards.[9] For example, workplace injury due to assault by a fellow employee has been found to be compensable if the nature of the work environment, its stresses and pressures, increased its likelihood.[9] Logical extension of this approach could include other hazards created by coworkers but not, strictly speaking, part of the employment task. Passive smoking in the workplace would provide one example. It has been estimated that as many as 3,200 nonsmokers may die of lung cancer each year as a result of workplace exposure to secondary cigarette smoke, making tobacco smoke one of the most dangerous and common hazardous substances to which workers are exposed.[10] It might be argued, in the interest of maximizing free choice by workers (not to mention disease prevention), that relevant employees must be notified of this risk under H.R.162. This example points out the wider role that the High Risk Occupational Disease Notification and Prevention Act could play in promoting disease prevention through the workplace setting.

Another difficult area concerns the ability of the system to deal with damage from paraoccupational exposures, injury or disease occurring in family members who might be considered in "privity of employment" with their exposed relatives who bring the hazard home with them or pass it on through reproduction.[9] For example, mesothelioma in the spouse who does the laundry for the asbestos worker and cancer in the child whose father is exposed to hydrocarbons are not strictly considered occupational diseases. Nevertheless, these individuals in their status as exposed and injured persons more closely resemble the employee than the general populace. We have elsewhere argued that this resemblance should perhaps entitle them to some types of compensation.[9] In the present context, H.R.162 clearly restricts notification to "individual employees" ("any individual employed by an employer, or any individual formerly employed by an employer").[1] However, two theories would require that the individual employee be informed of transmitted risk even if she is not herself at risk. First, the occurrence of disease in family members could produce increased psychologic burden and stress as a secondary disease in the employee from knowing that she was the agent of disease transmission. Second, when risk is transmitted reproductively from parent to child, the parent-employee should be notified on the theory that the condition in the parent is a chronic health effect, where health is defined as optimal functioning. This approach would foster not only increased prevention but also increased worker autonomy.

It is clear that H.R.162 represents a dramatic break with past efforts in the area of occupational health. Rather than attempting to eradicate disease through primary prevention, it places the onus on exposed workers to act to protect themselves. In so doing, it creates a more significant and responsible role for employees than that recognized by prior legislation. These moves toward secondary prevention and worker autonomy constitute major changes in the way the federal government approaches workplace health, moves that require thorough thought and analysis.

REFERENCES

1. H.R.162, 100th Congress, 1st Sess. (Jan. 6, 1987).
2. S.79, 100th Congress, 1st Sess. (Jan. 6, 1987).
3. Occupational Safety and Health Act, 29 U.S.C. § 651 (1976).
4. LONG, J. 1987. House passes worker notification bill in face of strong opposition. Chemical & Engineering News **65**: 19–20.
5. Freedom of Information Act, 5 U.S.C. § 552 (1982).
6. Toxic Substances Control Act, 15 U.S.C. §§ 2601–2629 (1982).
7. BRANDT-RAUF, P. W. 1988. New markers for monitoring occupational cancer. J. Occup. Med., **30**: 399–404.
8. LOCKE, L. 1985. Adapting workers' compensation to the special problems of occupational disease. Harv. Env. L. Rev. **9**: 249–282.
9. BRANDT-RAUF, S. I. & P. W. BRANDT-RAUF. 1987. Workers' compensation and occupational cancer. Sem. Occup. Med. **2**: 321–323.
10. APHA petitions OSHA to ban smoking in the workplace. 1987. The Nation's Health, July : 1.

The Worker's Place in Enforcing OSHA

ANTHONY MAZZOCCHI[a]

The Labor Institute
853 Broadway
New York, New York 10003

Sixteen years ago OSHA became reality. Seventeen years ago, on the behalf of my union, I filed complaint number one to OSHA concerning mercury exposure at Allied Chemical in Moundsville, West Virginia.

Many people were involved in the movement to develop the Occupational Safety and Health Act, and those of us who were involved in that effort had a fairly clear-cut understanding of the Act's intent. That the workplace should be free of hazards was the definitive congressional intent and it was the purpose of the Act to develop regulations and methods to achieve this goal.

Most of us will agree, however, that we have not achieved a hazard-free work environment during these past 17 years. A whole new generation of activists have grown up in that time who have become public health advocates. Something was wrong, and something had to be done about it. Those of us in the trade union movement did not possess the kinds of scientific skills that were necessary for advocacy.

Notification is an idea whose time has come. Workers must be told what might affect them. In the last 17 years, and especially in the last five years, I have seen a number of persons I worked with die of occupationally induced disease, an appreciable number of them from my own local union. And none of these persons panicked when he became aware that he was diseased beyond remedy. Their admonition to those of us who were well was to do something about what had afflicted them.

In hearing Dr. Millar I was a little disturbed by his elevating the right to know to almost a religious principle. I thought we were past discussing that. The law gives us the right to know. Under the National Labor Relations Act, our union filed a case against Minnesota Mining and Colgate-Palmolive. The law says a trade union has a right to know everything that is knowable in order to appropriately represent the persons they are certified to bargain for. That principle has been established. The question is how to implement what we have already agreed on—the concept of worker notification, which only has meaning if people are empowered to do something about what they know. So the question becomes one of power, and we have not made many advances recently because of our inability to "catalyze" people into action with respect to their health.

The question of smoking and passive smoking was mentioned earlier. I would submit that before you can even raise the issue of smoking, you have to deal with another occupational hazard that has not been discussed, namely, the requirement that a worker work continuously 35–36 hours at very dangerous jobs. It has become quite usual now for workers to work 17, 18, 19, even 20 hours straight. For the last seven years, one group at Minnesota Mining in New Jersey has worked a 70-hour work week and has worked about 7 days a week. I would not

---

[a] Present address: Oil, Chemical & Atomic Workers International Union, AFL-CIO, P.O. Box 2812, Denver, Colorado 80201.

want to work next to a person who did not have some method to relieve the tensions you develop working at an exhausting, boring, awful job for 12 to 13 hours straight or even for 24 hours straight, under very difficult conditions. While docking an 88,000-ton tanker or working for 20 hours unloading volatile cargo in the rain, you are not going to smoke, but the minute you are able to take a break, you are going to smoke. So the issue of that lifestyle hazard ought to be understood in a context of lengthy overtime and subcontracted work. Many advocates have come into the workplace who know nothing about those workers who are given responsibilities for extremely dangerous work, but who are not part of a bargaining unit or a skilled workforce.

I would suggest that the whole question of worker notification be placed within the larger context of how we think about what goes on in a workplace, and who has the ability to effect change. How we think about this question in the 1990s must evolve from the promise of the Act in 1970. It will soon be 20 years since Congress held out the promise of a workplace free from all hazard. What have we done over this generation? The 1990s must be a period where we attempt to empower those who best know how to effect change in the workplace.

Ever since the Industrial Revolution we have vested the power to regulate with the producer. But I believe that you cannot solve occupational health and safety problems while those who produce are given the responsibility to regulate themselves. That system does not work, and we ought to examine a new option. We ought to separate our responsibilities. Those who have production responsibilities ought to produce, and those workers who are the potential victims ought to regulate. Federal agencies ought to promulgate standards, and the workers ought to be trained. The cost of doing business should incorporate the cost of training, the outside consultants, and the public health community who are called in to assist us. It should be the worker who carries out the mandate of the law, the right to inspect, the right to cite, the right to bring about change based on what is known, the right to be notified, and the right to know. When we think about the subject in terms of empowerment, we will truly make a difference.

Notification of Workers at High Risk

Design and Implementation of a Program to Address Their Needs

DAVID K. PARKINSON

Department of Community and Preventive Medicine
SUNY at Stony Brook
Stony Brook, New York 11794-8036

Although the passage of the High-Risk Notification Bill is not finalized, this report assumes that the major provisions of the bill as passed in the House will be unaltered by the Senate. Although some provisions of the bill, such as the identification of clinical facilities to evaluate workers, need clarification, I believe that if implemented with sensitivity, it can be a major force in the prevention of occupational disease.

I intend to concentrate on practical issues that must be addressed if workers are to be given the facts on which they can make informed decisions. If this bill is enacted, the following issues have to be addressed:

1. Who will get the letter?
2. What will the letter say?
3. What role will unions have in determining the content of the letter sent to their members. Will union health and safety officers have access to the names of union members receiving the letter?
4. What should workers do when they get the letter?
5. What medical resources are available to provide workers with high quality medical examinations?
6. Who is responsible for paying medical fees?
7. How can a prevention component be integrated, because occupational medicine must be concerned with both primary and secondary intervention?
8. How can we evaluate whether the program has been "successful" or effective?

1. WHO GETS THE LETTER?

A. However high risk is defined, clearly a list of workers who fit the definition will have to be assembled. It is unclear from what sources these data will come, and how far back in time searches will be made for names to add to the roles of exposed workers.

B. Validation of available addresses from companies with exposed workers will have to be a part of this exercise. The list will presumably involve current, past, and retired workers. In my experience, attempting to obtain addresses of *current* workers revealed a large error rate. Identification of the addresses of past workers and retired workers will have an even larger error rate.

C. Will these lists be matched with death registries? It would be unfortunate if the same letter were sent to survivors and the spouses of those already dead. However, it is almost impossible for the ascertainment of death status to be 100% correct. This implies that the letter must be written with appropriate sensitivity.

D. How will the lists be ordered, that is, who will receive the letter during the first year of the program, who during the second, and so on? What are the consequences if NIOSH starts with their own records as the first pass in sending letters?

2. WHAT WILL THE LETTER SAY?

A. Will this letter provide technical information on the nature of the exposure and potential health consequences? Preparing such a letter using language that is understandable and not frightening to the recipient is an extremely difficult task.

B. How individualized will these letters be? It would seem medically unethical not to send out individualized letters. How specific will the letter be about the individual worker's length of exposure and risk associated with that length of exposure, or will, for example, the same letter be sent to a worker exposed to asbestos for 1 year as someone exposed for 30 years?

C. Similarly, will the letter explain that not all workers with the same exposure have the same risk of disease? For example, with asbestos exposure, smokers have a higher risk than do nonsmokers. Will the letter reassure nonsmokers about this issue or, conversely, stress the urgency of seeing a physician in the letter to a worker exposed to both asbestos and heavy smoking for 30 years?

D. Will the letter contain any information on preventive measures that might be taken? For example, a letter to a worker with high-lead exposure could suggest that removal from exposure or transfer to a low-head area is the option.

It is in the foregoing areas that I see a role for the health and safety departments of those unions, such as the United Steel Workers of America, who for many years have made a major commitment to their members in the area of health and safety. For many years the USWA has been involved in legislation designed to give their members access to information about their workplace environment. In addition, education programs have been developed for members in particularly hazardous operations such as coke ovens, lead smelters, and arsenic smelters. Although concerns in regard to confidentiality might prevent the union from having access to individual names, presumably there would be no problem with the union's knowing which plants were to be involved in the notification process.

E. What recommendations will be made in seeking medical care? My understanding of the bill is that the workers will be recommended to go to one of the designated centers of expertise. As most of you know, many of the Education Resource Centers do not have a clinical component to date. However, there are several excellent occupational medicine programs throughout the United States that could provide the highest quality care and consultation. If more flexibility is not built into the designation of evaluation centers, many competent occupational physicians who have already developed experience in handling occupational health issues would be excluded from an opportunity to help in these particularly emotive evaluations.

However, it is inevitable that the majority of workers will first seek advice from their primary care or family physician. Thus, the letter should include educational material for the person's physician, and serious consideration should be given to communicating with and arranging meetings of local medical societies in all areas to which the letters are sent. Thus, education programs should be presented for general practitioners who will probably be the first physicians consulted by a large proportion of notified workers.

There is another issue in this regard. Although the workers who receive letters are at high risk of contracting the specific disease, many of them will be older and possibly retired and will present with disease that requires attention, but that is not related to the exposure of concern. The evaluation must be comprehensive and would best be carried out in a center in which there is a close liaison between occupational medicine and general medicine clinics, so that efficient and high quality care is readily available for nonoccupationally related disease. Good liaison with the worker's family practitioner is essential; otherwise, it is almost inevitable that miscommunication and misunderstanding will occur.

Finally, I am concerned with the legal aspects of this notification program. Those of us who are involved in handling workers' compensation and toxic torts recognize that this bill potentially provides a bonanza for the legal profession. Unfortunately, too many incompetent lawyers are already involved in such suits, with a lack of preparation being common. Many lawyers take on too many cases and do not bother to evaluate the merits of individual suits. In the last year I have been involved in cases in which the lawyer, instead of dropping weak or nonexistent cases, has attempted to sell them to other unsuspecting colleagues. The opportunities from such practices with this bill are legion. I believe that it would be possible to establish a committee with representation from the legal profession, the medical profession, and the affected worker population that would develop a code of practice and criteria that should be used for legal cases developing from the notification process. The outcome of such a committee should be a model for an agreement between a lawyer and his client that can only be of benefit to the worker in these days of high contingency fees. I am sure my colleague, Professor Rothstein, will have more to say on this issue.

SUMMARY

I believe the high-risk bill is an opportunity to protect the health and well-being of the millions of workers who have been exposed to a myriad of chemicals that we know have the potential for disease. The practical details of implementing such a bill call for a high degree of sensitivity during the implementation of the program to the issues I have outlined; otherwise, its potential for good will possibly be swamped by frustration, miscommunication, and misunderstanding, and this will result in the provision of less than high-quality care for a group of people who deserve the best care and consultation available.

Predicting the Consequences of the High-Risk Occupational Disease Notification and Prevention Act

MARK A. ROTHSTEIN

Health Law Institute
University of Houston
Houston, Texas 77004

There are three areas in which the High-Risk Occupational Disease Notification and Prevention Act would be likely to affect both health and law. It is difficult to predict with certainty what the consequences of any new law will be. It is less difficult, but equally important, to identify the issues or questions that the new legislation is likely to raise.

The first issue is whether the High-Risk Notification Act will increase prevention of occupational disease. The second is whether the law will facilitate treatment of occupational disease. The third is whether the law will increase compensation for occupational disease.

Starting with the first issue, "prevention" is something that has been addressed to a great extent in the previous presentations. An issue that has not been discussed adequately, however, is whether the law, if enacted, would serve to increase, decrease, or perhaps have no effect on whether employers would be more or less encouraged to conduct epidemiologic studies.

Considerable evidence exists that some employers have, in the past, made a deliberate decision not to undertake such studies. There is currently no legal requirement that employers make any effort to correlate exposure data with mortality or morbidity data that they have. In fact, certain laws may even act to discourage employers from doing so. Many employers fear that if they discover new correlations, the regulators and personal injury lawyers will move in; and for a variety of reasons some employers believe that they may be financially worse off as a result of performing the studies. Would the new law further discourage employer studies or, perhaps under some other possible scenarios, encourage employers to do this?

A second question under the broad topic of prevention is: Will the monitoring of workers serve to prevent occupational disease? Although this specific question has been addressed already, a related question is whether increased monitoring of workers once they are hired will encourage employers to engage in more preemployment screening. Seemingly, every new development in occupational health surveillance and a variety of employment laws have encouraged employers to engage in more extensive preemployment screening. For example, section 510 of the Employee Retirement Income Security Act (ERISA), which prohibits employers from firing employees to deprive them of their health insurance and other benefits, encourages preemployment screening, because if sick workers cannot be fired, employers will want to avoid hiring people considered likely to become sick. Workers' compensation laws, where employers take workers "as is," also encourage preemployment screening. Will the High-Risk Notification Act lead to further screening because employers will want to avoid hiring people who later may be considered "at risk"?

Section 7(b) of the proposed law prohibits discrimination against an employee or applicant because the employee or applicant is considered to be within the "population at risk," *except* if the individual is being considered for a position with exposure to the same substance that generated the initial notification letter. This could possibly change state and federal handicap discrimination laws in the following way. Suppose an employee who was exposed to asbestos at employer number one's workplace now seeks a job with employer number two. If employer number two were to deny employment to an asymptomatic, otherwise qualified individual because of fear that the individual's prior asbestos exposure could result in illness during the term that the individual is working for employer number two, this may be considered discrimination on the basis of handicap in violation of state or federal law. Section 7(b) of the High-Risk Notification Act, however, would permit the second employer to refuse to hire the individual if the individual had received prior notice that he or she was at risk.

Finally, under prevention, will exposure levels be reduced? It is hard to say. Employees who know of risks in general or of particular risks arguably would be encouraged to engage in more aggressive collective bargaining to reduce levels even below those required by OSHA regulations. Perhaps employers knowing of scientifically valid data would be more likely to reduce levels and prevent further exposures. Perhaps employees would be more likely to wear personal protective equipment and take other measures for their own protection when they had been reluctant to do so in the past. Conversely, the law does not contain any direct regulatory provisions.

The second broad class of issues centers around whether the High-Risk Notification Act will facilitate the treatment of occupational disease. Certainly, it will increase the demand for trained occupational physicians as well as for occupational health training of all physicians. This raises the issue of how physicians, nurses, and other occupational health practitioners are trained. Medical school is merely the starting point. The High-Risk Notification Act would necessitate new programs of continuing medical education in occupational medicine. Many cases of occupational disease are currently not diagnosed as being occupationally related. The treatment of these diseases is likely to be helped if the associations between workplace exposures and the disease state were more clearly understood by the people who are examining and treating the current and former workers.

The third area of issues relates to whether the High-Risk Notification Act will have an effect on compensation for occupational disease. In the legislative history of the proposed Act, the statute is stated to be "liability neutral." For example, section 8(b) of the proposed law expressly provides that risk findings made by the Risk Assessment Board may not be introduced into evidence in any private lawsuit. Similarly, the notification form itself would not be admissible in any lawsuit.

Even if the law is intended to be liability neutral, it is certainly not litigation neutral. The question is not whether it will cause an increase in litigation. The questions are: (1) How much of an increase in litigation will it cause? (2) Will the increase be good or bad? and (3) What, if anything, should be done about it? It is likely that there are many exposed or formerly exposed workers who are currently suffering from an occupational illness who do not know the occupational nature of their illness and will only learn of this on receipt of a notification letter. In addition, some workers and former workers who currently have a nonoccupational illness, as soon as they get a notification letter, will be convinced that their illness is occupationally related. In either instance, these individuals are likely to get a lawyer to represent them and file a workers' compensation claim on their behalf or to sue under one of the numerous exceptions that are continually being carved out of the exclusivity principle of workers' compensation. These legal actions would include products liability lawsuits, actions for intentional torts, fraudulent concealment, dual capacity medical malpractice, and other theories.

Even if the plaintiffs were to lose some of the lawsuits, because it costs a lot of money to defend a toxic tort case and because there is always the possibility of a substantial recovery, even doubtful cases will have some settlement value. This reality of litigation encourages additional lawsuits.

Is occupational disease litigation a good or a bad thing? Certainly, workers' compensation benefits for occupational illness are too low either to provide adequate compensation or to encourage reductions in exposure levels. Thus, to the extent that companies may be faced with higher payments to workers, private lawsuits may serve as incentives for employers to clean up workplaces. They also may be viewed as a way of reallocating the costs of occupational disease. At the present time, the economic consequences of occupational illness are widely externalized from the employers in whose employment the occupational disease was contracted to the workers themselves, to private health insurers, to Medicare, to general welfare, and to other third parties. Arguably, personal injury litigation results in a redistribution of costs and a reallocation of responsibility back to the source of exposure.

Regardless of whether private lawsuits have these salutary effects, the system is woefully inefficient. It resembles a lottery in both fairness and payout. Most deserving claimants receive nothing; the "transaction costs" are so high that lawyers and expert witnesses receive most of the money paid out by the defendants, with relatively few claimants receiving all of the remaining money. It would be irresponsible to embrace and expand a system that encourages more employees to sue when plaintiff and defense lawyers take nearly two thirds of every dollar paid in compensation. It is also an act of self-delusion to believe that facilitating the recoveries of a relatively few workers eliminates the need for more fundamental reforms in overhauling the compensation system.

In conclusion, the proposed High-Risk Occupational Disease Notification and Prevention Act raises important questions about the way we attempt to prevent, treat, and compensate for occupational disease. The proposed law may be viewed as a beneficial, humane, and essential law; it may be viewed as a potentially complicating factor in a flawed compensation system; or it may be viewed as both.

Round Table 4: Discussion

NICHOLAS ASHFORD (*Center for Policy Alternatives, M.I.T., Cambridge, Mass.*): Mr. Rothstein, I am disappointed to hear your remarks about the adverse value of litigation. I think that tort litigation is, in fact, a bad idea, but an idea whose time has come. Indeed, it is the moving policy instrument in the area of hazardous waste clean-up, preventing the dumping of hazardous waste and forcing development of on-site technology for treating waste.

I have also looked extensively at the so-called insurance liability crisis and at the kind of behavior the tort law visits upon technological firms. I take issue with your observation that about 65% of every dollar goes to support litigation. Dr. Bill Johnson of Syracuse, who worked with Dr. Selikoff to look at asbestos insulation workers and at their recoveries under the tort system compared with their recoveries under the workers' compensation system, found that after subtracting the lawyers' fees and administrative costs, the workers still fare better under the tort system than under workers' compensation. I therefore challenge those comments. I do not understand the basis for your conclusions that tort is without value.

MARK ROTHSTEIN (*University of Houston Law Center, Houston, Texas 77004*): First, I did not say that workers do better under the compensation system than they do in private litigation, for it is not true. Nor have I said that the compensation system is fair, adequate, efficient, equitable, or to be desired. What I *have* said is that our current tort system, in which the worker gets so little out of every dollar that is paid, is simply not the most efficient way to compensate workers for a variety of illnesses. I am not just talking about occupational illnesses, but about medical malpractice and other sorts of problems in which the only people who seem to benefit are the lawyers and the witnesses. Finally, from a broad policy perspective, I recognize that private lawsuits have been extremely valuable in bringing about some forms of change. But consider a situation where two individuals develop cancer. One person is informed that he has cancer because of exposure in the workplace, while the other, who has the identical form of cancer and the same prognosis, is informed that his cancer is not work-related. Why should one person get nothing while the other receives a lot of money? Our system is crazy in this regard—it's like a lottery that just isn't working anymore.

ASHFORD: But you are not offering a system that is any better. We do not have a national health care system in the United States like that in Germany, where people do not spend time arguing about the source of the disease. In this context, giving fuel to the so-called tort-reform movement, as your remarks do, defeats the social purpose. There has been a massive campaign to persuade people that in medical malpractice, product liability, and worker litigation, the tort system is an inefficient way to compensate people, and so it should be eliminated. But the problem is that we do not have any other form of deterrent, particularly in the current era of "no enforcement." I think that we should stop blaming the lawyers; I am particularly disturbed about the notion of their being "ambulance chasers." It does not help our cause to attack the lawyers who file these suits.

ANTHONY MAZZOCCHI (*Institute for Labor Studies, New York, N.Y.*): The reality and the experience is that in Tyler, Texas, where this whole series of lawsuits began, the workers were not being compensated. They were dying, and lawsuits were the only remedy available to those workers. Through the discovery procedure in the course of these lawsuits, we discovered what was being kept from us. We had to use that particular device in order to advance the issue. It was the indignation that grew out of those lawsuits, and out of the evidence that we got from discovery—showing what the industry knew and when they knew it—that advanced the health and safety of people at risk to asbestos. Not a single law has helped us; a number of us worked to get a standard for asbestos, but it has never been implemented. In most workplaces, regulation has not been introduced. Lawsuits are the worst of the best and the best of the worst we have available. Until we have a system that eliminates the cause of disease, we will not eliminate the litigation. This is the reality of the way things work. Until you have something to replace lawsuits, you deal with fantasy.

DAVID PARKINSON (*SUNY at Stony Brook, Stony Brook, L.I., N.Y.*): The comments about the lawyers are very interesting. My experience is that lawyers have had very little impact upon getting workplaces cleaned up. I would like to know where they *have* had a major impact. As far as I can see, the attitude in many companies is to wait until suits are filed, and to settle them then. I do not see the commitment to clean up workplaces coming from lawsuits.

MAZZOCCHI: Look at what has happened in schools. We are removing asbestos now, simply because of lawsuits. Look at the removal of asbestos in workplaces and the fact that companies are not introducing asbestos into the workplaces. Those changes grew out of lawsuits. They have saved millions of lives.

PARKINSON: But in this bill—the High-Risk Worker Notification Bill—we are talking about issues where the chemical exposure has been identified. Everybody is agreed that the exposure is a hazard, and we are going to deal with that hazard by notifying workers. The lawsuits will come after that event has occurred. Surely we should be concerned about cleaning up workplaces, and using our efforts there, when we have already identified the hazard. I do not see how lawsuits in this situation are going to be effective in cleaning up workplaces.

KNUT RINGEN (*Workplace Health Fund, Washington, D.C.*): It is important to note that effectively designed demonstration research programs have a very strong impact in terms of changing things. What we are talking about here is *notification,* giving workers information that will provide them with a stronger weapon. There are many ways in which we can go about stimulating change.

ELIZABETH AVERILL (*Workplace Health Fund, Washington, D.C.*): In regard to Dr. Brandt-Rauf's statement about early mutagenic bioassays and the scientific ambiguity around them and their impact on worker notification, I would point out that, in fact, the scientific community can effectively communicate to workers their ambivalence about the information. Furthermore, workers have the right to know what assays will be done. It is really important to notify workers of these assays and of their potential implications.

PAUL BRANDT-RAUF (*Columbia University, New York, N.Y.*): Yes, but it is important to realize that the decision as to what you tell workers about these tests is not easy. You cannot be glib about it; ambivalence and uncertainty are difficult to communicate. Workers want to know the bottom line. You can tell them that the test is experimental and that we really do not know what we are doing in this study, but they will ask: Are we going to die? What are we going to die of?

AVERILL: We might disagree about how effectively workers can be informed about risk assessment and similar issues. But I stand by my point that with proper care and technique, uncertainty can successfully be communicated.

I have another point. I am very supportive of high-risk notification, but wary of the discrimination that may be inherent in the Bill. Although the right to know has a built-in antidiscrimination provision, I know of people who have been fired after exercising their right to know. Dr. Ringen alluded to the HIV-positive situation and the rampant insurance discrimination that exists against people found to be HIV-positive. This is an area that warrants a lot of consideration in terms of assuring that this Bill does not put people in jeopardy.

ROTHSTEIN: Let me note in reply that a tremendous number of employment practices are health-insurance-driven. Regardless of the liability issue or the compensation issue, many self-insured employers do not want people in their firms who may be rather severe insurance risks. That situation raises the specter of discrimination.

BARBARA BERNY (*Washington, D.C.*): I was concerned about the comments that OSHA was paternalistic and that somehow worker-notification was going to give workers a measure of free choice. The suggestion that primary prevention and collective protection (that is, regulation) are paternalistic, whereas individual notification and the right of free choice are somehow on a higher plane and more democratic, is a very dangerous notion. Individually, we cannot clean up the air, the water, the food, or the workplace. To suggest that collective remedies are paternalistic is a very dangerous position.

BRANDT-RAUF: I did not mean to suggest that. But in practice, the OSHAct has fostered debate between experts. Then once they have decided and the rules have been promulgated, there is relatively little impact that can be made by individual workers. If you had to put the Occupational Safety and Health Act and the High-Risk Notification Bill on a spectrum, the OSHAct would fall more on the paternalistic side and the other would fall more on the free-choice side. That is all I am suggesting. As I tried to indicate, if you push the free-choice argument, you may get some useful benefits out of it in terms of what you can do in the workplace.

PHILIP LANDRIGAN (*Mt. Sinai School of Medicine, New York, N.Y.*): This has been a fascinating session. We have moved from the philosophical consideration of the roots of the right-to-know, and from the fundamentals of Jeffersonian democracy and the Helsinki Declaration to consideration of the practical consequences of the right to know and of the gains that we hope it will produce in terms of disease prevention. I have learned a great deal; I hope you have as well.

Depoliticizing Occupational Health
Can It Be Done? Should It Be Done?

ANDREW MAGUIRE[a]

*North American Securities Administrators Association, Inc.
555 New Jersey Ave N.W.
Washington, D.C. 20001*

In 1987 two major books were issued by recent Secretaries of Labor. *Workforce 2000: Work and Workers for the 21st Century*[1] is an Administration study released by Bill Brock that seeks to identify the key issues in meeting global competitive challenges. *Unheard Voices: Labor and Economic Policy in a Competitive World*,[2] authored by Ray Marshall, argues that America's competitive survival depends on workers' playing a more important role in decisions from the shop floor to international economic policies. Marshall's 306-page book contains one passing reference to occupational safety and health in the context of a discussion of the role of labor unions. Brock's volume outlines six policy challenges for workers in the workforce for the next century, but it does not mention occupational safety and health.

Meanwhile, according to the Industrial Union Department of the AFL-CIO, an estimated 100,000 workers die and a third of a million more are disabled each year from occupational diseases caused by hazardous exposures. We do not need to accept any particular set of numbers in the numbers sweepstakes—even if yours are a fifth of those, or some other number—to recognize and agree that the promise of the 1970 Occupational Safety and Health Act "to assure so far as possible that every working man and woman in the nation has safe and healthful working conditions," and its goal that "no employee should suffer material impairment of health or functional capacity," are and will continue to fall far short of what was intended unless major changes occur.

Recent analysis of our official national efforts through OSHA and NIOSH to control hazards are contained in reports done by the Department of Labor itself, by the General Accounting Office, by the Administrative Conference of the United States, and by the Office of Technology Assessment. The Department of Labor sees "a pattern of systemic weaknesses" in OSHA management, regulation-setting, and enforcement. The GAO highlights the lack of a credible rule-making process. I am sure you are familiar with these numbers: an average of three years or more for making a rule up to about 1981, and then after that even longer—up to 5 or 7 years.

Some 160 NIOSH criteria documents have produced something like half a dozen standards. And when these are produced they are almost always less stringent than what had been proposed. If you look at the recent OTA study on carcinogens, again you find something like 71 NIOSH recommendations or criteria documents, but only 21 actions. Among the 50 awaiting action at the time that the OTA report was written in 1987, only one was the subject of a final rulemaking proceeding and there were no proposals whatsoever on 46 of the other 49.

---

[a] Present address: The Washington Financial Group, 1400 Eye Street, N.W., Suite 1155, Washington, D.C. 20005.

The American Conference of Governmental Industrial Hygienists recommends exposure limits for 615 or more items and these are updated yearly. But OSHA retains essentially the 1960 ACGIH-recommended exposure limits on only 400 or so substances and it has issued standards of its own in only a handful of cases in the 17 years since its founding. Eula Bingham rehearsed the list yesterday; we are all familiar with it.

There was an innovative attempt to develop generic standards, including the cancer policy in the late 1970s. Some of us worked hard trying to promote a more systematic and rational approach through generic standards, rather than starting the entire evaluative process from scratch in every case—with the duplication of already available information, additional costs, and harmful delays that result. But even after the adoption of the generic cancer policy, no carcinogens to the best of my knowledge have ever been regulated under it. The Administrative Conference of the United States says OSHA faces "total paralysis" unless it regains control of rule making, which is now buffeted about by the demands of petitioners, standard-setters in the private sector, the OMB, the White House, Congress and the courts. In the words of the Office of Technology Assessment, "OSHA's regulatory agenda has increasingly been set by outsiders through petitions, court orders, referrals and congressional directives." In its study, OTA suggested 30 options for improvement, but few if any have been acted on in any serious way.

The problem, of course, goes well beyond OSHA, as we know. OTA's multiagency study on identifying and regulating carcinogens makes the situation clear. You will forgive me if I refer to the Annual Report on Carcinogens, which has been prepared episodically since 1978 as a result of an amendment I succeeded in writing into law. Some 144 chemicals appearing in the annual report tested positive in the National Toxicology Program or in other tests so that they can be identified as human carcinogens or as reasonably anticipated to be carcinogens. According to the OTA report, of those 144, no agency—and we are talking here about FDA, CPSC, and EPA as well as OSHA—has regulated more than a third of those having positive test results. Typically, only 30 to 50 of the 144 or so substances have received regulatory attention. And EPA's Toxic Substances Control Act activities and OSHA share the worst record of the lot.

But you are familiar with this litany. Now the question is where do we go? Eula Bingham has referred here to two realities. First there is no substitute for control measures: that is to say, regulation and enforcement is what we must be about. The second major reality to which Eula Bingham referred was that the movement against regulation is a well-organized, well-funded, ideologically motivated political movement.

I might quote NIOSH's J. Donald Millar when he said somewhat plaintively, "I wish OSHA would take our recommendations and just put them into place. But the real world doesn't operate that way." If the answer is that we *should* depoliticize occupational health, the fact is that it would be very difficult to do so. In an ideal world in which the findings of science were accorded the utmost respect and were not subject to interpretation or dispute, one could depoliticize. In an ideal world in which politicians and administrators would act immediately on the best and the most up-to-date scientific findings, rolling over any special-interest-motivated opposition, it would be possible to depoliticize. Then workers would, in fact, be better protected, more disease would be prevented, and workplaces would be closer to the safe healthy places envisaged by the 1970 Act. Then, and only then, it would be safe to depoliticize occupational health.

Since we do not live in such a world, we cannot depoliticize occupational safety and health, even if we should. Furthermore, we should not depoliticize it even if we could, because to do so would mean, in effect, that we were giving up. Irving Selikoff is one of the articulate people on this subject. In the absence of a level playing field, if you are not out there and in the game to win you are just kidding yourself and you are conceding to the opposition.

Where are we then in the real political world and what should we be doing? The Marshall and Brock books tell us, by what they don't say, where we have been and where, unfortunately, we still are: occupational safety and health is a side issue for many people, including key decision makers, authors of important books on the workplace, experts on the future of the economy, and even for those who recently have led the Department of Labor.

Then, of course, there has been the overall deregulatory push of the 1980s. Let me invoke some images of deregulation to clarify still further where we are on the political and policy scales:

Image number one: Interior Secretary Hodel, in response to the threat to the ozone layer, calls for massive voluntary administrations of suntan lotion, dark glasses and hats. This illustrates the preposterous nature of adopting a protective device strategy when control strategies are available.

Image number two: The Council of Economic Advisors, testifying before a Senate committee just before the October 19th stock market crash, says that hostile takeovers and the activities of high-rolling Wall Street manipulators, though nonproductive in any traditional economic sense, and while generating enormous profits for a few at the expense of the many, are nevertheless great for capitalism and great for America. So, buyer beware if you want to participate in the market!

Image number three: The OMB kills occupational safety and health standards affecting the health, and indeed the lives, of countless numbers of workers—in order to do what? To reduce paperwork. Surely this is the ultimate uncivilized and barbaric extension of a bureaucracy run amok!

But the tone is changing. Secretary Hodel's preposterous proposal was treated with the ridicule it richly deserved and EPA and the State Department went ahead to negotiate the first truly preventive international protocol regarding a worldwide threat to health and the environment. After a few months at the Securities and Exchange Commission, and after the Brady Commission recommended strong new regulation to avert in the future what was almost a total collapse of the market last October, Chairman David Ruder now is strenuously projecting the image of someone who is concerned about the small investor and describes himself proudly this week in the *New York Times* as a regulator. Can you imagine that? Someone heading an agency in this administration proudly describing himself as a regulator and one who apparently is prepared to regulate!

As for OSHA, it finishes the year with a small burst of activity: rules on formaldehyde and on field sanitation—after more than a decade of struggle, let us recall, on the field sanitation issue. I remember working on that when I was in the Congress in the 1970s and also on employee health records and employee access to hazards information. Finally, after years of effort it appears that workers will be notified of the existence of hazards and to some extent the nature and degree of their risk. Many of us worked on this in the 1970s, but it took even the Carter Administration far too long to act.

For years there has been virtually no activity by Congress on OSHA. Until 1987, the last oversight hearings were held in 1981. Over these years Congress has been mainly engaged in the business of granting all sorts of exemptions under OSHA. It has been a race to exempt, to get political credit at home with local pressure groups. But now, with some more aggressive and far-sighted leadership on key committees, an effort is being made not only to strengthen and extend the important notification divisions, but also to thoroughly review OSHA's performance and mandate and to legislate improvements. Congress now appears ready to act.

You know what the substantive agenda should be. I do not have to add to that. You know the litany of failures and shortcomings and qualified, very qualified, successes. But let me propose here some modest strategies and tactics.

First, get as much scientific work done as you possibly can. There is nothing in the end that is more important. Whatever passage of time has to be involved to get political "nonleadership" to follow with appropriate policies what science has clarified, action still depends upon facts: marshalling and presenting them impressively.

Second, press the decision makers to respect and act on scientific data or be subjected to tough questioning as to why they are not doing that. There needs to be consciousness in the Congress and outside that scientific findings ought to be taken very seriously—more seriously than some other considerations that are often more prominently on a Congressman's mind.

Third, get thoughtful members of Congress to act not only on OSHA's mandate and operations, but also on getting the OMB under control. Just as I was leaving the Congress in 1980, I helped to launch a series of hearings that the Oversight and Investigations Subcommittee of the House Energy and Commerce Committee began at that time to examine the peremptory role the OMB assumes: even secretaries of cabinet departments were told what they could or couldn't do; these presidential appointees could not even set their own priorities within a given budget allocation. As if this were not enough, the OMB is now deeply involved in the regulation business. Congress has begun to look into this, but something must be done because the present situation, which results from the OMB's inappropriate role, is totally intolerable. And change will have to come from Congress.

Fourth, push consensus-building. You will notice that this precept has a certain overtone of depoliticizing, and I admit that this kind of effort can play a very useful role. Let's have advisory committees, as Eula Bingham suggests, to hammer things out in quasi-official capacities. Let's make sure there are occupational and environmental health experts in the National Cancer Institute and on other advisory boards. Let's make sure that outside professional groups put together task forces and get experts to participate in panels at conferences like this. And wherever possible, let's have tripartite labor, business, and public participation along with scientists to create the broadest base of support for what needs to be done.

There are forums and opportunities for depoliticizing issues and for building consensus. That happened with the cotton dust standard, and with pesticide negotiations over the last couple of years, although the whole effort finally flew apart in the political process. But let's keep clearly in mind that such efforts succeed only within a politicized environment. Only when the contending interests have to deal with each other and entertain the idea of compromise are compromises actually achieved. And then, of course, the factual material that the scientific community can introduce becomes a key determinant of what those compromises actually look like.

Fifth, intervene and encourage others to intervene. Encourage people to sue. When there is a regulatory administrative proceeding or when something is on the floor of the Congress, the people who are there day after day are people representing special interests, persons with a financial stake in the outcome. So if the people representing the public interest are not there, and if the scientific persons are not there, the outcome is skewed against us. Last year I testified at a hearing called by David Rall and the NIEHS to hear views on the Annual Report on Carcinogens. And who testified at that meeting? A stream of industry witnesses all day long talked about what was wrong with the annual cancer report, and what was wrong with having things listed this way as opposed to that way, or requiring only two positives when there should be four positives, and so on. And almost nobody was there from the public interest side.

Sixth, organize. Organize as scientists to get information into the hands of people that can use it if you decide that you cannot directly use it yourself. Get the information to public interest groups who are in a position to follow up. And may I suggest even calling on your Congressman? When was the last time one of you called on your Congressman? Take a group of people from the university working on an issue, or colleagues with special expertise and concern, and go in and talk about something that is important to the public. You have the right to do that and you have the special expertise and you ought to do it. Congressmen respond to those kinds of initiatives. Some few are going to look at the issue on its merits. A lot more are going to try to be interested if it works out okay in the public relations context. Then there are a lot of others—let's be honest about this—whose daily activity is to figure out how to position themselves with respect to the interests bearing down upon them. Their notion of a compromise is that which makes the fewest people unhappy. But you can be among the people that they will have to reckon into that calculation!

I don't know whether the New York Academy of Sciences can set up any kind of national policy committee that would track and work on some of these occupational health issues, but I would invite them to think about that kind of strategy.

Seventh, train and educate more and more people. There is no substitute for skills and expertise, widely distributed. I understand that there has been a tremendous fall-off in training in recent years. What a disaster! In the 1970s we pushed for more money for more training to prepare more qualified people. We have to get back on that track. Engineering schools and business schools and labor studies institutes and law schools have to understand that occupational safety and health issues are central issues to the workforce and to the economy of this country, now and in the future. And that understanding has to be reflected in the curriculum. Scientists can help make such changes happen.

Eighth, get into the public relations business. You have heard the saying that everything is sales. It's true; after you do the scientific work you have to sell your ideas to the public. As Eula Bingham said, you have to create an atmosphere that mobilizes pubic opinion so that public officials will be making decisions within that context and so that those decisions will result in control strategies rather than in rhetoric.

Maybe in the end we could achieve a political process in which issues could be depoliticized. It would be a Promised Land in which the perceptions of all the actors' self-interests had so shifted that unanimity would reign. The Manville Corporation has a letter supporting the Metzenbaum Bill now on the table. Whatever the strengths or weaknesses of the bill, whatever the reasons for Manville's support, however belatedly that support comes—never mind! There is something here that is important to note. Science has indeed accomplished something when we get to the point where the Manville Corporation and Senator Metzenbaum are sitting down to break bread together over his latest bill to strengthen OSHA.

As someone once said in commenting on the role of scientists: "Scientists have reduced the number of calamities we may blame on God." Let me close by expressing the hope that as scientists you can continue to work and to organize yourselves to reduce the number of calamities, period.

REFERENCES

1. U.S. DEPARTMENT OF LABOR. 1987. Workforce 2000: Work and Workers for the 21st Century. William B. Johnson, Project Director, and Arnold E. Packer, Co-Project Director. Hudson Institute. Indianapolis, IN.
2. MARSHALL, RAY. 1987. Unheard Voices: Labor and Economic Policy in a Competitive World. Basic Books. New York.

PART IV. WORKSITE INSPECTION AND DISEASE PREVENTION

The Insurrection of Vestigial Failures against OSHA[a]

SHELDON W. SAMUELS[b]

Industrial Union Department, AFL-CIO
Washington, D.C. 20006

SOCIAL TRANSACTION

Sixteen years ago, at a session of the American Society of Safety Engineers, I delivered a paper entitled "OSHA as a Social Transaction." Many in management, and some in government, especially the Southern Industrial Council, who characterized the OSHAct as a Marxist plot, attacked the paper because it viewed the passage of that law as a stage in broad social change in America. They did not accept the overwhelming mandate of the Congress that not only ratified a change in the workplace, but also broke ground for a new genre of environmental law that empowered the citizen as an environmental decision maker.

Anyone who has followed the proliferation of "right to know" legislation and rule making knows that the current wave of activity grew out of labor's successful effort to achieve implementation of participatory rights explicated in the OSHAct. This effort in itself was largely the consequence of deeply vested change among workers and their families. Environmental risks perceived to be unnecessary became increasingly rejected. Smoky stacks and workrooms were no longer accepted as a condition of employment. These factors—the perceived need by the workers for participation in decisions affecting their well-being and the rejection of traditional hazards of work—were the critical changes that moved both the Clean Air Act and the Occupational Safety and Health Act higher on the legislative agenda of the environmentally activist unions.

OSHA still serves well the social purposes for which it was created—regulatory action and enforcement, research, and education—and a benefit we did not anticipate, the curious trend (going against the general trend) in reduced labor-management strife over health issues.

Social change, like all forms of biologic development, is often burdened with vestigial remnants of earlier stages. Left without function, these at times disrupt the development of the individual, if not the evolutionary process itself.

Within the bureaucracy charged with implementing the environmental protection laws of the United States, there is a state of civil insurrection by vestigial elements, an insurrection both insidious and (seemingly) innocuous, its perception obscured by the opacities of the multiple moral cataracts that plague us as a society.

There is a clear parallel in history. When the expansionists of ancient Athens failed to extend their power and conquer Syracuse, they, then left without a function, conspired to persuade the citizens of Athens that the system of govern-

---

[a] This paper was inspired by Billy Wilson, a meat cutter, and Les Reid, a machinist, whose struggles should encourage workers' representatives everywhere.

[b] Address for correspondence: I.U.D./AFL–CIO, 815 16th Street N.W., Room 301, Washington, D.C. 20006.

ment was at fault, that democracy ought to be abandoned, and that the citizens ought to embrace these failed vestigial leaders as their rightful oligarchic rulers. They succeeded. They succeeded because there were no other leaders persuasive enough to untangle the alleged deficiencies of a system of laws from what Michael McCloskey, Chair of the Sierra Club, correctly identifies as "ministerial failure."

In our time, those who have failed to extend their power in the legislatures and in the courts nevertheless have found some success in fostering the abandonment of our democratic and democratically derived system of environmental laws. They have done this through manipulation of what the people must perceive as labyrinthine mysteries of administration. Others can find examples in the administration of the laws intended to protect our air, water, food, and the land itself. Here we point to the administration of the Occupational Safety and Health Act of 1970, a law beset by maladministration from the day it was enacted.

Documentation of this charge is found in the proposal that the United States Department of Labor substitute the efforts of its own standard-setting mechanisms for those published by a private organization, the American Conference of Governmental Industrial Hygienists. Hundreds of environmental values would be replaced by numbers that would often be smaller than those now in law and thus are perceived to provide greater protection for workers.

The fundamental issue is not whether adoption of the updated TLVs (threshold limit values) is the most effective means of increasing the level of protection afforded by OSHA standards. Such protection cannot, in any case, be expected to occur. And protection is not the issue. The question is whether the Act should be rewritten by administrative decree and, secondarily, if the Act is defective, why the Secretary of Labor has not brought the defect to the attention of the Congress.

The fact is that a faction of civil servants and industry employees never accepted the decision of our Congress as to how standards ought to be developed and promulgated, with the consequence that the methods prescribed by the legislation have never been fully implemented and tested.

The TLV Committee of the ACGIH was replaced by the National Institute for Occupational Safety and Health, a decision that was no minor action or accident of legislative drafting. Before the passage of the Act, the ACGIH earned and deserved the respect of workers in this and every other country for developing a system of environmental values that became enforceable, internationally recognized standards. The Bureau of Occupational Health, predecessor to NIOSH, supported that effort with funds and personnel. Those who participated, especially the industry members (including an occasional labor hygienist), must be remembered and commended. They met a need in the best way available during times characterized by ignorance, apathy, and usually unfettered manslaughter in the workplace.

I do not believe that anyone has been a more persistent critic of the TLV committee than myself. Yet I must reject criticisms of their work that do not take into account the severe social, political, and economic handicaps endured by environmental scientists and managers before 1970.

The questionable scientific basis, the dollar-driven compromises in deriving the values, and even the lies about the existence of "thresholds of protection" and the actual levels of protection afforded were justified.

Yes, as activists as different as Galileo and Jaspers would affirm, lies are justified when they clearly and directly serve to extend human life and freedom. In this case, thousands of lives must have been extended, a conclusion as certain as the law of probability itself. There were no feasible alternatives to the work of the TLV committee before passage of the Act. The federal government did not move to create an official national standards development body for the work environment, as they did for other environmental issues in the preceding decade.

When the TLV Committee was created, the environmental movement as we now know it did not exist. The public health movement then, as now, placed the health of workers in a special category characterized by inaction. The labor movement was mired in its long struggle to accomplish what it could do best: achieve the legislative remedy initiated in 1949 by Hubert Humphrey.

Those of us who were in government at the time worked without effective public support except during moments of trauma. Air pollution incidents and mine disasters resulted in air pollution control and mine safety legislation. The need to control toxic chemical contamination of the workplace was not widely accepted even among medical scientists, with the exception of Selikoff, Mancuso, Hueper, Case, Hardy, Bouhuys, Nelson, and a few others. They were notable, not only because they were exceptions, but also because they acted to bring the problem to the attention of the labor movement, the professional community, and the Congress.

In 1965, the National Advisory Environmental Health Committee, chaired by Norton Nelson of New York University with George Flaccus of Jones and Laughlin Steel Corporation, James Sterner of Eastman Kodak Company, and George Taylor of AFL-CIO as members, submitted a Special Report to the Surgeon General of the United States Public Health Service which was adopted as public policy. That policy made clear the enormity of the need and the inadequacy of the existing institutional arrangements, including those used in the development of standards.

The report recommended that the "Division" [of Occupational Health, USPHS] should be empowered to develop Federal criteria upon which standards . . . could be based. . . . This is an area of . . . protection which is at present outside the jurisdiction of any Federal agency." (p. 5)

After exhaustive hearings, standards development was made the focus of a consensus between labor and the leading medical scientists of the day both within and outside government. Management was part of this consensus insofar as the establishment of a federal system for developing standards was concerned.

It was a Senator from New York—Jacob Javits—who crystallized the specific need and remedy.

Andrew Biemiller and George Taylor of the AFL-CIO had testified on the issue before the Senate Subcommittee on Labor on November 26, 1969. "We oppose any legislation," they stated, "which would, in effect, make any private standards-producing organization an arm of the federal government. . . ."

The scientific and congressional records provided, and continues to provide, ample justification for this position. The Act represented an opportunity for reform so that lies and distortions of science did not have to continue. Indeed, their moral justification came to an end with an essential congressional observation: "But don't you think a good case could be made," asked Jacob Javits of New York, " . . . for some kind of institute of occupational health and safety, some really classy autonomous agency . . . something which would be as fine an organization as the National Science Foundation . . . to be like the National Institutes for Health, which would be the fundamental agency to which we would look for the development of standards."

The Conference report (*Congressional Record*-House, December 16, 1970) reflected the answer of both houses of Congress: " . . . the Secretary of HEW [is required] to consult with the Secretary of Labor to develop a research plan in order to develop criteria to assist in setting standards" (p. 42). "The Conference agreement provides for the creation of the National Institute (for Occupational Safety and Health)" (p. 43).

The private standards, such as those of ACGIH, were to be "interim" measures replaced through the development and promulgation of permanent standards as a joint venture of the Secretaries of Labor and HEW. The TLV Committee was replaced. Eighteen years later, the joint venture exists in name alone and the Administration proposes to change the law through publication in the *Federal Register*.

STANDARDS AS SYSTEMS OF CONTROL

The attention given to the ACGIH environmental values obscures the fundamental redefinition (by the Congress of the United States) of the concepts and term "standard." Our law makes of a standard a total system of use and enforcement: an environmental value or work practice or process containment or personal protection—or any combination of these—in concert with a system of employer-employee education, environmental monitoring, medical surveillance, warning devices, recordkeeping, protection for the complaining or medically removable worker, and the right of the worker to participate in the interpretation of and compliance with the standard. The OSHA standard is not an environmental value. It is a matrix of scientific, technical, social, and economic values. OSHA standards are not goals, as ACGIH values are meant to be (albeit inadequately). They are enforceable, mandated prescriptions for control. They are systems of control. Only the "interim" values can be less.

To adopt the current ACGIH values, even as supplemented with a few NIOSH-recommended exposure limits, would fail then to meet the mandate of the law. The NIOSH exposure limits, generally more stringent on the basis of the numbers alone, are published in criteria documents that provide OSHA with all of the elements of a complete standard, although NIOSH leaves the feasibility issue to be decided by OSHA as provided by law.

The Secretary of Labor has failed to consider, as required by law, the recommended systems of control developed by NIOSH to accompany those few NIOSH recommendations that have been integrated with the OSHA "update."

Moreover, the Department of Labor has had before it since May 8, 1975 (40 FR 20202) a joint OSHA/NIOSH proposal to supplement the TLV list so that real protections, rather than illusory measures, are obtained. This is the Standards Completion Program developed by NIOSH to lend meaning, that is, actual protection as envisioned *correctly* by the Congress, in the form of a complete system of control.

The Congress correctly concluded, and experience has verified, that changing the environmental values, even to what appear to be stricter limits, does not in itself result in more-protective standards. Permanent standards are meant to be more protective and must include all of the protective elements prescribed by the Congress. If the administrators believe that the congressional judgment, signed into law by the President and in effect for nearly two decades, is incorrect, then it is incumbent on the Secretary of Labor to apply to the Congress for a change in the law. To do otherwise is a ministerial failure—without moral or legal justification—that subverts the constitutional role of our elected representatives.

The proposal reverses the decision of the Congress on who will develop standards and what should be contained in such standards. The alleged compensation of higher levels of protection to be afforded by the proposed incomplete standards is a chimera that was rejected by the Congress and by the premises of the Standards Completion Program recommended 13 years ago by the National Institute for Occupational Safety and Health.

RESOLUTION THROUGH EMPOWERMENT

Insurrections that take the form of subversion through conscious ministerial failure need not be dealt with, in our society, like the Whiskey Rebellion. Court, legislative, and mass media pressures are adequate to generate the political action by which our democratic institutions can be protected. That is our strength. Unlike the Athenian parallel, the vestigial failures in our society are not likely to succeed. They have been identified and will be dealt with by citizens never before so empowered through social change.

Round Table Papers: 5. Worksite Inspection and the Control of Occupational Disease

Worksite Inspection and the Control of Occupational Disease

The OSHA Experience

JOHN R. FROINES

Southern Occupational Health Center
Division of Environmental and Occupational Health Sciences
UCLA School of Public Health
Los Angeles, California 90024

Passage of the Occupational Safety and Health Act in 1970 has without doubt had a major impact on occupational health in the United States. The Act and its subsequent implementation made occupational safety and health a national issue in the 1970s and focused a considerable degree of public consciousness on the problems of health in the workplace. It is generally accepted that as activities in occupational health across the country have grown, significant progress in improving workplace conditions has been made. Unfortunately, it is also apparent that significant workplace health issues continue to exist. The historical problems of lead and silica exposure, for example, continue today; recent work indicates that industrial exposures to these materials are still excessive.[1,2] During the past decade new workplace-related diseases resulting from chemical exposure have also been noted. Neurologic disease derived from exposure to dimethylaminopropionitrile or Lucel-7, reproductive impairment from dibromochloropropane (DBCP), and carcinogenesis associated with certain industrial chemicals, such as vinyl chloride, are all examples of disease discovered since passage of the Act.

Thus, examples of both success and failure in the control of occupational disease are numerous. The question before us today is: How effective have OSHA onsite inspections been in achieving control of workplace exposures and thereby reducing occupational disease? A corollary question is: What complementary efforts might be instituted to enhance the efficacy of workplace inspections?

A BRIEF REVIEW OF OSHA INSPECTION DATA FROM 1979–1985

A brief review of OSHA inspection results may be of value in assessing the value of workplace inspections in the control of occupational disease. We used the OSHA Integrated Management Information System (IMIS) to review the results of OSHA compliance activity. This system contains a record of each inspection conducted over the course of OSHA's history.[3] In 1979, OSHA began to include actual exposure measurements in the IMIS. Before 1979, the exposure information was collected and entered as a proportion of the permissible exposure limit (PEL). This paper reviews a data tape covering inspections over the period 1979–1985. Previously published work[1,3] describes research conducted by the author and colleagues analyzing OSHA inspection data from 1979–1982.

From 1979–1985 OSHA collected samples for 546 different chemicals during the course of inspections. Measurable exposures occurred for 389 substances, and there were overexposures (over the PEL) for 201 chemicals. Fifty-five substances had only one overexposure, and 88 substances had fewer than 10 overexposures. Our analysis of inspection data reveals that OSHA focuses its primary sampling efforts on fewer than 15 substances. Substances with more than 100 test samples having exposures greater than the PEL were silver (109), toluene (142), coke oven emissions (164), styrene (231), arsenic (272), asbestos (275), chromium (275), coal tar pitch volatiles (310), carbon monoxide (373), iron oxide (388), copper (534), nuisance dust (919), silica (1,971), and lead (3,693). Lead and silica had more than 1,000 test samples greater than the PEL. Several of these substances have limited evidence of significant toxicity; only a few of them have adequate OSHA standards. The actual number of overexposures in any given Standard Industrial Classification (SIC) was extremely limited with the exception of those of lead and silica. Overexposures for these 14 substances occurred over a period of years and across a significant number of SIC codes. For example, there were 40 SICs in which 275 overexposures to chromium were detected, an average of one overexposure per SIC per year.

BREADTH OF COMPLIANCE ACTIVITY

These summary statistics are incomplete, because data from the majority of state-plan states are not included in these numbers, but they do suggest that the breadth of OSHA compliance activity is very limited. OSHA's ability to identify hazardous worksites apparently is inadequate. The limited number of substances studied and overexposures identified derive in part from the use of the 1968 American Conference of Governmental Industrial Hygienists Threshold Limit Values, many of which are clearly outdated. The lack of breadth also appears to result from a failure to identify where agents of concern are actually used and violations of the standards anticipated. OSHA has not developed a successful inspection strategy based on analysis of actual use and predictions about potential worker exposures. In addition, OSHA's inspection pattern of emphasizing complaints may not be entirely appropriate when it comes to identifying overexposures to chronic hazards.

OSHA appears not to have considered how information from EPA's Toxic Substances Control Act (TSCA) or from OSHA's Hazard Communication Standard can be used to identify potential exposures that could broaden the inspection base, and NIOSH Health Hazard Evaluations (HHEs) are not used for scheduling purposes. The newly completed National Occupational Exposure Survey (NOES) conducted by NIOSH may be of particular value in the future. In this regard, OSHA has not had success in applying the National Occupational Hazard Survey (NOHS), but the new survey is undoubtedly more reflective of current use patterns.

A variety of factors may explain the lack of breadth in OSHA inspections including: an inadequate process for selecting inspection sites, systematic failure to develop data on chemical use and exposure, failure of the complaint system to identify existing health hazards, and standards that are not reflective of current biomedical knowledge. In addition, because there is currently no mechanism for collection of environmental monitoring data mandated in 6(b) standards, OSHA

TABLE 1. Temporal Trends in Lead Exposure (1979–1985)

Year	No. of Inspections	No. of Test Samples	% Samples >0.05[a]	Median Inspection Severity[b]
SIC = 2816 Pigment Manufacture				
1979	7	82	52	1.2
1980	6	23	65	0.5
1981	4	39	62	3.4
1982	2	5	80	4.9
1983	8	47	45	0.7
1984	7	33	60	1.3
1985	5	26	73	2.0
SIC = 3341 Secondary Lead Smelting				
1979	26	415	69	1.2
1980	20	163	47	0.7
1981	23	193	53	0.5
1982	15	90	73	1.8
1983	24	201	62	1.1
1984	15	110	50	0.2
1985	17	138	39	0.3
SIC = 3362 Brass-Bronze Foundries				
1979	16	142	65	0.9
1980	25	197	49	1.0
1981	28	211	55	0.8
1982	16	146	58	1.6
1983	20	169	32	0.5
1984	26	139	45	0.6
1985	28	198	38	0.7
SIC = 3691 Battery Manufacture				
1979	17	217	62	1.2
1980	26	287	68	1.1
1981	16	155	77	1.9
1982	20	150	67	1.1
1983	15	217	69	1.5
1984	20	141	59	0.9
1985	23	297	38	0.8

[a] mg/m^3.
[b] Severity levels are levels of lead exposures expressed as a proportion of the PEL, that is, a severity level of 2.0 is twice the PEL. The median severity level is the overall median of inspection median exposure levels expressed as a proportion of the PEL.

cannot use the data to trigger its own inspections. Analytic evaluation of OSHA inspections is beyond the scope of this report, and a more in-depth analysis of OSHA compliance activities will be reported elsewhere.

EVALUATION OF INDUSTRY COMPLIANCE

From 1979–1985, OSHA conducted 3,934 inspections in which lead was sampled. Of the 14,168 test samples for lead collected, 3,693 (26%) were over the PEL. OSHA adopted a new standard for lead in 1978, and it was implemented during the period of our evaluation. TABLE 1 illustrates the degree of compliance with the standard for industries with high lead exposure over that period. There appears to be improvement in battery manufacture (SIC 3691), and, to a lesser degree, secondary lead smelting (SIC 3341). However, at least 38% of the test samples exceeded the standard for these industries. In the other industries little or no change in exposure levels has occurred. Anecdotal information from both industry and labor also suggests that the battery industry may have made significant strides in implementing controls since the advent of the standard.

Unfortunately, OSHA has no systematic way of measuring the success or failure of its own compliance effort. There is no ongoing evaluation process to determine if the agency's inspections are reducing the hazards associated with chemical exposure. One of the major problems with the OSHA approach to self-evaluation is that the agency measures success on the basis of input variables, such as the number of inspections or the penalties levied, as opposed to an evaluation of compliance, which is the abatement of the hazard through the use of engineering controls. OSHA has no means to assess outcome variables, reductions of exposure through control technology implementation. There is no record on whether controls have been instituted as a result of a compliance process. Anecdotal information suggests that extensions to abatement orders are given repeatedly when engineering controls are mandated. OSHA has little in-house ability to assess claims of technical infeasibility. In addition, follow-up inspections are limited.

LEAD AND SILICA OVEREXPOSURES

As described earlier, the number of overexposures to lead and silica is significant. In the case of lead, there were more than 3,600 test samples greater than the limit. There were 52 four-digit SICs with at least one third of their inspection medians greater than the PEL. In previously published research we identified 9 two-digit SICs that have evidence of substantial exposure to silica (TABLE 2). In the following three-digit SICs, 325, 326, and 332, more than 60% of the inspections had silica test samples greater than the standard. The data for lead and silica suggest that overexposures are occurring in overwhelming proportions. Respirator use has undoubtedly had an effect in preventing an epidemic in silica- and lead-related disease, but reports from state registries that assess blood lead levels and compliance with the biologic monitoring requirements of the OSHA lead standard suggest that there is significant noncompliance with the standard (Dr. Linda Rudolph, personal communication). Because of overexposures and noncompliance with the biologic monitoring aspects of the lead standard, a special effort should be made to assess the health status of workers in the lead industries as well as workers exposed to silica. In promulgating the lead standard, OSHA suggested that there were five industries with high lead exposure: primary and secondary smelting, battery manufacture, lead pigment manufacture, and brass-bronze foundries. Our analysis of the OSHA data appears to indicate that at least 47 other industries require scrutiny.

TABLE 2. Major Silica Exposures by Industry; OSHA Inspection Data 1979–1982

SIC	Industry	No. of Inspections/ No. of Samples	% of Inspections with Test Sample over PEL	Mean Severity Level[a]	Median Severity Level[b]	Median Exposure over PEL[c]	SICs with Highest Exposure
16,17	Construction: heavy construction and special trades	55/131	51%	4.6	0.9	9.1 (59)[d]	1622,29 1721,99
28	Chemical manufacturing	78/225	30%	1.4	0.3	3.3 (59)	
2816,9	Inorganic chemicals	7/33	57%	1.0	0.3	2.0 (16)	
2821,41,44	Resins, soaps, cosmetics	12/39	50%	6.0	0.1	5.5 (16)	
32	Stone, glass, clay manufacturing	155/636	42%	1.2	0.4	3.2 (187)	
3211,21,29	Glass manufacturing	27/57	22%	1.3	0.2	6.6 (7)	
3251,3,5,9	Structural clay	35/221	66%	1.2	0.9	2.2 (78)	
3261,4,9	Pottery products	26/161	73%	1.7	1.0	2.4 (64)	
3281	Cut stone	5/25	40%	1.0	0.8	1.2 (9)	
33	Primary metal industries	259/2,044	52%	1.1	0.5	2.8 (564)	
3321,2,4,5	Iron and steel	154/1,531	67%	1.3	0.6	2.9 (490)	
3361	Aluminum	29/98	14%	0.4	0.3	1.5 (7)	
3362	Brass, bronze, and copper	34/199	32%	0.5	0.4	1.7 (34)	
34	Metal fabrication	54/161	46%	1.8	0.6	4.1 (44)	3441-3 3471,9
35	Machinery (nonelectric)	50/279	56%	2.2	0.7	4.7 (93)	3523,3553, 355,3599
37	Transportation equipment, manufacturing	34/84	50%	9.7	0.9	23.2 (37)	3751
39	Miscellaneous, manufacturing industries	11/32	64%	2.1	1.1	3.6 (16)	3959,3996

[a] Severity levels are levels of silica exposures expressed as a proportion of the PEL, that is, a severity level of 2.0 is twice the PEL. The mean severity level is the overall mean of the mean level for each inspection, an average of all test samples taken in that inspection.
[b] The median severity level is the overall median of inspection median exposure levels expressed as a proportion of the PEL.
[c] The mean of median severity levels of overexposures in each inspection.
[d] Number of test samples over the PEL.

Data indicating continuing overexposures to lead and silica raise the important question of why OSHA has no means to assess the reasons behind continuing high exposures. Analysis using OSHA IMIS data for lead indicates that when the data are analyzed by job title, consistently high exposures are demonstrated for certain jobs in the battery manufacturing industry. Unfortunately, there are no data to assess whether the continuing high exposures are a result of economic or technologic factors or simply employer recalcitrance. OSHA inspection and evaluation strategy apparently fails to ask for—or answer—the following questions: Why were there more than 3,600 overexposures to lead during 1979–1985 (even without including data from most state plan states)? Why are these exposures ongoing, and why does OSHA not have a means to evaluate the temporal trends in its data, to establish a means to ascertain the basis for the trends, and to devise strategies that will result in reduced exposures?

The problems just reviewed can be summarized as follows:

1. OSHA's inspection effort lacks breadth. The agency focuses on a few substances, there is limited application of data on chemical use that would broaden the inspection base, and the current system results in continual reinspection of industries and substances previously identified.

2. A positive aspect of the reinspection of industries with known exposures to certain highly toxic agents is that it identifies real problems. It also shows, however, that OSHA has not been successful in implementing control technology to reduce exposures. Moreover, there is no evaluation mechanism in place that would facilitate an assessment of why high exposures continue to occur.

3. OSHA's evaluation process focuses on input variables (e.g., number of inspections) instead of actual compliance through implementation of control technology.

NEW APPROACHES TO FACILITATE OSHA's INSPECTION EFFORTS

The key issue is how OSHA, with its limited resources, can achieve compliance with its standards. A program of inspection, citation, penalty, and abatement is never going to work for those industries with significant continuing exposures unless OSHA can determine a means to identify reasons for the ongoing problems, with appropriate follow-up to ensure that positive changes have occurred.

It is essential that OSHA, in cooperation with NIOSH, create a means for ongoing surveillance of industrial exposures. Relying solely on data from inspections overly narrows the scope of the data available. What is required is an expansion of efforts in the area of hazard and medical surveillance including biologic monitoring. An appropriate surveillance strategy would be to require industry to collect data on inplant exposures for selected substances. The data would then be collected by OSHA, computerized, and used as a basis for developing intervention activities. The data collected would be exposure measurements, biologic monitoring results, and, possibly, certain medical surveillance information. To avoid an overburdensome requirement, the data could be collected over time intervals from selected industries chosen at random. The 6(b) standards promulgated by OSHA already contain monitoring requirements, but these provisions were not envisioned to be used for surveillance purposes and may require modification. The 6(b) standards, however, form the basis for beginning such a surveillance effort. An effective surveillance strategy can prompt subsequent intervention when controls are nonexistent or inadequate. The OSHA inspection program would review industry-gathered data to assure that it is being effectively collected. An example of this approach is the required monitoring of dust levels in the coal mines by operators and subsequent follow-up by MSHA.

HAZARD SURVEILLANCE RECOMMENDATIONS FOR OSHA

1. Collect, analyze, and use data currently required to be collected under existing 6(b) standards: acrylonitrile, arsenic, asbestos, benzene, coke oven emissions, cotton dust, formaldehyde, ethylene oxide, lead, and vinyl chloride. Set up an appropriate surveillance strategy for subsequent follow-up.

2. Promulgate a generic standard that requires industry to conduct environmental monitoring for a wider range of substances. Biologic monitoring data need to be collected also, but within that context the complex issues of rate retention and medical removal protection would need to be addressed. Data collected in this generic standard would be collected by OSHA, analyzed, and used as a basis for intervention.

3. Consider how data from the Hazard Communication Standard can be collected, evaluated, and used as a basis for setting inspection priorities. Up to now that information has been considered as data for workers, but there is no reason it could not be used more extensively. The use of the data from the Hazard Communication Standard would enable OSHA to expand the breadth of compliance activities especially when coupled with data from NOES and TSCA.

4. Some states have enacted laws that require reporting of occupational disease such as silicosis or excessive blood lead levels. Additional consideration should be given to how these data can become incorporated into the overall surveillance strategy. It would be appropriate for the data to become included in the OSHA IMIS and used as a basis for setting inspection priorities.

5. OSHA needs to establish an evaluative mechanism to determine the effectiveness of its compliance effort. In particular, when certain jobs or processes in industry continually demonstrate overexposure, the basis of those violations must be evaluated. This should include engineering review as well as other factors that might influence employer compliance.

6. Focused enforcement activities are entirely appropriate when continuing overexposures are occurring, but they do not represent a valuable effort unless effective evaluative efforts are simultaneously conducted. These and other surveillance activities need to be considered if the limited resources of OSHA can better be used to identify and ultimately control workplace disease.

REFERENCES

1. FROINES, J. R. & D. H. WEGMAN. 1986. An approach to the characterization of silica exposure. Am. J. Ind. Med. **10**: 348–361.
2. FROINES, J. R., S. L. BARON, D. H. WEGMAN & S. O'ROURKE. 1989. Characterization of the airborne concentrations of lead in U.S. industry. J. Occup. Med. Submitted for publication.
3. FROINES, J. R., C. A. DELLENBAUGH & D. H. WEGMAN. 1986. Occupational hazard surveillance: A means to identify work related risks. Am. J. Pub. Health **76**: 1089–1096.

The Role of the Worksite Inspection under the Occupational Safety and Health Act

Reflections on 17 Years of OSHA Experience

MORTON CORN

Division of Environmental Health Engineering
School of Hygiene and Public Health
The Johns Hopkins University
Baltimore, Maryland 21205

Safety inspection is deeply rooted in the history of the field of occupational safety and health; its origin was concern for equipment performance, resulting in equipment inspections.[1] There is a longer history of equipment and facility inspection in the field of loss control as well.[2] In addition to periodic oversight inspections by organizational headquarters staff or insurers, first-line supervisors were usually assigned a more frequent inspection role for their immediate jurisdiction, as they are today in the vast majority of U.S. corporations.[3] Safety in the United States is a line manager responsibility under the Occupational Safety and Health Act, for the line manager is viewed as the agent of the employer who, under Section 5 of the Act, is accountable for providing a safe and healthful workplace. Criteria for inspections have traditionally been established by staff professionals, that is, safety and health specialists, but correction of deviations from inspection criteria is the responsibility of line management. In the past, records of inspections were not conscientiously maintained, but recent OSHA emphasis on record keeping has substantially improved this practice.

The workplace inspection process can also be traced to professional recognition of the risks of work. Inspection was a technique used by the concerned employer and was adopted throughout the organization. The technique was subsequently officially assigned to Federal and local regulatory agencies when legal safety requirements for the workplace, namely, railroads and mines, were first adopted. For many years inspections in these sectors focused exclusively on equipment and rolling stock. When the inspection process was transferred to the regulator, it became a device to insure adherence to specific promulgated regulations for the workplace. Deviations from requirements were cited, and civil penalties were assessed early on. The Occupational Safety and Health Act of 1970 also provided for criminal penalties. The transfer of informal inspection procedures within an organization to operating procedures of regulatory agencies has served to define very specifically the conduct of inspections and the rights of employees and the regulatee.[4] Thus, under OSHA, employees have established certain rights regarding the inspection. Employees can:

☐ Initiate an inspection through written request to OSHA;

☐ Accompany the compliance officer during inspections of the establishment;

- ☐ Bring an action in the Federal District Court for a Writ of Mandamus to compel the Secretary to act in an alleged imminent danger situation;
- ☐ Be immediately notified by the compliance officer of any imminent danger discovered during his or her inspection;
- ☐ Request a conference with the employer and the compliance officer at the end of an inspection;
- ☐ Receive notice from an employer contesting a violation;
- ☐ Contest the reasonableness of the abatement period provided by the Secretary;
- ☐ Have party status in any review commission proceeding;
- ☐ Participate in any variance proceeding brought by the employer.

The OSHA inspection process is highly codified.[5] The behavior of the compliance officer, procedures for checking compliance officer suggested citations, and issuance of these citations are all delineated in the Field Operations Manual of the Occupational Safety and Health Administration.

In summary, the inspection procedure, without question, has withstood the tests of time in the safety field. It is widely regarded as an effective safety management tool. However, it behooves us at this point to examine the manner in which this safety management tool has served us as a regulatory instrument.

CRITICAL AREAS OF INSPECTION EFFECTIVENESS

To Inspect or Not to Inspect

Some will ask if the philosophy of safety inspection is appropriate to the OSHAct. I believe inspections are necessary. Voluntary programs for compliance by employers, the responsible party under the OSHAct, are admirable and should be encouraged, but the regulatory agency should never relinquish the right to inspect, even for prescribed protracted periods. Inspection is a form of auditing; the latter is universally accepted as an effective operating business tool. Management philosophy stresses planning, organizing, implementing (leading), and controlling.[6] The auditing process is associated with evaluation of all that precedes it. The safety or health inspection is, for all intents and purposes, a manifestation of auditing, as Lees and I have indicated with regard to the Industrial Hygiene Audit.[7] Those in the private sector should recognize it as such and should appreciate that for the government to relinquish its prerogative to inspect is analogous to corporate headquarters relinquishing its prerogative to review the bookkeeping accounts of a corporate division or individual production facility. The latter would be strange indeed to any business manager. Therefore, all of the lovely acronym programs of the Occupational Safety and Health Administration, instituted during the last 8 years, which are thin veils for excusing the involved organizations from inspections, should be curtailed. That is *not* to say that in these cases inspections of firms with good records might be infrequent; they might be, depending on the judgment of the regulatory agency. But the right to inspect should not be relinquished in any formally specified interregnum built into a set of guidelines for voluntary programs.

Targeting of Inspections

A major concern of OSHA during the last 10 years, and one that I dealt with 11 years ago as Assistant Secretary of OSHA, was the efficient use of the limited resource of Compliance Safety and Health Officers (CSHOs). The recent report by the National Academy of Sciences indicates that OSHA gathers a great deal of work-related safety and health data, but it does not effectively utilize these data to establish priorities, including inspections.[8] The emphasis on record keeping by OSHA may be an effort to improve its targeting effectiveness. With approximately 1,000 inspectors now at OSHA, and approximately 5,000,000 workplaces to oversee, the need for targeting is evident. This targeting process must be improved. It is not merely an issue of identifying the Standard Industrial Classifications (SICs) that need targeting; it is necessary to identify individual firms within these SICs. Why cannot the safety/health records that OSHA is attempting to improve be forwarded to the agency to permit OSHA to better utilize inspection resources? With inspections somewhere in the range of 60–70 thousand per year, the contrast between needed inspections and performed inspections is stark.

Civil Penalties

One has a sense of déjà vu when the topic of fines associated with inspection citations is discussed. OSHA fines have never been of a magnitude to capture the attention of the *majority* of cited employers. Fines will have to be increased to be effective for the small to medium-size business. In my consulting practice with companies in the private sector, I have emphasized that, in the long run, the presence of serious citations will build a persuasive record of negligence on the part of the employer. There is a tendency of many employers to pay minimal fines rather than expend a larger sum of money to contest a poorly supported OSHA citation. I urge the employer to spend more money to contest if he has any evidence that the citation was not valid. Cumulating a record of serious citations will work against the employer, because safety is really a probability function involving minimizing risk. Each risk has an associated probability of occurrence. We minimize risk or the probability of an unwanted event occurring, but the event will occur. We do not know when and where. As Lowrance has stated, "safety is an acceptable risk."[9] When the event occurs, the previous record of attention to minimizing risk will be scrutinized and a string of serious citations, all of which were settled at relatively modest cost, will serve to formulate a view of the employer's sincerity in addressing safety and health in the workplace.

However, to smaller businesses, the money for citations *is* important and increased fines will help. Needless to say, some well-placed criminal citations will rapidly get the attention of employers charged with responsibility for the workplace.

The foregoing are old topics of discussion that have surfaced at numerous meetings such as this one. Perhaps it is time to think about some innovative solutions to the inspection process. In my opinion, the safety function will not succeed at a high level, that is, reduction of risk to a minimum at the workplace, until the employee is an equal partner in the effort. The majority of employers I have encountered in the United States indicate that, because the law holds them totally responsible under Section 5a of the OSHAct, they will dictate policies and procedures to be used in the establishment, through the appropriate line managers who are their agents. Many organizations do not have joint labor-management safety and health committees. Because 80% of our work force is unorganized, many establishments exist in which the employee is told what to do but does not participate in the decision-making of what is to be done. The Hazard Communication Act and individual state right-to-know laws should make many of these procedures more comprehensible to employees, but they do not give the employee a share in the decision-making for standard operating procedures in safety. Why can we not mandate joint labor-management safety and health committees in the workplace? I am well aware of the controversy associated with safety committees among safety professionals and managers,[10] but my experience with joint safety and health committees composed of labor and management representatives has been almost uniformly positive. Once the employee is drawn into the process of minimizing risks in the work environment, he or she is committed to it.

Professionalism

In the early days of OSHA, professionalism of the inspectorate was a major topic of agency criticism. The OSHA inspectorate is now functioning at a much higher level of professionalism, but what is not clear to the public is that the administrative process of the agency carried out through regional and area directors flavors the inspection process. Regional directors reporting to field coordinators and appointees of the agency are told (not found in written records) how vigorously or leisurely to conduct inspections. These administrators, in turn, make their wishes known to individual compliance officers. Much of this is quite subtle, but the language of superiors is clearly understood in the agency. For almost 8 years we have had a period of minimal enforcement of workplace safety and health standards. OSHA, if released to do so, could perform far more vigorous and meaningful inspections. This would not eliminate the need for better targeting, for increased fines, and for greater involvement of the workforce. Remember, the inspection process is an audit function. It should feed back to improve matters; therefore, the structure must be in place to improve that which is identified through the inspection process. The improvement of inspection efficiency will, by itself, measurably contribute to the creation of private sector organizational attention and structure to remediate deficiencies. A great deal depends on the inspection process.

SUMMARY

The inspection process has its counterpart in other areas of safety, namely, automobile safety, airplane safety, truck safety, structural safety, and the like. That we are less than pleased with the results in measures of workplace safety performance during the last decade and a half is not a reason to forsake the inspection process. There are ways to greatly improve the inspection process. The current dialogue should focus on extensions and improvements of inspections rather than relieving regulatees of the inspection experience. The inspection process has demonstrated its value as a safety management tool.

REFERENCES

1. HAMMER, W. 1985. Occupational Safety Management and Engineering, 3rd Ed. :177–179. Prentice-Hall, Inc. Englewood Cliffs, NJ.

2. Factory Mutual Engineering Co. Staff, 1967. Handbook of Industrial Loss Prevention. :14–1. McGraw Hill Book Co. New York, NY.
3. National Safety Council. 1970. Supervisors Safety Manual, 1970. :183. National Safety Council. Chicago, IL.
4. FELLNER, B. & D. W. SAVELSON. 1976. Occupational Safety and Health-Law and Practice. :27–28. Practicing Law Institute. New York, NY.
5. OSHA Instruction CPL 2.45A Ch-11. General Inspection Procedures. Office of General Industry Compliance Assistant. Washington, DC.
6. HODGETT, R. M. 1982. Management: Theory, Process and Practice. The Dryden Press. Chicago, IL.
7. CORN, M. & P. S. J. LEES. 1983. The industrial hygiene audit: Purposes and implementation. Am. Ind. Hyg. Assoc. J. **44:** 135–141.
8. POLLACK, E. S. & D. G. KEIMIG, Eds. 1987. Counting Injuries and Illnesses in the Workplace: Proposals for a Better System. National Academy of Sciences, National Academy Press. Washington, DC.
9. LOWRANCE, W. W. 1976. Of Acceptable Risk. William Kantmann, Inc. Los Altos, CA.
10. DeREAMER, R. 1980. Modern Safety and Health Technology. J. Wiley & Sons. New York, NY.

Is Regulation Effective?

A Case Study of Underground Coal Mining

JAMES L. WEEKS

Deputy Administrator
Occupational Health
United Mine Workers of America
Washington, DC 20005

With the passage of the Federal Coal Mine Health and Safety Act of 1969 and the Occupational Safety and Health Act of 1970, we initiated a significant experiment in primary preventive medicine in the nation.

"Primary preventive medicine" is a carefully chosen term. The Occupational Safety and Health Administration (OSHA) and the Mine Safety and Health Administration (MSHA) (and its predecessor, the Mining Enforcement Safety Administration, MESA) are regulatory agencies and, as a consequence, are frequently analyzed together with other regulatory agencies whose principal functions are to regulate economic matters. The result has been that analysis of these agencies has been conducted most prominently by economists and lawyers. Public health professionals have "dropped the ball," as Eula Bingham observed at the close of her tenure as head of OSHA. Yet the mission of both agencies is a public health mission and should be analyzed as such.

The basic structure of these two Acts is similar. Both mandate two primary functions: setting standards and enforcing them. The question raised at this conference is whether this approach has been fruitful. Most health standards are based on Threshold Limit Value (TLV) lists published by the American Conference of Governmental Industrial Hygienists. Most safety standards were likewise adopted from existing consensus standards and safety codes. The Mine Safety and Health Act also embodies numerous statutory (as opposed to regulatory) health and safety standards. Enforcement involves inspection of worksites by trained inspectors who have authority to enter workplaces and write citations when they observe violations of standards. Both Acts also create workers' rights to participate in inspections and litigation and to participate in standards setting.

By now, there should be sufficient data and experience to ask the important question raised in this workshop: Are these experiments successful?

The subject of this paper is the historical experience with the Mine Safety and Health Act, but its focus is whether regulation as constructed by both OSHA and MSHA has measurable positive effects.

The experience with coal mining, underground coal mining in particular, presents us with a laboratory-like experiment concerning whether this approach is effective. The experiment began with the Coal Mine Health and Safety Act of 1969 and continued with its successor, the Mine Safety and Health Act passed in 1977. The 1977 Act preserved the structure and function of the 1969 Act, so that for all practical purposes we have had consistent statutory authority to intervene in the coal mining industry since 1970.

To interpret this experiment, I wish to draw an analogy between it and experiments in toxicology. Experiments in toxicology have several important features that make it possible to isolate variables of interest. These features are as follows:

1. To produce an observable effect, doses are "high." Toxicologists usually have to make a trade-off between exposing a large number of animals to a small dose or a small number of animals to a large dose of whatever is the focus of the experiment. Questions of economy and feasibility usually dictate the latter option, resulting in "high" exposure levels.

2. Experimental animals are homogeneous in important ways such as species, sex, age, and genetic endowment, unless any of these variables are a concern in the experiment.

3. The difference between experimental groups is well defined and carefully controlled in order to isolate variables of interest.

4. All variables are measured and recorded, a feature common to all experimental sciences.

The purpose of these features in toxicology is to enable the toxicologist to focus attention on specific variables. Once the relation between exposure and outcome has been established in a well-designed experiment, we can conclude that there is an effect. The well-designed epidemiologic investigation should attempt to mimic these features of experimental science.

The historical experience in coal mining is close to mimicking an experiment in toxicology in the following ways:

(1) Exposure to workplace health and safety hazards is high. Underground coal mining regularly has the highest fatal and nonfatal injury rate of any industry in this nation and continues to have the highest fatality rate among other industrial nations.[1,2] Occupational respiratory disease is likewise common among miners.

Regulatory intervention has been aggressive, that is, exposure to the variable of interest is "high." For example, *every* underground coal mine is *required* to be inspected four times each year. There is no such requirement for mandatory inspections of workplaces under OSHA's jurisdiction. MSHA inspectors have the authority to close all or parts of mines; under OSHA, the inspector must seek a court order. Mine operators must submit a mine plan (i.e., a detailed plan showing how they will operate their mine so that it meets all pertinent standards) to the agency before they begin operations, effectively having to obtain a permit. Mine operators are required to provide miners with 40 hours of training before work and to provide annual retraining. Exposure to respirable dust in coal mines is monitored on a regular basis by both mine operators and MSHA. Mine operators are also required to provide miners with regular chest x-rays to control the progression of pneumoconiosis. Miners with positive chest x-ray films may transfer to so-called less dusty areas.[3] Under OSHA, workers exposed to some hazards (e.g., lead) also have similar medical removal protection.

The difference between OSHA and MSHA may seem too great to permit applying lessons from one agency to the other. Rather than treat these differences as problems, however, I choose to treat them as opportunities to raise the generic policy question of whether regulatory intervention is an effective means of preventing occupational injury and illness. Or, to put the matter differently, if regulation in this high hazard industry is ineffective, less aggressive regulation, such as that by OSHA, is even less likely to be effective.

(2) The work environment and the population of miners are relatively homogeneous. Industrial practices are common throughout the industry and, as a consequence, so are health and safety hazards. Although some technologic innovations have been made in the industry not required by the Act, over the last 20 years, the pace of change has been relatively slow with few dramatic changes such as have occurred in other industries (e.g., robotics and the use of computers). Moreover, enforcement of the Act has forced some technologic change that has had a direct

bearing on mine safety. For example, MSHA requires that all pieces of equipment used at the mining face (where coal is cut) be "permissible" (i.e., able to operate in explosive mixtures without generating a source of ignition), have cabs and canopies to protect miners in the event of a roof fall, and likely will soon require the use of automatic temporary roof supports (ATRS) when working beyond permanent supports. Technologic change has been forced by the Act.

(3) The 1969 Act was a significant departure from prior federal or state government intervention concerning miners' health and safety. The first efforts of the federal government concerning mine safety came with the organization of the Bureau of Mines in 1910. The Bureau has limited authority to investigate mine catastrophes, but it was not until 1941 that it had authority to enter and inspect mines. Even then, however, there were neither mandatory standards nor penalties. In 1952, the Bureau acquired the authority to inspect and close "dangerous" mines employing more than 15 persons. Amendments in 1966 extended coverage to all mines. These efforts were designed principally to prevent mine fires and explosions. Little attention was paid to other causes of injury or to health matters, and surface mines were not included.

The 1969 Act adopted existing comprehensive health and safety standards, made them mandatory, and provided for inspections and stiff penalties for noncompliance. This Act was a clear shift from an era of voluntary compliance to one of enforcement. It created a schedule for lowering exposure to respirable dust. It also created an innovative program for compensating miners with "black lung," which was the subject of a similar New York Academy of Sciences symposium nearly 20 years ago.[4]

Because of this rather abrupt change, we have, in effect, a clear difference between experimental groups before and after the implementation of this Act. Conveniently, the Act was passed on the next to the last day of 1969, facilitating a neatly divided "before and after" analysis of data by calendar years starting with 1970.

(4) Data have been gathered and can be used for analysis. Mine operators are required to report certain accidents (regardless of whether an injury occurred), all injuries, and all fatalities. MSHA also investigates and is required to issue a report for all fatalities. Although MSHA compiles and makes available these data, the primary source for fatal and nonfatal injuries is the mine operator. Data gathering is more complete under MSHA than under OSHA.[5]

Mine operators are also required to measure exposure to respirable dust. They must take a minimum of five samples in each section of each mine six times per year. This resulted, in fiscal year 1987, in approximately 100,000 samples taken by mine operators and another 20,000 taken by MSHA inspectors. There are also provisions for measuring exposure to free silica.

To measure the effects of the Act, I examined two outcome variables: industry-wide fatality rates, and exposure to respirable dust. I also make passing reference to trends in the prevalence of coal workers' pneumoconiosis. These variables are examined for a period of time before the Act was passed and after its passage, from 1970 to the present.

Consideration of fatality rates, as opposed to nonfatal injury rates, is used for several reasons. Nonfatal injury rates are age dependent, and without information about the age distribution of the mining population, it is impossible to compute age-adjusted nonfatal injury rates. MSHA does not collect this information and it is not easily obtainable elsewhere. Second, there is doubt about the reliability of nonfatal injury reports in any event. Fatality rates in the coal mining industry are not age dependent, and reporting of fatalities is more reliable and complete.[1]

To consider health outcomes as opposed to safety, I measured trends in exposure to respirable coal mine dust, the causative agent of pneumoconiosis. In the process, I will comment on the occurrence of pneumoconiosis among miners.

MATERIALS AND METHODS

Data to compute annual fatality rates (number of fatalities per 100 worker-years) among underground miners were obtained from MSHA's Health and Safety Analysis Center (HSAC) for the period 1933 to 1987.[6-8] A simple linear regression of fatality rates on years was conducted for equal time periods before and after the Act.[9]

Fatalities by mine size and by accident classification were obtained from MSHA for the years 1970 to 1987 for the purpose of assessing recent trends. Since hours worked, by mine size, are not yet available for the industry for 1986 and 1987, we are unable to calculate size-specific fatality rates and have instead conducted a proportional mortality analysis of fatalities classified by mine size. We conducted a similar analysis for type of accident for each year from 1970 to 1987.

Different summary measurements of exposure to respirable coal mine dust were taken from published reports for years before 1983 and from regular reports issued by the Department of Occupational Health and Safety at the United Mine Workers Association (UMWA) for later years.

Estimates of the prevalence of pneumoconiosis were obtained from the National Institute for Occupational Safety and Health (NIOSH) using two data sets. First, since 1969, NIOSH has been conducting the National Study of Coal Workers Pneumoconiosis (NSCWP) and has recently summarized results of this study.[10] Second, according to the 1969 Act, mine operators are required to provide miners with periodic chest x-rays in order to control the progression of coal workers' pneumoconiosis (CWP). Data from this chest x-ray surveillance program were recently summarized and published.[11]

None of these data sets is ideal. It would be an improvement, in reporting all occupational injuries, to have more information on working populations in which injuries occur, that is, information about the denominators, in order to make adjustments for age, experience, hours of work, and other variables.[1]

Most data concerning exposure to respirable dust are derived from the dust monitoring program. This program is designed to determine compliance with the respirable dust standard of 2.0 mg/m^3 by having mine operators take dust samples. The purpose of taking these samples is not to make a scientific survey of exposure in the industry. Mine operators also have a clear vested interest in the outcome of samples. There have been several cases of fraud. Because of these problems, there is widespread skepticism among miners concerning the reliability of this program. One analysis of data from this program showed that exposure to dust is underestimated.[12] The magnitude of bias for industry-wide data is likely small,[13] and in any case, it is probably consistent so that comparisons are possible.

Estimates of the prevalence of pneumoconiosis are likewise flawed. Originally designed as a longitudinal study, the NSCWP has experienced a high rate (80%) of miners lost to follow-up, and NIOSH has not included measurements of exposure to respirable dust in their analysis of medical data. Therefore, it has not been possible to calculate incidence rates and progression or to evaluate directly the current dust standard. Rather than a longitudinal study, we have a series of cross-sectional measurements of prevalence. These problems are currently being addressed by NIOSH. Participation by miners in the surveillance program has steadily declined. Participation varies significantly between mines, with an industry-wide average participation rate of 32% in the third round, in 1981.[12] This weakens our ability to make reliable estimates of the prevalence of CWP in the whole population of miners.

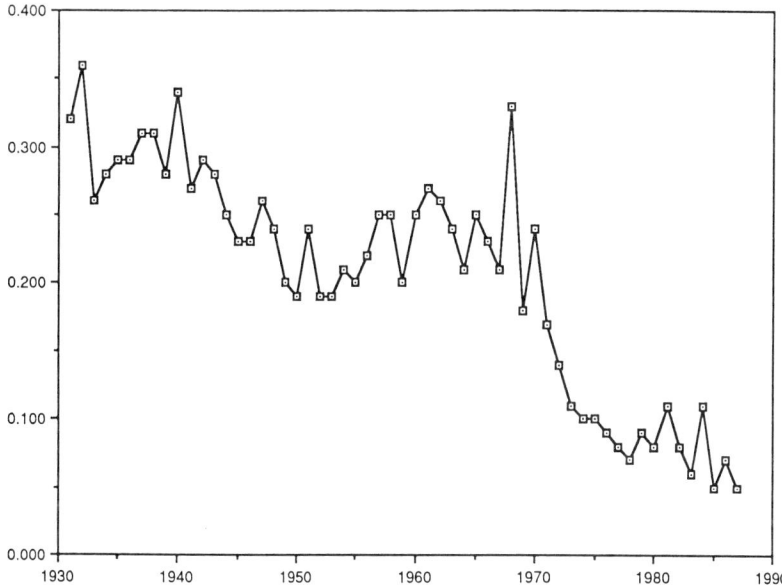

FIGURE 1. Underground fatality rates: 1931–1987. *Horizontal axis:* year; *vertical axis:* fatality rate (fatalities per 100 full-time workers per year).

RESULTS

1. *Fatality Rates.* Regression analysis clearly shows that before the Act, fatality rates showed no trend. In the decade following the Act, rates declined consistently.[9] Observation of fatality rates since 1933 showed little improvement until 1970 (FIG. 1). Some disasters (by convention, a disaster is defined as any accident resulting in five or more fatalities) may have biased this regression. Therefore, we did simple linear regression of fatality rates on years both with and without disasters and came to the same conclusion.

By 1980, the fatality rate was less than half the rate for the period before the Act. Since about 1980, this decline has slowed considerably; there is a slight downward trend that is not significantly different from zero.[14]

To evaluate the recent lack of progress in reducing fatalities, we evaluated fatalities both by accident classification and by mine size for the period 1970 to 1987. The proportion of fatal accidents classified as roof falls, powered haulage, machinery, fires and explosions, and others was calculated for each year and then classified into two time periods: 1970–1979 and 1980–1987.

The proportion of fatalities from roof falls, powered haulage, electrical hazards, and others remained essentially the same for both periods, accounting, averaged over the whole period, for 38%, 22%, 7%, and 11%, respectively. The proportion of fatalities associated with machinery declined from 13% of all fatalities in the 1970s to 7% in the 1980s. Those associated with fires and explosions increased from 8% in the 1970s to 16% in the 1980s (TABLE 1A and 1B).

Fires and explosions, which are relatively infrequent, are more likely to be disasters, which accounts for the wide range (from 2 to 31% for the period 1980–1987) of proportions of fatalities from these causes.

It has been well known for many years that the rate of fatal injuries at small mines is significantly greater than that at large mines.[1] Therefore, we calculated the proportion of fatalities by mine size for each year from 1970 to 1987 and then for the two time periods 1970–1979 and 1980–1987. Classified in this way, there is an increase in the proportion of fatalities in very small mines (19 or fewer miners) and a decrease in the proportion in large mines (100 miners or more). However, if we confine our attention to the last 3 years, 44% of fatalities occurred at very small mines, compared with 21% for the period 1980–1984. Thus, for the last 3 years, a much larger than expected proportion of fatalities has occurred at very small mines (TABLE 2A and 2B).

Proportions can rise or fall either because underlying causes rise or fall or because the remainder of the universe (in this case, all other fatalities) is expanding or contracting. With respect to the increase in the proportion of fatalities from

TABLE 1. Mine Fatalities by Cause 1980–1987 (%)

Year	Cause						
	Roof Fall	Powered Haulage	Fire, Explosion	Electrical	Machinery	Other	Total
A. 1980–1987 (%)							
1980	31 (31)	24 (24)	5 (5)	10 (10)	16 (16)	13 (13)	99
1981	37 (31)	20 (17)	36 (30)	9 (7)	6 (5)	13 (11)	121
1982	49 (46)	17 (18)	7 (7)	6 (6)	4 (4)	12 (13)	95
1983	19 (37)	9 (18)	8 (16)	6 (12)	1 (2)	8 (16)	51
1984	30 (31)	16 (16)	30 (31)	4 (4)	8 (8)	10 (10)	98
1985[a]	16 (31)	12 (23)	3 (6)	5 (10)	4 (8)	12 (23)	52
1986[a]	26 (45)	8 (14)	1 (2)	8 (14)	8 (14)	7 (12)	58
1987[a]	19 (44)	13 (30)	2 (5)	6 (14)	2 (5)	1 (2)	43
Totals	227 (37)	119 (19)	92 (15)	54 (9)	49 (8)	76 (12)	617
B. 1970–1979 and 1980–1987 (%)							
1970–79	456 (38)	277 (23)	91 (8)	81 (7)	161 (13)	128 (11)	1,194
1980–87	227 (37)	119 (19)	92 (16)	54 (9)	49 (8)	76 (12)	617

$x^2 = 38.70$, 5 df, $p < 0.001$.
[a]Preliminary data.

TABLE 2. Mine Fatalities by Mine Size

	Size			
Year	19 or Fewer	20–99	100 or More	Total
A. 1980–1987 (%)				
1980	17 (17)	20 (20)	62 (63)	99
1981	26 (21)	45 (37)	50 (41)	121
1982	29 (31)	26 (27)	40 (42)	95
1983	10 (20)	16 (31)	25 (49)	51
1984	17 (17)	18 (18)	63 (64)	98
1985[a]	30 (57)	9 (17)	13 (25)	52
1986[a]	18 (32)	15 (26)	25 (43)	58
1987[a]	19 (44)	15 (35)	9 (21)	43
Totals	166 (27)	164 (27)	287 (47)	617
B. 1970–1979 and 1980–1987 (%)				
1970–79	220 (18)	314 (26)	660 (55)	1,194
1980–87	166 (27)	164 (27)	287 (47)	617

$\varkappa^2 = 19.70$, 2 df, p <0.001.
[a]Preliminary data.

fires and explosions, both forces appear to be at work. For machinery-related fatalities, the cause of this decline is unclear. For the changes observed in small mines, the increase in the proportion of fatalities is explained by fewer fatalities at larger mines. The number of fatalities per year at small mines is relatively constant from 1980–1987, but the number at large mines shows a steady decline.

To summarize, compared with the period 1970–1979, there were more fatalities than expected from fires and explosions and fewer than expected from machinery-related accidents. The proportion of fatalities from all other causes remains the same. There were more than the expected number of fatalities at small mines, especially in the last 3 years. Therefore, we conclude that the lack of progress in reducing the risk of fatal injuries is in part explained by excess fatalities from fires and explosions and in part by excess fatalities at small mines.

2. *Respirable Dust.* Exposure to respirable dust before 1969 was rarely measured. One survey of 29 mines was undertaken by the Bureau of Mines for three periods: 1968–1969, the last 6 months of 1970, and the first six months of 1971.[15] The average MRE-equivalent dust concentration for continuous miner operators was about 6 mg/m^3 in 1968–1969, then fell to about 2.5 mg/m^3 in 1970. (MRE refers to the Medical Research Establishment in the United Kingdom. Because it was data from the MRE that formed the basis of the dust standard in the United States, and because dust concentrations are measured differently in the United Kingdom, measurements in the United States have to be converted to their "MRE equivalent" with an empirically derived conversion factor.)

From 1971 to 1980, average concentration of respirable dust for continuous miner operators declined from 2.8 mg/m^3 to 1.3. In 1987, it was 0.98 mg/m^3. Similar progress was not evident for certain jobs on longwall mining sections. In 1980, the average concentration for the shear operator was 2.2 mg/m^3 and for the tailgate operator, 2.6 mg/m^3.[16] In 1987, it was 2.0 mg/m^3 for the shear operator.

At the United Mine Workers, we calculate annual average for specific mine sections in order to identify those mines that have persistent problems in controlling exposure to respirable dust (TABLE 3). These data demonstrate two factors. First, only a small percentage of continuous mining operators are exposed to annual averages in excess of 2.0 mg/m^3, illustrating that achievements in controlling exposure to respirable dust with this type of mining technology persist. Second, a significantly larger proportion of longwall sections have annual averages over 2.0 mg/m^3, and there is no progress in reducing dust with this type of mining for this period.

This type of analysis can conceal some important problems. First, use of industry-wide averages obscures particular mines with persistent dust problems. Second, even though the percentage of continuous mining sections with annual averages over 2.0 mg/m^3 is very low, because this is the most common mining technology in the industry, this low percentage accounts for the largest number of sections with excess exposure to dust. In fiscal year 1987, for example, there were 76 continuous mining sections, 46 longwall sections, and 20 other sections with annual averages over 2.0 mg/m^3. Third, exposure to respirable dust is not randomly distributed. If one section of a mine is out of compliance, we have found that other sections are more likely to be out of compliance also, and certain mines regularly report excess exposure to respirable dust.[17]

In comparison with limited data on dust exposure before the Act, current exposure is clearly lower and, on average, below the standard of 2.0 mg/m^3. Most progress appears to have occurred within 2 years after the Act was passed. Problems persist with certain mines and with longwall mining methods.

Experience with dust problems on longwall mining suggests a historical trend that runs counter to the need to control dust. That is, each new generation of mining technology seems to produce more dust. In 1982, for example, ordering the practiced mining technologies from oldest to newest, that is, hand loading, conventional mining, continuous mining, and longwall mining, also ranks from the least to the most dusty (TABLE 4).[18]

3. *Pneumoconiosis.* Despite nearly 20 years of epidemiologic research, it has not been easy to demonstrate that the occurrence of pneumoconiosis among U.S. miners has been reduced, largely because of the aforementioned weaknesses in research and monitoring programs. It has barely been possible to agree on terminology.[19] A recent summary of the NSCWP concluded with the disappointingly ambivalent statements that, "The prevalence of [coal workers' pneumoconiosis] appears to have declined over the three rounds [from 1970–1981] of the [surveillance program] and the NSCWP. The main cause of the decline in CWP, seen between round 1 and 3, lies more with population changes than with the effects of preventive measures."[10] The population changes referred to are a substantial reduction in the average age of active miners.

TABLE 3. Percentage of Sections with Annual Average Dust Concentration Greater than 2.0 mg/m^3

Fiscal Year	Continuous Mining	Longwall Mining
1982	—	33.7
1983	—	35.5
1984	3.6	32.8
1985	4.3	37.7
1986	3.1	32.7
1987	3.8	38.4

TABLE 4. Percentage of Dust Samples Greater than 2.0 mg/m^3 by Mining Method, 1982

Method	Percentage Greater than 2.0 mg/m^3	Number of Samples
Hand loading	1.9	1,758
Conventional	10.3	10,058
Continuous	13.4	63,258
Longwall	33.2	2,777

Results from the surveillance program, even though based on a defective data base, show that the prevalence of CWP category 2 declined from 13% in round 1 (1970–1973) to 7% in round 3 (1980–1981) for workers with 35 years' experience. Prevalence of category 1 CWP, for the same population, changed from 14% in round 1 to 23% in round 2 to 17% in round 3, indicating no trend.

DISCUSSION

Regulation under MSHA has been effective. It has reduced the risk of traumatic death in the industry. It has reduced exposure to respirable dust. It appears also to have reduced the occurrence of pneumoconiosis. At the very least, those trends are consistent with the purpose of the 1969 Act and have occurred since its implementation.

Regulation does not occur in a vacuum, however. Fatality rates and trends in exposure to respirable dust rise and fall with many other factors. Some of these other factors include the federal black lung program, government-subsidized research for mine safety, and the presence of the United Mine Workers of America. Current payments to beneficiaries under the black lung program average about $1.6 billion per year and are a direct consequence of neglecting exposure to dust in years past. The federal black lung program may be a rare instance in which compensation is an incentive to control hazards.

In addition, the Bureau of Mines devotes a substantial proportion of its resources to practical research on safer mining technologies. The Bureau was formed in 1905 specifically to promote mine safety and other matters, but many of the products of its research had to wait until change was compelled by regulation. Thus, much of the early success in reducing fatality rates and exposure to respirable dust was made possible by requiring "off the shelf" technology developed by the Bureau.

Another factor is that a large proportion (approximately 75% by hours worked) of underground miners are organized by one union, the United Mine Workers of America. As a union, we have a substantial commitment to the health and safety of our members, with the largest per capita staff and budget of any international union in the United States. We also have extensive contract language with coal mine operators with provisions for training, and workers' rights to refuse unsafe work and health and safety committee rights to shut down sections of mines in the event of imminent danger. Rank and file miners also played a significant role in developing compensation for "black lung."[20]

A recent study that examined the place of unions in occupational health and safety found that workers at unionized plants generally fared better than did their nonunion counterparts, an association strongest in the mining industry. Organized workers succeeded in obtaining more frequent and higher quality inspections and other measures of enforcement activity.[21] Thus, the union is a significant incentive supporting the enforcement of MSHA regulations.

However, significant problems exist with this agency that were brought to light most clearly in the Senate oversight hearings held in March 1987.[22] During the hearings and at other times, it became evident that there were signficant efforts to "deregulate" safety and health in the mining industry, just like there have been at OSHA.

This case study of underground coal mining shows that regulation is effective in achieving the public health objectives of controlling safety and health hazards in the mining industry. Other important factors in the mining industry include a program for compensating workers with black lung, government-subsidized research concerning workplace safety, and a highly organized workforce prepared to exercise its rights through both using regulations and negotiating strong contract language.

REFERENCES

1. National Research Council, Committee on Underground Coal Mine Safety. 1982. Toward Safety Underground Coal Mines. National Academy Press. Washington, DC.
2. U.S. Public Health Service, National Institute for Occupational Safety and Health. 1987. National Traumatic Occupational Fatalities, 1980–1984. NIOSH, Morgantown, West Virginia.
3. 30 U.S.C. 801 *et seq.*
4. Annals of the New York Academy of Sciences. 1972. p. 400.
5. National Research Council, Panel on Occupational Safety and Health Statistics. 1987. Counting Injuries and Illnesses in the Workplace. National Academy Press. Washington, DC.
6. U.S. Department of Labor, Mine Safety and Health Administration. 1984. Summary of Selected Injury Experience and Worktime for the Mining Industry in the United States, 1931–1977. IR 1132. U.S. Government Printing Office. Washington, DC.
7. U.S. Department of Labor, Mine Safety and Health Administration. 1978–1984 (published annually). Injury Experience in Coal Mining. U.S. Government Printing Office, Washington, DC.
8. U.S. Department of Labor, Mine Safety and Health Administration. 1985–1987 (published quarterly). Mine Injuries and Worktime Quarterly. U.S. Government Printing Office. Washington, DC.
9. WEEKS, J. L. & M. B. FOX. 1983. Fatality rates and regulatory policies in bituminous coal mining, United States, 1959–1981. Am. J. Pub. Health **73:** 1278–1280.
10. ATTFIELD, M. 1987. Past, Present and Predicted Future Levels of Coal Workers' Pneumoconiosis in Working U.S. Coal Miners. National Institute for Occupational Safety and Health, Morgantown, West Virginia.
11. ALTHOUSE, R. B. 1985. Ten Years' Experience with the Coal Workers' Health Surveillance Program, 1970–1981. Centers for Disease Control. CDC Surveillance Summaries **34:** 33SS–37SS.
12. BODEN, L. I. & J. GOLD. 1984. The accuracy of self-reported regulatory data: The case of coal mine dust. Am. J. Indus. Med. **6:** 427–440.
13. ATTFIELD, J., R. REGER & R. GLENN. 1984. The incidence and progression of pneumoconiosis over nine years in U.S. coal miners. II. Relationship with dust exposure and other potential causative factors. Am. J. Ind. Med. **7:** 417–426.
14. WEEKS, J. L. (letter). 1986. Trends in fatality rates in bituminous coal mines, 1970–1985. Am. J. Pub. Health **76:** 1151–1152.
15. JACOBSON, M., P. S. PAROBECK, & M. E. HUGHES. 1971. Effect of Coal Mine Health and Safety Act of 1969 on Respirable Dust Concentrations in Selected Underground

Coal Mines. U.S. Department of the Interior, Bureau of Mines. IC 8536. U.S. Government Printing Office. Washington, DC.
16. COSTANTINO, J. 1983. Dust control accomplishments in U.S. underground coal mines. *In* Proceedings—Symposium on Control of Respirable Coal Mine Dust. J. Barrett, J. Jacobson, W. H. Sutherland, G. R. Tinney, & P. M. Turcic, Eds. U.S. Government Printing Office, Washington, DC.
17. WEEKS, J. L. 1984. Mine associated variation in the concentration of respirable coal mine dust in underground bituminous coal mines. *In* Proceedings, Fifteenth Annual Institute on Coal Mining Health, Safety and Research. M. Karmis, W. H. Sutherland, J. R. Lucas, D. R. Forshey, & G. J. Faulkner, Eds. Virginia Polytechnic and State University, Blacksburg, Virginia.
18. WEEKS, J. L. 1983. Survey of current problems in respirable coal mine dust control. *In* Proceedings—Symposium on Control of Respirable Coal Mine Dust. J. Barrett, M. Jacobson, W. W. Sutherland, G. R. Tinney, & P. M. Turcic, Eds. U.S. Government Printing Office. Washington, DC.
19. WEEKS, J. L. & G. R. WAGNER. 1986. Compensation for occupational disease with multiple causes: The case of coal miners' respiratory diseases. Am. J. Pub. Health **76:** 58–61.
20. DERICKSON, A. 1983. Down solid: The origins and development of the black lung insurgency. J. Pub. Health Policy **4:** 25–84.
21. WEIL, D. 1987. Government and labor at the workplace: The role of labor unions in the implementation of federal health and safety policy. Unpublished Ph.D. Thesis. Harvard University, Cambridge, MA.
22. U.S. Congress, Senate. 1987. Committee on Labor and Human Resources. Hearings: Oversight of the Mine Safety and Health Administration. 100th Cong., 1st Sess. U.S. Government Printing Office. Washington, DC.

Occupational Disease Prevention in Canada

A Change of Direction?

GORDON ATHERLEY

President and Chief Executive Officer
Canadian Centre for Occupational Health and Safety
Hamilton, Ontario L8N 1H6, Canada

Worker's health and safety in Canada has made remarkable progress in the past decade. A distinctively Canadian approach has emerged, and important legal and social frameworks have been created. Yet, despite extensive activity directed at prevention, occupation-related disease[a] remains a risk for some working Canadians.

Occupation-related musculoskeletal aches and pains such as back problems reach epidemic proportions. Infectious diseases, notably AIDS and hepatitis B, loom threateningly in the occupations of many workers. Diseases of the skin and respiratory system caused by sensitization to materials in the workplace continue to disable workers. The true incidence of occupation-related cancer remains unknown.

In deciding how to respond to the trends, decision-makers involved in workers' health and safety in Canada are faced with deciding whether the way forward lies with more of the same activity (on the grounds that the situation would have been much worse without the activity of the last decade) or something different (on the grounds that radical change is required).

IMPORTANT INFLUENCES ON WORKERS' HEALTH AND SAFETY IN CANADA

Workers' health and safety in Canada is influenced by the broader community. The environmental movement demonstrates that the public no longer needs convincing about the importance of action on acid rain, PCBs, and all the other industrial chemicals and physical agents that contaminate the natural world. Public opinion surveys confirm that the public expects action. Issues of contamination and pollution wind up on the agendas of politicians and not just the desks of officials. The need to solve problems by elimination of contaminants encourages the ideas that tough anticontamination standards are not necessarily economically retrogressive and that consistent, pan-Canadian approaches may be required.

AIDS exerts a powerful influence on thinking about community health. Health promotion emphasizes provision of information to equip individuals to take better

---

[a] As more diseases are associated with occupation, more multifactorial etiologies are revealed. The qualifier, "occupation-related," seems broader than "occupational," because the latter tends to limit the category to the classical diseases of occupation, which by no means represent the gamut. Occupational deafness increases as a problem, judging from a recent analysis of workers' compensation claims in Alberta.[1]

control over their lives. So far, information is the principal AIDS strategy that governments direct towards the wider public. The strategy aims to give the public greater awareness of the need for control over normally rather private aspects of their lives.

Substance abuse attracts public concern. The extent to which it affects the workplace is unknown. Controversy raised by proposals for mandatory drug testing of workers leads to a broadening consensus that it is not the solution to problems of substance (or alcohol) abuse in Canada, and that it should not be instituted as a general routine.[2] As a byproduct, further questioning is evoked about mandatory biomedical surveillance, which has become an issue in Canada.[3,4] Questions focus on the quality of the defense offered by medical surveillance when used as a backstop; whether the defense is offered to employer or worker; and whether the defense is sufficient to justify the use of law to compel workers to subject themselves to it, to oblige employers to provide it, and to require regulators to enforce it. The issue turns on concerns about whom the data go to, what these are used for, and whether the medical focus that mandatory biomedical surveillance gives to occupation-related disease diverts attention from engineering control.

Influences acting on and generated by governments, employers, and labor within the Canadian world of workers' health and safety currently create contradictory and inconsistent pressures. Fears of the costs of occupational disease, for example, constitute one such pressure.[5] The fear of costs of compensation vies with the fear of costs of prevention. Pressures resulting from disquiet at the nonsolution of problems and the apparent worsening trends are inconsistent because of controversy about the way forward. Labor seeks greater power for workplace health and safety committees. Employers see such proposals as erosion of management's right to manage. Both express impatience with governments' performance as regulators and as operators of the workers' compensation system.

Labor, employers, and governments, however, hail the recent Workplace Hazardous Material Information System, federal-provincial-territorial legislation equivalent to the U.S. Hazard Communication Standard, as an outstanding success in tripartite cooperation in creating forward movement.

STRATEGIES IN REGULATORY ACTIVITY IN CANADIAN OCCUPATIONAL HEALTH AND SAFETY

Regulatory activity aimed at workers' health and safety in Canada is a multijurisdictional responsibility in which the federal government counts as 1 among 10 provincial and 2 territorial governments. The activity invokes technical and social strategy.

Technical strategy in Canada, as elsewhere, produces regulations with detailed and performance specifications for engineering control, personal protection, and, in the case of several disease-related hazards, biomedical surveillance. Technical strategy can reasonably be credited with much of the decline in the "bloody" occupational injuries and certain categories of fatalities, such as trenching collapse. Exactly where the credit should go for the overall favorable trend in fatalities is less clear, because the graph of fatal accidents at work closely follows the ups and downs of fatal transportation accidents. In Canada, as elsewhere, the regulatory responsibilities for the two are separate and distinct.

For the period 1969–1985, the two sets of accident data correlate highly (Spearman's rank correlation coefficient, $r_s = .9$, $z = 3.60$). The data still correlate highly ($r_s = .82$, $z = 3.29$) when allowance is made for year-by-year changes in the employed workforce. The high correlation is a mathematical fact, but it could also be a meaningless association. Until this and other uncertainties are resolved, it is difficult to draw firm conclusions from the workplace fatality data about the general effectiveness of the regulatory activity relative to any other.

The increase in occupation-related disease speaks to a need for evolution of technical strategy. Social strategy reflects the distinctively Canadian element. It is expressed in laws as three rights for workers: to know, to refuse, and to participate. The right to know is legislated in the Workplace Hazardous Material Information System. This important development follows the call by labor union activists during the 1970s to workers to "find out what hurts you in your plant."[6] Like the public at large, the working public is no longer satisfied to leave everything to the experts. Workers want to know for themselves and to equip themselves with trustworthy, intelligible, timely, and relevant information to participate in committees that plan actions to rid workplaces of dangers. And it is not just workers; managers and supervisors often feel that they are inadequately informed on occupational health and safety problems for which they are held responsible.

Right-to-know appears in legislation, actual or proposed, concerned with protection of the environment as well as protection of workers. As a likely and constructive outcome, Canada will develop a well-informed industrial public, wanting cleanup of contamination as the means to prevent and avoid disease linked to environment and occupation. Right-to-know laws help make information a major impulsion in occupational health and safety, one that is facilitated by the electronic information revolution.

The right to refuse means that a worker can expect legal protection if he or she decides not to work with some substance, on some equipment, or in some place because he or she believes that to do so would be dangerous. At first, this protection covered only situations of imminent danger. Subsequently, it began to extend to danger of a continuing nature.

Few data are available from which to judge the impact. Existing impressions suggest that refusal actually occurs only in extreme situations. But the knowledge that it is available to workers seems to stimulate constructive action before situations become extreme. Its true success might not be revealed by the raw data on the number of times it is formally invoked; its real strength may lie in its silent influence.

The right to participate is realized in the joint labor-management health and safety committees that most worksites (other than the smallest) are required to have in nearly all the jurisdictions. These committees are generally regarded as useful developments that need to be well served with information if they are to reach their full potential.[7] Although employers find controversial some government and labor proposals to give committees more power, the committees' continued importance is not in question.

The right to participate is also realized in the tripartite and bipartite structures that govern regulatory activities and, in some instances, workers' compensation. Examples are New Brunswick, Quebec, and soon, the federal Government. Although tripartism grows increasingly attractive owing to its acknowledged achievements (the Canadian Centre for Occupational Health and Safety provides one example), labor-employer bipartism is also being developed in connection with hazardous substances.

As social strategy develops, the niceties of the two isms emerge. Government is not always a partner equal to the other two because officials are seldom completely free to commit their governments to courses of action, whereas representatives of labor and employers may come to the table with full negotiating rights.[8] Impatience with government may be a factor that favors labor-employer bipartism.

INFLUENCE OF THE SOCIAL ON THE TECHNICAL STRATEGIES

The social strategy, whose influence continues to grow, encourages reflection and discussion that foreshadow effects on the technical strategy.

Some proponents advocate what they term the neutral ground, situated well away from the various controversies of employers, labor, and government. They characterize it as objective, excellent, independent, and "good" science.

Criticisms that this ground is scientist-dominated, closed-shop punditry have been responded to with increased openness of the scientific process, notably to labor. But surprise and disappointment ensued with the dissatisfactions that emerged with some of the "open" studies.

The dissatisfactions may signal prerequisites for success when the two isms oversee research into occupation-related disease. Participants may need to share clear understandings of just what the research can and cannot be expected to yield in the way of data and conclusions and with what degree of uncertainty. "Further research is required" may be completely justifiable scientifically, but it is a conclusion that carries a high risk of frustration in tripartite and bipartite projects.

Other proponents advocate the common ground. They define it as what labor, employers, and sometimes governments accept as common ground. What these two or three stakeholders (according to the ism involved) finally identify as the common ground tends to be solution-seeking action on problems. What they always seem to stress in retrospect is the importance of confidence and mutual trust. What seems always to surprise them, if the Workplace Hazardous Materials Information System and the Centre's workshops are any general indication, is how broad the common ground really was when they got right down to it.

Enthusiasts characterize the common ground as dominated by common sense, consensus, and trustworthiness. They point to the way information causes disquiet with the status quo, so that the need for change itself becomes the common ground. Skeptics see the search for a common ground as too unscientific and altogether too "social."

Because they rely to such an extent on information, stakeholders exploring for the common ground tend to become impatient with scientific research, although their own vehicle of discovery is often cumbersome and slow. Some professionals and scientists view information as not quite the "real thing" of occupational health and safety, unlike research. Yet analyzing and interpreting scientific information reveals gaps in knowledge and opens up opportunities for research.

Emphasis on information creates a prerequisite for information parity, in which all stakeholders come to the table equally well briefed with excellent, impartial information. The prerequisite puts a premium on excellent, impartial information providers. With the experience of exploring for the common ground has arrived some understanding of its nature and the factors that the search for it involves.

Common ground and consensus, although closely related terms, should probably not be used as synonyms. Common ground is something that preexists, that awaits discovery, and that can be extended by exploration. It is not threatened by acknowledgments that it is bordered by territory that is not common. Consensus is concord or agreement of opinion often arrived at after discussion in which participants move position. "Failure to arrive at consensus" carries an unsuccessful implication.

Demanding that participants reach a consensus may be inhibiting, especially when troublesome issues are on the agenda. Requesting them to identify and describe any ground that they have in common may be a more encouraging start to a process that could well lead to consensus if allowed to run its natural course.

The terms stakeholder and participant probably should be separated cautiously. Stakeholders hold a stake, defined as something at risk. Participants have a legitimate interest in participating, but have nothing major to lose in the way that stakeholders have. In an arena as diverse as workers' health and safety, it can be difficult to establish clear-cut rules and procedures to limit involvement to stakeholders, who understandably resist the intrusions of parties whose interest seems not to qualify them for stakeholder status. In informal processes, progress may result most rapidly when everyone is referred to as a participant. "Stakeholder" is probably best confined to formal, highly structured processes that lead directly to decision-making.

Some of the factors for success in tripartite and bipartite searches for common ground include: (1) multiway and reciprocal sensitivities to the constraints acting on participants; and (2) wide recognition that the common ground is finite and limited and that pushing too hard threatens the process and ultimately reduces the chances of arriving at consensus. Despite these seeming constraints, experience with the process suggests that the common ground expands rather than contracts as the process develops.

RESEARCH AND SCIENTIFIC ACTIVITY

An important difference emerges between gatherings of researchers and bipartite or tripartite workshops. The former naturally enough see ideas for further research as an outcome of prime importance, whereas the latter seek solutions to problems.

Calls for action on solutions to workplace problems, which seem likely to increase as bipartite and tripartite processes spread, may move research and scientific development into an increasingly technical and engineering orientation. For example, the common ground at a 1987 workshop on workplace back injury included a clearly worded statement that the problem was to be solved by changes in the workplace.[9]

Movement of the orientation of research highlights a divergence of direction for research and scientific activity aimed at occupation-related disease. In one direction, the epidemiologic approach focuses on disorders of bodily constituents and functions, diseases, and deaths of persons contaminated by noxious factors of the workplace or the general environment. In the other, the environmental approach concentrates on the contaminants and the contaminators rather than the contaminated persons. In theory, the two approaches complement each other, because it seems useful to correlate the consequences and the contamination.

But the limitations of real-world data, which epidemiologists are the first to acknowledge, are such that uncertainty may well be irreducible even with the most refined epidemiologic technique. Epidemiologists rightly qualify their conclusions and call for further data. But the almost constant need to continue or enlarge studies may just be starting to diminish enthusiasm for correlation-seeking.

Efforts to combat the problem of the irreducible uncertainty diverge. One stream moves to more localized data, that is, data that focus on specifics. With computers, narrative and descriptive information, as distinct from purely numerical data, can be stored, searched for, and analyzed with increasing facility. The other stream flows towards greater data bulks, through record linkage. For examples see the Appendix.

Administrative processes, largely workers' compensation, provide most of the vital statistics related to occupational health and safety in Canada. Localized data are seldom available from these sources, even as a byproduct. Collecting localized data often requires new procedures, which can be expensive to create and operate.

Data linkage among the data collected as byproducts of administrative or regulatory purposes occasionally runs afoul of public concerns about privacy of medical and personal data. Canada possesses increasingly strict laws to maintain privacy of such records against unauthorized intrusion, electronic or otherwise.

OVERVIEW

Early in 1988, it is possible to say that support in Canada for the idea of the common ground could impart sufficient momentum to alter technical strategies underpinning regulatory effort and to reorient research and scientific activity. It is arguable that worker-employer knowledge has emerged as the single most influential factor in Canadian occupational health and safety today.

REFERENCES

1. ALLEYNE, B. C., R. M. DUFRESNE, N. KANJI & M. R. REESAL. Costs of workers' compensation claims for hearing loss. 1989. J. Occup. Med. **31:** 134–138.
2. Drug testing in the workplace: Proceedings of the Workshop, Hamilton, Ontario, June 9 and 10, 1987. 1987. Canadian Centre for Occupational Health and Safety, Hamilton, Ontario.
3. Occupational medicine, medical surveillance and human rights: The way forward: Proceedings of the Workshop, Hamilton, Ontario, March 19–21, 1986. 1986. Canadian Centre for Occupational Health and Safety, Hamilton, Ontario.
4. Health surveillance of workers: The report of the Task Force on Health Surveillance of Workers. 1986. Can. J. Pub. Health **77:** 91–99.
5. Study calls for public inquiry: WCB costs bankrupting small business, CFIB. 1988. Can. Occup. Health & Safety News **11:** 1–2.
6. BOUDREAU, E. 1988. Personal communication.
7. Advisory Council on Occupational Health and Occupational Safety. 1987. Ninth annual report: April 1, 1986 to March 31, 1987. Vol. 56. Queen's Printer for Ontario, Toronto, Ontario.
8. O'CONNELL, M. 1987. Personal communication.
9. Workplace back injuries: Proceedings of the Workshop, Hamilton, Ontario, November 12–13, 1987. 1988. Canadian Centre for Occupational Health and Safety, Hamilton, Ontario.

APPENDIX: EXAMPLES OF DATA COLLECTION FOR EPIDEMIOLOGIC PURPOSES

1. Localized data. These capitalize on the storage capabilities of computers and present at least three variations.

a. Narrative descriptions. These are recorded in considerable detail for defined categories of accident. Examples are the MINING INCIDENTS and FATALITIES data bases currently being built by the Centre in cooperation with the Chief Inspectors of Mines in the various Canadian jurisdictions and the provincial coroners, respectively.

b. Comprehensive data on workplace contaminants and the steps taken to control them. These are numerical and narrative and can be highly detailed. An example is the NOISE LEVELS data base being developed by the Centre. It stores noise levels measured at specific machines, together with data on engineering noise control and the use of hearing protectors.

c. Exposure data. These would be recorded so that individual workers' exposures to hazardous chemical and other agents could be logged throughout their working lifetimes. The data bases would be used to evaluate occupational histories with far greater reliability than is presently possible. The data bases would be logical developments of (a) and (b) and obvious candidates for record linkage, but they would create legal issues of individual privacy. At the time of this writing, no operational example could be identified in the public domain in Canada.

2. Record linkage. Canada possesses a unique resource in the form of a machine-readable mortality data base with records dating back as far as 1950, plus a system for linking them to other files of personal or medical information. Although several studies have successfully focused on occupation-related disease, linkage with occupation is acknowledged to need further development. For further information see: D. B. Petrie. 1986. "Computerized record linkage, long term follow-up and Statistics Canada. In proceedings of the Workshop on Computerized Record Linkage in Health Research. University Press, Toronto.

Occupational Health Sciences and Practice in the 1990s

International Perspectives

M. A. EL BATAWI

*World Health Organization Collaborating Center
Department of Occupational Health Sciences
New York College of Osteopathic Medicine of the
New York Institute of Technology
Old Westbury, New York 11568*

The rapidly changing work environment and methods, increased dependence on automation, success in hygienic control of many chemicals by bringing them to lower concentration levels, and the demographic shift of working populations from production to services in industrialized countries are all factors influencing the scientific trends in research and development in occupational health and its practice.

These changes are occurring at a time in which an increasing number of countries are starting primary health care and health promotion in the workplace to deal with long-standing health problems of underserved working populations in small industries and agriculture; these have largely been unattended in many parts of the world, including some highly industrialized countries. These factors, in addition to industrialization of developing countries, are reformulating occupational sciences and approaches.

This paper presents a brief review of the highlights of modern and future trends in occupational health. This review can in no way be comprehensive of the vast areas that need to be addressed.

MAJOR TRENDS FOR THE 1990s

Protection and Promotion of Workers' Health

Despite the traditional understanding of health protection *and promotions* as the primary objectives of occupational health (ILO/WHO, 1950), some countries, such as the United States of America, identify "health promotion in the workplace" as a separate discipline on its own to be carried out by completely independent groups of health workers other than occupational health personnel. Some other countries have initiated a number of essentially preventive health programs such as cessation of smoking among working people and control of alcohol and drug abuse as "health promotion" activities. In some countries, such programs are almost nonexistent.

As for health protection of workers including preventive occupational hygiene measures, placement health examinations, and health education, the scope of coverage in many industrialized and developing countries is limited to large and some medium-sized industries. The quality of health protection measures leaves much to be desired. For example, the application of ergonomics is limited to a small proportion of workplaces. Job enlargement as a means of preventing monotony and psychologic stress is rarely found in real practice.

Workers are becoming more aware of their rights to health and safety in the workplace. Many developing countries have instituted occupational health as a component of health care systems. Industrialized countries are discovering more evidence that investment in health protection and promotion is morally and economically rewarding. The 1990s will witness a new era in occupational health practice.

Emphasis on Workers' Participation and Life-Style

As worker's health problems are increasingly becoming recognized as multifactorial, and with the diminishing role of specific occupational hazards in disease causation, the role of the workers themselves in preventive health care will become essential. Their knowledge about work processes and hazards, as well as safe work practices, is presently a priority in vocational training and in safety education. Workers' life-style, including diet, exercise, and smoking and drinking habits are key factors in health. The workplace has always been a good setting for workers' education on these aspects.

The Underserved Working Population

The health problems of a major sector of the labor force throughout the world, particularly those employed in small industries, agriculture, and small mining operations, will continue to be of serious magnitude. More knowledge about the magnitude of their complex health problems, particularly in the Third World, may become available as more surveys and service units progress. An easy solution to health and safety problems will not be readily available, particularly in view of the following factors:

1. The long-standing heritage of occupational health as a discipline of labor administration with a limited role or no role for national health systems. Although this is gradually changing, the recognition of workers' health as a priority in public health will probably take time in many countries;

2. The limited effectiveness of occupational health legislation and workplace inspection;

3. The shortage of trained personnel in occupational health coupled with the need to improve and upgrade the training objectives and content that are available at present; and

4. The economic difficulties in many Third World countries that are likely to continue during most of the next decade.

Trends in Training of Occupational Health Personnel

Present training and education programs have to be adapted to the new dimensions of occupational health practice and science. Clearly, there are major changes that require reconsideration of training objectives and content. These changes include: (a) new policies on primary health care strategies insofar as underserved workers are concerned; (b) new needs resulting from modern technology development; and (c) new approaches to health promotion at work.

Occupational health resources are also in need of strengthening almost everywhere. Undergraduate medical training should include occupational health as an essential component; an increasing number of medical schools are providing more hours to occupational health.

In a recent survey by WHO and its collaborating center in the Republic of Singapore, of 532 medical schools in different parts of the world, it was found that the developing countries are probably more keen about "obligatory" courses in occupational medicine than are many industrialized countries (TABLE 1). At the postgraduate level, however, the number of departments of occupational health in the schools of medicine or public health has more than doubled in the last 10 years in developing countries. These presently exist in no less than 40 countries in the Third World.

TABLE 1. Teaching of Occupational Health in Medical Schools[a]

Region	No. of Schools Surveyed	Occupational Health Obligatory	
		No.	%
Africa	34	28	82.3
Asia	214	156	72.9
Europe	155	109	70.4
Middle East	17	10	58.8
North America	112	54	48.2
Total	532	357	

[a] Data from the Department of Community Medicine, University of Singapore.

Occupational Health Sciences

Occupational Toxicology

The most outstanding expected evolution will concern internationally recommended *health-based* occupational exposure limits of toxic substances. The old methods for setting these standards may gradually disappear. Instead, as initiated by WHO, exposure limits will become a two-step procedure. The first is international agreement on health-based exposure limits, taking into account all internationally available scientific, experimental, and epidemiologic information in east and west, north and south, for examination by international committees in which East European countries will be represented. The second step is to be undertaken by national authorities in each country who will decide on *operational* limits suited for their own technologic, economic, and other factors.

Neurobehavioral Toxicology

The central nervous system is the most complex functional entity. Much is known about it, particularly in the behavioral and emotional areas. Neurotoxins constitute hundreds of thousands of chemicals about which limited information is available in spite of much advanced modern research. Even less is known about early or delayed behavioral changes due to chemical exposure. The next decade will build on the present findings, with a view to detecting and evaluating neurobehavioral toxicity at an early stage.

Occupational Toxicology of Reproduction

The fact that many chemicals have been found to produce reproductive damage in males and females is alarming. Much has been learned about chemical carcinogenesis and occupational cancer; much less is known about genotoxicity, teratogenicity, and mutagenicity in humans. There is increasing evidence of an existing relation between chemical exposure and sterility in males and females, fetotoxicity leading to abortion or stillbirth, congenital malformation, and childhood cancer. The scope of epidemiology here is obvious, although difficult, but such research must start now and grow before the turn of the century, probably through well-organized registers.

Immunotoxicology

This new field is concerned with the study of adverse affects on the immune system resulting from interaction with toxic chemicals. These adverse effects may result as a consequence of: (1) a direct or indirect action of the compound and/or its metabolite on the immune system; and (2) an immunologically based host response to the compound or its metabolites, or the host antigens modified by the compound or its metabolites. Much more knowledge is needed in the study of altered immunologic events associated with exposure of humans and animals to toxic chemicals, the study of allergy and autoimmunity caused by xenobiotics, and the study of techniques used in immunocytochemistry.

Work-Related Diseases

To what extent do work and occupational factors play a role in causation of multifactorial health problems of mankind? What is the relation between adverse psychosocial stress and coronary heart disease, hypertension, back syndrome, and allergic manifestations? To what extent does so-called "inert" dust in the workplace affect the respiratory system and the course of chronic obstructive pulmonary disease including occupational asthma? How can ergonomics be applied to prevent musculoskeletal health problems, so highly prevalent among working populations? What are the extra-auditory effects of noise and of total body vibration on the various vital systems of the body? Is it possible to quantify stress in the workplace and its health effects in a manner that would allow for monitoring and early intervention to prevent advanced health damage and even suicide? These and many other questions on work-related diseases must be addressed to elucidate where the causal relationship is *in part* rather than *in toto*, as in the case of specific and classical occupational diseases. The application of epidemiology is a foremost necessity in the study of work-related multifactorial health problems. No occupational health professional may be qualified without adequate epidemiologic experience.

CONCLUSIONS

The 1990s will witness an ascent and increased priority for occupational health in all aspects: broader and more challenging areas of research, attention to the long-neglected working populations in developing and industrialized countries, much more self-reliance and workers' participation with an impact on life-style of workers and consequently their families, and new approaches to workers' health care that are more coordinated and interactive with community health.

These challenges and approaches require the vigorous and dynamic efforts by leaders of occupational health and the close international cooperation in research and training with the noble objective of preventing disease and promoting health of working populations in the world.

Lessons from the UK[a]

MORRIS GREENBERG[b]

74 North End Road
London NW11 7SY, England

The lesson that may be learned from the United Kingdom is that for establishing, developing, and maintaining programs for the promotion of occupational safety and health, the following features are required: (1) the appropriate political philosophy, will, and power; (2) effective legislation; (3) adequate resources and organization to be provided for its implementation; (4) the recruitment and support of persons of outstanding caliber with a variety of talents required for devising and operating the programs involved; (5) the collection of adequate data and their systematic analysis for evaluating the effectiveness of control measures and to determine areas for priority action; (6) periodic review of the adequacy of provisions for health and safety at work in the light of technologic change and expectations. In the process, revolution and evolution within the law were required.

In support of this thesis a brief summary of key political events over the past three centuries in the United Kingdom and stages in the development of occupational safety and health policy will be presented. It would be presumptuous to pretend to be offering new insights; however, some comfort and moral support are to be found from the observation that they do not necessarily do these things much better abroad and that the constraints on arriving at the birth of an occupational safety and health millenium are universal in nature.

In 1688 the Stuart dynasty was expelled, and James II, replaced by William and Mary, headhunted from the Netherlands. The Whig party then aimed onwards for the subordination of the power of the Crown to that of Parliament and the upper classes. The first attempt at reform by William Pitt in 1785 failed, as did the second by John Russell in 1831. The following year saw the successful passage of the Reform Bill under the Earl of Grey. One of the first actions of the Reform Parliament was to set up a Commission in April 1833 to report on the conditions of employment in textile factories. The Commission reported promptly and Government acted no less promptly to place on the statute book on August 29, 1833, "An Act to regulate labour of children and young persons in Mills and Factories of the United Kingdom." This included regulation of minimum age of employment, hours of work, and education. It marked the beginning of effective legislation for occupational safety and health. Prior to this, at the end of the 18th century, there had been a proliferation of factories producing textiles, mostly away from the center of government. The political and economic philosophy was that of laissez-faire: government intervention in conditions of employment was considered inexpedient in practice and wrong in principle. Poor Law, going back some 200 years to Queen Elizabeth I, still operated: young paupers who were a charge on the parishes in the South were transported to the North as "apprentices" in the textile mills. As a result of the itinerant investigative journalists of the late 18th

---

[a] The contents of this article represent the author's views alone and in no way reflect those of the Department of Health or the Health and Safety Executive.

[b] Address for correspondence: Division of Environmental and Occupational Health, Mt. Sinai School of Medicine, New York, New York 10029.

century, the depraved conditions under which children worked and lived in the mills were revealed.

An Act was passed in 1802 to do something about their health and morals. It being recognized that legislation without means for reinforcement was ineffective, it was arranged for a magistrate and clergyman to make regular visits to factories. The ignorance or complacency of these visitors was considered responsible for the worthlessness of such visits that were made. Some attempts were made subsequently to improve the Law by extending its benefits to "free" children. It remained, however, for the political reform of 1832 and the will to action for a proper start to be made on an effective program of occupational safety and health legislation, the development of which still continues.

The 1833 Act was an enabling one that permitted the King to appoint four persons of equal status to be Inspectors of Factories and places where the labor of children and young persons under the age of 18 years of age may be employed. They had powers of entry at all hours, could require any person to give evidence under oath, and for a short period had powers of judging and sentencing.

The Civil Service at the time had still to undergo reform. It was small, and appointment was made by political influence: an independent body of Commissioners and entrance examinations were for the future.

Nevertheless, although loyal Whigs were appointed, they were of such outstanding caliber that they pitted themselves against the resistance of the manufacturers. (There were, of course, a few employers such as Robert Owen who demonstrated that humane conditions of employment were compatible with a prosperous enterprise.) When one of the original four found the pressure too great, he was promptly replaced by another Whig of impeccable loyalty: a James Stuart of truly outstanding character, whose curriculum vitae included killing a political rival in a duel (acquitted—"death by misadventure"), followed by a period of financial embarrassment, relieved by a stay of a few years in America, from whence he returned to the UK to edit a newspaper before being recruited as an Inspector. Of two of his colleagues no records remain, but they were believed to be men of substance and education who had held positions in the world before their appointment. The other was Leonard Horner, a gifted man of humble origins who was elected Fellow of the Royal Society for distinguished work in geology. A fervent Benthamite (the highest morality lay in the pursuit of the greatest happiness of the greatest number), he was chosen to be the first Warden of University College London, from which post he was recruited as Inspector. He continued as Inspector for 26 years, evolving into Chief Inspector in due course.

With no rules or precedents to guide them, the quadrumvirate first set out to contact the owners of all 3,000 textile factories to explain the new legislation. Many of the owners were surprisingly cooperative and eager to understand the interpretation of the Act. A system of Regional Superintendents and sub-Inspectors was set up to carry out the day-to-day inspections. Travel was hard and employers and workmen could be hostile: in 1836 one sub-Inspector sustained a broken leg in the course of inspection and another was mobbed by workmen en route. (The difference in reception between the various members of the hierarchy may have depended on differences in their social class. Effectiveness as an Inspector, whatever the social class, has always depended on the exceptional caliber of the individual. Slight young Inspectors of gentle nurture can be as persuasive and forceful and effective as older, more robust-appearing individuals.)

Amendment to the 1833 Act was soon under discussion. The 1844 Act required the fencing of dangerous machinery and the reporting of dangerous accidents. With the expansion of legislative provisions, the organization of the Inspectorate also developed. In 1879 a new Factories Act gave comprehensive cover to some 110,000 factories and workshops with 44 Inspectors, and set the seal on an organization based on divisions and districts that lasted into the 1970s when 379,000 factories were served by 564 Inspectors. Apart from relatively minor changes in organization and the enlargement of the scope of the Factories Acts which were carried out piecemeal, with the provision of special controls for certain specific industrial activities, and a great proliferation of statutory instruments, for some years consolidation was the order of the day. Study of the Annual Reports of HM Chief Inspector of Factories gives a fascinating view of the problems and successes of a remarkable band of men and women, increasingly including engineering, scientific, and medical specialists to deal with the complexities of industry, safety, and health.

Although considerable progress had been made, discontent with the level of persisting accidents and disease led in May 1970 to a further Commission being established (Robens) to review the provision made for health and safety at work and to consider whether changes were needed in the scope or nature of the legal requirements, and the nature and extent of voluntary action. They also considered whether any further steps were required to protect the public from hazards arising from activities in industrial and commercial premises and construction sites, other than from environmental pollution. They consulted widely and investigated the situation abroad. They concluded that there was too much law, too much of which was intrinsically unsatisfactory and which now comprised nine main groups of statutes, some 500 subordinate instruments containing in detail provisions of varying length and complexity, growing at the rate of 100 a year. The elaboration, detail, and complexity, coupled with the language and style, rendered it repellent and unintelligible to those it was intended to influence. Many provisions were out of date with modern technology and knowledge. Interpretation was presenting problems even to Inspectors and industrial experts.

People became conditioned to look on health and safety at work as being effected by developing detailed rules imposed by outside agencies with higher standards to be achieved by more frequent factory inspections. The Commissioners held that the primary responsibility for doing something about current occupational accidents and disease lay with those who created the risk and those who worked with them: they recommended that less reliance be placed on state regulation and more on personal responsibility and personal effort.

They also considered that the fragmentation of administrative jurisdiction, with nine separate groups of statutes (factories; commercial premises; mines and quarries; agriculture; explosives; petroleum; nuclear installations; radioactive waste disposal; alkali emissions), divided among five government departments and seven separate Inspectorates, was inefficient.

The Commissioners concluded that a more unified and integrated system was required for the State's contribution to health and safety at work, but more fundamentally they stressed the severely practical limits to the effectiveness of negative regulation by external agencies and the desirability for a more effective self-regulating system.

Among the various recommendations made were the following critical ones:
1. The establishment of an autonomous National Authority for Health and Safety at Work unifying the current separate inspectorates.
2. New statutory arrangements should be made to increase the effectiveness of the State's contribution and to provide a framework for better self-regulation in the form of a new enabling Act, giving a clear statement of the basic principles of responsibility, supported by regulations and greater reliance on nonstatutory codes of practice.

3. Industry level organization linking management and union, with each devoting more resources to safety and health.

4. The National Authority to be composed of people drawn from the relevant fields of experience and interest.

The report was presented to Parliament in July 1972, and within a relatively short period the Health and Safety at Work Act of 1974 came into being. In view of the extent and complexity of the perceived problem, the execution was in no way inferior to the 1832 reform. The Act clearly stated that it should be the duty of every employer to ensure, so far as is reasonably practicable, the health, safety, and welfare at work of all his employees. That duty extended to include: provision of plant and systems of work; safe handling, storage, and transport of articles and substances; and provision of appropriate information, instruction, training, and supervision. Employers were to be required to prepare a written statement of general policy on health and safety at work and the organization and arrangements for carrying out that policy and bringing it and any reasons to the notice of all employees. Provisions were made for employees to be represented on safety committees. A requirement to conform to the Act was also placed on self-employed persons. Persons designing, manufacturing, importing, or supplying any article for use at work were required to make it safe, to test it, and to provide adequate information about use and maintenance.

There was also a duty placed on employees to take care of themselves and others. A standing Health and Safety Commission was established by the Secretary of State for Employment, to comprise no less than six and no more than nine commissioners that he would appoint, three from employers' organizations, three from employees' organizations, and others as appropriate. A three-man executive was created to exercise, on behalf of the Commission, its functions as directed. Under the Executive were gathered together a group of Inspectorates from the various Ministries. The Commission was empowered to set up advisory committees. It has established 7 subject advisory committees, including 1 on toxic substances and another on medical matters, and 11 industry committees. All of these are tripartite with membership agreed by both sides of industry.

This latest initiative on Safety and Health at Work was developed in the heady days of the 1970s. Its success depends on the extent to which the six features listed at the start of this paper are implemented. In providing for the 1990s, as for the 1830s and 1970s, a review of the shortcomings of the current system and proposals for their remedy is called for, supported by the political will for their remedy, the provision of the appropriate resources for tackling the problems, and the recruitment of outstanding persons to devise and operate the system.

Worker Safety

A Role for the Court?

T. ALEXANDER HICKMAN
Chief Justice
Supreme Court of Newfoundland
Trial Division
Newfoundland, Canada

It is, for me, both a pleasure and a privilege to address this distinguished and important Conference. Some of you may have known, prior to my introduction, that I am from Newfoundland; some may even know where it is. I suspect that few of you have heard of, let alone can place, my home town of Grand Bank, a long-established fishing community on Newfoundland's Burin Peninsula. The hazards of the workplace are well known to anyone from Grand Bank. Indeed, it may be difficult to visualize a workplace more fraught with danger than the ice-slick deck of a dragger as she challenges the North Atlantic in winter. When the ocean claims a dragger and her crew, as has happened on too many occasions, it is also difficult to appreciate the bonds of grief that draw together the members of a community, and indeed all residents of Newfoundland, into a sorrowing family.

I speak to you then from a background in which working men routinely and knowingly risked, and indeed still risk, their lives to pursue their calling. I speak to you also from a background of 20 years in the practice of law, 13 years in Government, and, since 1979, the judiciary. More recently, the experience of chairing the Royal Commission on the Ocean Ranger Marine Disaster has added substantially to my awareness of issues relating to the safety of the workplace. I propose to discuss with you what I perceive to be the appropriate role of the courts in dealing with issues relating to the safety and well-being of the worker.

It is my view that when a matter relating to worker safety reaches the court, it is generally an indication that one or more of those persons or organizations primarily responsible for maintaining a safe working environment have failed—a mistake has been made, a regulation has been broken, someone may have been negligent, and a human being has suffered. As an aside, when we gather in distinguished company to discuss and debate issues as important as these, it is all too easy to lose sight of the injured worker.

If the court is to play any role in dealing with employment-related injuries and safety of the worker, it is necessary that the court be accessible to the injured worker and other interested parties. I had occasion to consider recently whether or not our new *Canadian Charter of Rights and Freedoms* enabled a worker to sue his or her employer, notwithstanding provisions in the workers' compensation legislation that precluded recourse to the courts. The *Charter* section in question, s. 15 (1), came into force on April 17, 1985 and reads as follows:

> 15.(1) Every individual is equal before and under the law and has the right to the equal protection and equal benefit of the law without discrimination and, in particular, without discrimination based on race, national or ethnic origin, colour, religion, sex, age or mental or physical disability.

It was argued that the removal by legislation of the right of recourse to the court and of the right to perhaps greater compensation than would be available under the legislation, created an inequality that was discriminatory. I ruled that in the circumstances and under the provisions of the *Charter,* the right to sue could not be abrogated. My ruling was later overturned by the Newfoundland Court of Appeal. Since this case, or at least the issues raised by it, will in all likelihood come before the Supreme Court of Canada, it would be most inappropriate for me to comment further on the issue it raises. I mention it only to point out that behind all the evidence, behind all the legal argument, behind all the scholarly debate lies a father and husband electrocuted on a bakery floor.

Following my decision, a Superior Court Justice in Alberta concluded that because an injured employee was precluded from suing *any* employer covered by the compensation scheme, the equality provisions of the *Charter* were offended. This decision was made on narrower grounds than mine, but as I have said, I believe and indeed hope that the whole question of workers' recourse to the court will soon be considered by the Supreme Court of Canada.

Although I cannot debate the legal issues involved in these cases, I can say that historically, workers' compensation legislation was enacted in response to a social need and did not initially eliminate the worker's right to go to court. However, in the United Kingdom, the courts had difficulty in accepting the concept of liability without fault, with the result that absolute jurisdiction was given to the Workers' Compensation Boards. In Ontario, the first compensation legislation was enacted based on the report of the Honourable Sir William Ralph Meredith, Chief Justice of Ontario. Because of the difficulties encountered by workers in meeting the common-law defenses of *volens*, common employment, and contributory negligence, Chief Justice Meredith recommended that workers be precluded from suing their own employers in return for guaranteed compensation funded by all employers. The legislation was subsequently amended to prevent actions against any employer or employee covered by the compensation scheme, and this is now the practice across Canada. This system, however, is one of two compensation schemes. In the United Kingdom and some other jurisdictions, the right of court action coexists with an absolute right of recovery of established workers' compensation benefits.

The evolution of the compensation scheme has been described as a trade-off between employees and employers. Historically, this is not correct. Employees were never involved or consulted, and it cannot be said that they agreed to give up their common-law rights.

However, even if full access to the court were available, it must be remembered that the court is not a guarantor of safety. Although there are mechanisms in law that allow judges to establish and require increasingly high standards of conduct from those in the workplace, it is a fallacy to believe that the availability of access to the courts will ensure a safe workplace. What the courts can do, and in my opinion should do, is to appreciate and understand the differing roles of those whose actions affect the workplace, and to reflect appropriately the values of society in establishing acceptable levels of conduct from those participants.

The relative roles of those responsible for safety in the workplace have changed considerably over the years and are continuing to evolve as workers and society in general look for greater assurance that a workplace presents an acceptable level of risk. The responsibilities of the worker, the employer, unions, and government have been and are being defined both by government and by the courts, as they respond to tragedies such as the Ocean Ranger disaster, to technologic change, and to societal pressures.

Just as it is a mistake to view the court as a guarantor of safety, so is it to look to governments to provide a detailed regulatory regimen that will govern every facet and aspect of the workplace. Not only would such a regimen be complex, cumbersome, and all but unenforceable, but also it would foster the illusion that, through the exercise of its regulatory jurisdiction, the government is representing any given workplace as safe. No government can or should do this.

In Report Two of the Royal Commission on the Ocean Ranger Marine Disaster, we stated, and I quote:

> There are those who seek reduction of risks through increased regulation. During the past few decades, there has been a great increase in regulatory control without comparable discernible benefit. Regulations do not of themselves ensure safety and may be counterproductive in their consequences. Responsibility for safety may become a complacent acceptance of rules and regulations, and the evolving technology that is applied may be only as good as the rule and the rule formulators. Those who argue for greater regulatory control ignore the ever-present human element. The human element in safety in this context has two basic dimensions. It is expressed in the judgments that determine the characteristics of the equipment of the personnel coming together to constitute a MODU operating at a particular time and place. Designers, builders, owners, operators and regulators working as part of an evolving industry all influence this outcome. Second, the human element is expressed in the quality of the judgments made in resolving the balance between safety and productivity during operations. These judgments are guided by a fabric of safe practices carried out by the personnel on board. Thus, here too, safety depends fundamentally on human integrity, judgment and competence. Regulation can establish performance standards in critical areas of technology and operating practices but it cannot encompass the many dimensions of human behaviour that contribute to or detract from safety.[1]

Although this was written in the context of the offshore oil industry, I believe it is applicable to any endeavor.

Human behavior is the key to safety. The mere fact that a regulation exists will not ensure actual behavior in compliance with that regulation. A regulation or statute expresses government's opinion on a particular practice or item of equipment. The regulation may or may not reflect society's opinion or values, and it may or may not coincide with what is considered appropriate by workers and employers. Because regulations cannot cover every foreseeable circumstance, and because in certain situations compliance with regulations may in fact fall short of an acceptable standard of conduct, it follows that the primary responsibility for the maintenance of a safe workplace must rest on those whose judgment daily influences the worker. I speak of the worker and the employer.

Having sat through numerous trials involving an assessment of human conduct, having participated in the dissection of the Ocean Ranger accident, and even now listening to evidence analyzing a mishap in the administration of justice in Nova Scotia, I remain convinced that accidents and mishaps are more often than not attributable to lapses in the judgment of those directly involved. Furthermore, it is not uncommon for a number of unrelated shortcomings, through unfortunate coincidence, to form a chain leading to an avoidable accident.

There is no substitute for the unwavering application of sound judgment by individual workers and employers. If there is indeed anything that will approach a guarantee of worker safety, this is it.

When an accident does occur, it is, I believe, a proper role for the courts to assess whether or not the judgments exercised by those involved paid due regard to safety. This, of course, requires a court to understand what safety is—what is the goal to be achieved? Again, with your permission, I quote from the Ocean Ranger Report:

> But, what is safety? The term in its human context has no meaning except in relation to potential risk of harm. It is essentially a relative term, the complement of risk. Risk is not new to our times and place. It has been a pervasive and persistent factor of man's condition since the beginning of life. It remains a constant companion, since man is daily at risk whether at home, at work, or on the highway. It is a feature of everyday life nor can it be avoided. There is no such thing as absolute safety; all that is achievable is a state or condition that can be deemed to be "safe enough"—acceptable to society and capable of being tolerated by those directly involved.
>
> Human perception of risk varies whether the perception is individual or public, whether the risk is voluntary or imposed. The perception also varies with time, with place, and with the context of the activity. Man, individually, takes risks voluntarily and routinely that would cause a collective uproar if imposed to the same degree by a corporate or public body. We are loath to have others do unto us what we consciously do unto ourselves. Perception of risk is highly colored by the culture of a society and the context within that culture in which the activity takes place. Risks accepted as normal in some cultures would not be tolerated in others. The risks faced by a roustabout on an oil rig or a sailor on a ship are peculiarly different from those of an office worker on land. The risks encountered by those who earn their living on the sea or as steelriggers on high-rise structures may appear highly dangerous and recklessly undertaken to a prairie farmer. Perceptions change over time, and risks of years ago would not be acceptable to society today.
>
> Many factors influence our perception of risk. One of the most potent of them is fear of the unknown—of the future side effects of current scientific enterprises and of new technologies; of radiation, for example, undetected by any of the senses, the effects of which may be long delayed even to the next generation. Another factor is the size of the disaster, real or apprehended. The crash of a large aircraft, the loss of a semi-submersible, the collision of a school bus at a railroad crossing cause shock and an outcry for improved safety measures. And yet, hundreds more people are killed in automobile accidents and die unnoticed except for those close to them. It is also a curious feature of human nature that a society which balks at heavy expenditures to prevent possible accidents and which permits, for example, a lack of protective covering over a well will spend unlimited sums to rescue a child who has fallen into one.[2]

A court should, I believe, try to reflect the standards of society when establishing an acceptable standard of conduct. One of the hallmarks of the common law is that it remains infinitely flexible. In any given set of facts—and I can assure you that, despite protestations from many able counsel, no two situations are alike—a court can assess whether or not the standard of conduct is currently acceptable. Ever since the lady found the snail in her bottle of ginger beer, courts have imposed ever higher standards on those whose actions may, given a reasonable application of foresight, cause harm to others.

A court, of course, can only react. It cannot search out cases on its own initiative—it cannot call conduct and standards into question unless someone complains. But in ruling on the complaint that is brought before it, a court is able to give an indication of the standards of conduct that are considered acceptable, and in so doing, it hopefully influences for the better those who would engage in similar activities in the future.

The conduct of others in the future is of little consequence to the complainant who appears before the court. He or she wants "justice," usually in the form of monetary compensation. The ability to seek justice, to argue for redress before an individual who is totally independent and who is bound only by the law, is a cornerstone of our freedom and our democratic system. However, as I have said, it would not be proper for me to direct any comment to the legal issue of loss of access to the courts for workers covered by legislative no-fault compensation schemes. However, I think that I can say, and this point in no way relates to any argument under the *Canadian Charter of Rights and Freedoms*, that in any case in which a potential complainant is prevented from going to court, an opportunity is lost for conduct to be assessed and for guidelines for future conduct to be established.

In conclusion, permit me to reiterate my concern that the rights of the injured employee must not become submerged in academic debate and concern for the global picture and common good. The common good is surely no more than respect for the rights of each and every individual, and it was because of the desire to protect such rights that many of our courts and legal principles were fashioned. The *Canadian Charter of Rights and Freedoms* enshrines the right of the individual to be free from legislative discrimination. The realization that a worker has been injured or that a family has been bereaved does, I believe, help one to interpret such legislation in a manner consistent with accepted legal principles, yet tempered with compassionate concern for the individual.

REFERENCES

1. Royal Commission on the Ocean Ranger Marine Disaster. 1984. Report Two: Safety offshore eastern Canada. :16–17. Supply and Services Canada, Ottawa.
2. *Ibid.*: 14–15.

Round Table 5: Discussion

RAY ELLING (*University of Connecticut, Farmington, Conn.*): This is a panel on experiences in various countries, and much has been said about political will and worker involvement. The case of Sweden is particularly interesting in this regard. In Connecticut, we have had a New Directions program for six years, and we have succeeded in educating 350 or so "trainers," persons who could go and pass their knowledge on to others. Now Connecticut is a state with three million people and Sweden is a country with eight million people and they have 110,000 or more such trainers. Those people have the right to stop a production process if they see a hazard. They have considerable influence on the joint union—management Health and Safety Committee. So Sweden to a great degree has a worker-based system of control; Connecticut, by comparison, probably has a deficit of some 41,000 trainers.

ROD LAIRD (*Manitoba Federation of Labor, Winnipeg, Manitoba, Canada*): Too often we use Sweden as an example of a country we would like to emulate in terms of worker education, occupational health and safety, and workers' rights. In making some comparisons between Canada and the United States, I see that, regrettably, Canada is a little closer to the Swedish ideal than is the United States. That situation may result from a variety of reasons, but it does primarily reflect the fact that the concept of the right to know is insufficient in itself. If the right to know gives a person nothing more than information about the likelihood of developing cancer and his options are either to work under those conditions or be unemployed, it seems that the right to know is a pretty hollow "right." It must be coupled with the ability to do something about the condition.

In the labor movement in Canada, we have talked about three rights in occupational health and safety: the right to know, the right to participate, and the right to refuse. The right to participate usually gets embodied in participation in joint management–worker workplace health and safety committees, but it is not limited to that. We need to participate in committees that develop standards, and in those that develop legislation; in Canada, we more or less succeed in this endeavor. It is not as successful in some places as in others. There are different jurisdictions, but we do have these processes; in Manitoba, that is the way it works.

In addition, we like to participate with persons who possess a lot of medical expertise. However, we don't just want a judgment from the top. Rather, we want to use your expertise and work with you. We don't want you to just tell us what's good for us, for we feel that we know a great deal as well.

The third right is the right to refuse. The right to refuse to perform unsafe work without incurring negative consequences is the essence of this right. In nearly every jurisdiction in Canada, legislation guarantees the right to refuse unsafe work. Such legislation is generally underutilized, although when it first came out employers were very much concerned that it would be abused. That has not been the experience.

In general, refusal occurs in individual cases where the unsafe condition is fairly obvious. However, right now in Toronto there has been a massive work refusal involving more than 3,000 workers at McDonnell-Douglas. These workers discovered, through their own initiatives, rather than by any cooperation of their employer, that they are all being exposed to a wide spectrum of hazards, including lethal amounts of carcinogens. Today there are still more than a thousand people at McDonnell-Douglas who are being paid a full day's pay to sit in the lunchroom and do nothing else. This is significant because for years the workers suspected that they were being exposed to lethal hazards. But their concern amounted to naught: nobody paid any attention; nothing was ever done. The right to refuse brought the matter to a head, however. McDonnell-Douglas is losing millions of dollars. The loss is not sufficient for them to close down. They are not threatening to do that. But it is sufficient to force them to clean up their act, which they are now doing. But until the clean-up is completed, those workers will continue to be paid for not working.

Now that hits an employer where it really hurts—in the pocketbook. So I would suggest that without coupling other rights to the right to know, the achievements of labor will be insignificant.

There is one other right that is important to include here: the right for workers to organize themselves into unions. In Canada, our experience has been that where we have good legislation, such as the right to know, the right to participate, and the right to refuse, it is most effective and, in fact, almost only effective where there are unions in place to make it work. Where there are no unions, the legislation is totally ignored.

The rate of unionization in Canada is substantially higher than it is in the United States, and it is continuing to increase. In the United States it is substantially lower than in Canada and it is continuing to decrease. At this workshop we have heard the exhortations for unions to join together to create a public atmosphere to ensure the passage of good legislation, but because of decreasing unionization this is unlikely to come to fruition. Workers and unions must first concentrate their resources on survival, and that means organization.

Fortunately, in Canada we are able to devote more of our resources to things like occupational health and safety; and I believe that that is one of the reasons why we are a bit better off than you are.

JOHN R. FROINES (*University of California School of Public Health, Los Angeles, Calif.*): With reference to Dr. Weeks' presentation, Mort Corn and I were just looking at some figures. We have determined that although OSHA and MSHA have similar numbers of inspectors, they have responsibility for vastly different numbers of workplaces. OSHA would need to have 750,000 compliance officers it if were to provide a level of coverage per workplace comparable to that provided by MSHA. From the point of view of reducing unemployment in America, that's a very good idea, but from the point of view of practicality, it is not. One of the important questions we need to address is the enormous difference between the resources committed to OSHA and those committed to MSHA in terms of developing a more effective policy for controlling occupational disease.

A major priority for the future will be to generate information that will give us a better sense of the scope of the problem of occupational disease, as well as better information on the distribution of exposure levels. Inspections are not going to ever be able to fully accommodate that task.

My own view, and that of the National Academy of Sciences and of NIOSH, is that we need to expand our surveillance efforts in this country. As discussed yesterday, we need to develop generic standards, which would include environmental and biological monitoring programs, as well as medical surveillance.

One of the problems with OSHA today is that despite a number of 6(b) standards which contain provisions for environmental monitoring, medical surveillance and biological monitoring where it is appropriate, the information obtained by those programs nevertheless stays in the repositories of the industries that collect it.

Linda Rudolph at the Department of Health Services at the University of

ROUND TABLE 5: DISCUSSION

California has just completed a very important study in which she has looked at implementation of the OSHA lead standard as assessed by biological monitoring. She finds the situation similar to that which we found in looking at the compliance with the OSHA lead standard in terms of exposure levels. In essence, she found that a large number of companies are not complying with the biological monitoring provisions. Battery manufacturing firms are complying, but other industries are not.

So we first need to gather information where it exists. OSHA must collect it and NIOSH must collect it. Further, these data must be analyzed and evaluated so as to provide a means to set inspection priorities, to improve the quality of the inspections, and to improve our understanding of the scope of exposure and biological monitoring. We need a generic standard that requires industry to collect information on existing exposure levels for a large number of chemicals. We must require increased biological monitoring and increased medical surveillance as part of generic standards. This must be done in the context of enforcement strategies, but, more importantly, we also must insist that this information become part of an overall surveillance effort such that information is made available to regulatory agencies, to researchers, and to the workers themselves.

In summary, we need to discuss the mechanisms that can take us beyond our current situation, in which individual inspections occur infrequently, cover a small number of chemicals, and are poorly followed up. We need a more highly coordinated surveillance effort. The ultimate question is not whether workplace inspections are effective, but how we can create strategies for controlling occupational disease.

Round Table Papers: 6. A Blueprint for Effective Workplace Inspection in the United States

The Future is Now

Developing Effective Workplace Inspection in the United States

DAVID H. WEGMAN
Department of Work Environment
University of Lowell
Lowell, Massachusetts 01854

In 1970, the Occupational Safety and Health Act (OSHA) held great promise for worker health protection. It proposed to remedy the problems that were present in the fragmented and unequal enforcement that resulted from a state-based system. Many expected that the Act would herald a new era, that there would be dramatic reduction in the number and distribution of work-related accidents and illnesses among U.S. workers. In many respects OSHA's impact has been substantial, and benefits have accrued even where a direct role is not identifiable. Workers and employers are more aware of risks and the need for their control, and structures now exist in plants, corporations, and unions that are a positive response to the existence of OSHA.

But any new agency must struggle to determine the manner in which it will fulfill its mandate. This includes creation of an administrative structure, employment and training of staff, and development of rules and regulations through which to function. OSHA experienced these developments with the expected false starts, failures, and slow evolution of a new national program. Even though most interested people were aware of the politically sensitive nature of regulations that apply to the workplace, no one appears to have guessed just how sensitive an area it would prove to be. This was borne out when OSHA made the political decision to set the initial asbestos standard without regard to cancer risk. Even so, this standard had to be demanded by legal petition, taking advantage of the requirements that existed for special emergency rule-making procedures. This experience was followed by the intensive battle over a new standard for vinyl chloride, another emergency standard. In fact, almost all of the original new substance-specified standards and the majority of the existing ones were set using the emergency and not the routine standard-setting procedures. These, and other battles, took place against the backdrop of four different administrations, seven directors of OSHA, and a number of changes in Congressional committees providing oversight.

To date, then, the picture that OSHA presents to the public is comprised of conflicts between various interest groups, several new occupational standards, and little evidence that there has been a substantial change in risks experienced by the worker in the factory or the office. Is this evidence of an agency that has failed? I would suggest rather that it is evidence that real change is generally slow, often painful, and inconstant. As an optimist I propose that today the task is to consider what should be done so that we can observe the evolution of OSHA into an effective and forceful regulatory agency.

This panel is confronted, in particular, with the task of examining where OSHA should direct its attention in the sphere of inspection as the agency strives for adulthood. This examination is of particular interest to OSHA watchers, because so little public attention has been directed to the role of inspection in regulating the risks in the work environment. For the most part the public battles regarding OSHA have been around standards. To the extent that they have addressed inspection they have been focusing on which industry is, or should be, subject to inspection. But little attention has been paid to the objectives of the actual inspection including targeting, level of detail, possible penalties, effective followup, and appropriate monitoring by workers, management, and government.

It is presumptuous for this panel to actually suggest a blueprint for inspection. But it is not presumptuous for the panel to identify key areas to consider in developing inspection programs. We should recognize that it is unlikely that OSHA could ever have as comprehensive an inspection program as that discussed earlier by Jim Weeks concerning coal mine health and safety. Therefore, we will attempt to focus our attention on the key issues in maximizing the impact of OSHA's inspection effort within reasonable expectations.

Les Boden will address the importance of and means to greater worker involvement in the inspection process. Peg Seminario will address considerations for how OSHA can and should refocus and redefine the task of inspection. Had Joe Canella been able to attend, as originally planned, I would have asked him to characterize those areas where inspection might best be left to voluntary compliance and those that should be emphasized or newly created as requiring the special attention of government enforcement. I would like to take a moment here, however, to address issues included in two related areas: information needs and inspection targets.

To examine OSHA's inspection experience and what OSHA might wish to accomplish in the next 5 years, there is an obvious need to turn to data on the impact of inspections to develop the answer. This includes determining the magnitude of the different disease and hazard problems in industry as well as developing information on trends in these problems. This information could then be placed in the context of inspection practices to identify where inspections have made a difference and where they need to be improved or redirected.

What is striking is that such a search would lead to the discovery that there is essentially no reliable information for such an evaluation. Barney Frank's Congressional oversight committee decried this fact and called for immediate action to change the situation.[1] The response of the administration to this call led to an intensive effort by the National Institute for Occupational Safety and Health (NIOSH), the Bureau of Labor Standards (BLS), and the National Center for Health Statistics (NCHS) to respond to the need. The recent National Academy of Science (NAS) report, "Counting Injuries and Illnesses in the Workplace," proposed some ways to address the problem and it should prove useful reading to those who have not yet seen it.[2] In the main, however, it focuses on injury. It was unable to address the problem of disease at anywhere near the depth that it addresses injury.

The NCHS has responded by incorporating questions in several of the different national survey systems planned for the near future. These should give some improved estimates on work-related problems in the general population but without regard to the source of the problem. NIOSH embarked on a renewed effort at developments in disease surveillance and should be reporting on these efforts and proposing a number of new initiatives in the near future as well. Although this effort is expected to enhance recognition and reporting of disease, the problem of assigning actual cause to a specific case remains and will always be quite difficult.

A proposal in both the NAS report and the NIOSH effort suggests that development of hazard surveillance information may offer a means to estimate disease burden, to monitor changes in that burden, and, most importantly, to target specific areas that should receive priority attention for inspection and control of hazards. It is hoped that special attention can be paid to this area because it should provide significant and useful information on risks and how to target control of future disease burden for regulators, health professionals, planners, and the public as a whole.

Even if the knotty problem of estimating and monitoring disease and injury burden were to be solved, there remains the major task of determining how actually to carry out inspections. To this end it is important to consider the purpose of an inspection and the expected outcome. Much discussion of inspections is directed at the need to identify and punish infractions. Many complaints about OSHA identify the failure to do this. But OSHA will never have enough inspectors to accomplish even this end. Furthermore I suggest that this is not the appropriate way to characterize the task. For if it were, then attention would be directed at the inspection to *accomplish* the control rather than to *verify* its presence.

How might the latter objective be made more central to OSHA's efforts? One way is to design a program so that inspections are directed toward increasing the *risk* of inspection. In this way the deterrent nature of an inspection can be better utilized. For example, if 1,000 inspectors are given the task of visiting three workplaces a day with employment of 25 or more and of being in the field three quarters of the time, then 600,000 workplaces of this size can be visited each year. The result is that an employer of 25 or more can expect to be visited more than once a year.

This accomplishes the end of increasing "risk" of inspection and promotes voluntary compliance. It would be short-lived in actual effect, however, unless the inspection actually presents a risk of penalty and if workers are not included as integral to the abatement process. The inspection needs to be designed so that if an infraction is found, a penalty assessment is highly likely, the penalty is substantial enough to be a deterrent, and the workers are carefully informed of the circumstances, the abatement plan, and their rights under the process.

To accomplish this goal several steps need to be taken. Most of these will be the topics of other panel members. Suffice it to say here that without a plan to increase inspection numbers by improved targeting and reduced paper work, and the willingness to readily impose penalties after initial warning (and to penalize to the maximum, not the paltry average $200 at present), compliance inspections can at best be considered cheap consultant visits.

An often forgotten step, however, is that some substantially improved monitoring system must be developed together with record keeping designed for rapid and efficient perusal. It would be possible, in fact, to require standardized record keeping on exposure assessment, medical monitoring, worker training, and ventilation effectiveness which are forwarded regularly to an OSHA area office so that these could be perused prior to a visit. The visit, in turn, could review basic compliance, examine recognized problem areas, and carry out a walk-through in search of new or unrecognized problems.

For example, if an OSHA area office is responsible for a secondary lead smelter, then there should be blood lead monitoring, air lead monitoring, a medical surveillance program, a respirator program, and a worker educational program all directed at the one substance—lead. Similar information would be available on other hazards, carbon monoxide for instance. If there were rules on keeping and forwarding of records to OSHA on these items (using forms and data management systems designed to focus attention on sentinel events or trends), then the OSHA compliance officer would be well informed and properly oriented to accomplish the maximum when entering the plant for a quick walk-through.

The record review and the walk-through would provide the basis for immediate compliance action, for a decision to call for a more complete evaluation, or for a decision that there was sufficient evidence that the plant was in compliance. Such an approach would miss some problems that were not readily evident, were purposely hidden, or were intermittent. These would be susceptible to a separate program designed to improve worker input to problem identification and compliance. Even still, the approach briefly mentioned could greatly increase the coverage of OSHA inspections, reduce some of the unfocused detailed industrial hygiene activities that are expensive in time and dollars, and also permit the construction of a data system that would provide much better estimation of the distribution and magnitude of potential risk and the success in its control.

Experience in the coal mine compliance activity suggests that privately collected data needs to be considered with care and not always taken at face value. However, such data are far superior to no data, and can be randomly checked by OSHA compliance officers to identify evidence of misleading reports.

Inspections in the future, in any event, must include consideration of a data base that permits surveillance of compliance activities, an inspection plan that greatly increases coverage, and a targeting system that is flexible and directed at both important acute and long-term risks.

REFERENCES

1. U.S. CONGRESS, HOUSE OF REPRESENTATIVES. 1984. Report on Occupational Illness Data Collection: Fragmented, Unreliable, and Seventy Years Behind Communicable Disease Surveillance. Subcommittee of the Committee on Government Operations, 98th Congress, 2nd Session. Washington, DC. U.S. Government Printing Office.
2. POLLACK, E. S. & D. G. KEIMIG, Eds. 1987. Counting Injuries and Illnesses in the Workplace: Proposals for a Better System. National Academy Press. Washington, DC.

Unlocking OSHA'S Potential

An Inspection Strategy for the 1990s

LESLIE I. BODEN

Boston University School of Public Health
Environmental Health Section
Boston, Massachusetts 02118

OSHA's IMPACT ON HEALTH AND SAFETY

Studies of the Occupational Safety and Health Administration (OSHA) consistently indicate that OSHA inspections have had little or no impact on workplace injury rates. Studies by Smith[1] and Viscusi[2] were unable to detect significant improvements in injury rates after OSHA was established. Even positive studies indicate only small reductions in injury rates related to OSHA enforcement. Mendeloff,[3] in an analysis of California's state-enforced program, estimated that safety regulation led to a 2 to 3% decline in lost-workday injuries. Smith[4] compared 1973 rates of firms inspected early in the year with those inspected near the end of the year and found that the early inspections were associated with a 7% decline in injury rates. However, early inspections apparently produced only a 2% decline in 1974. McCaffrey[5] repeated Smith's study for the 1976–1978 time period and was unable to detect any decline in injury rates associated with early inspection.

It is more difficult to evaluate OSHA's impact on health hazards. Mendeloff's analysis of inspectors' measurements of exposure to trichloroethylene and silica suggests that they have not changed over time, and evidence on lead exposures is mixed. Exposures to vinyl chloride and asbestos have declined since the promulgation of OSHA standards for these substances.[6] However, the vinyl chloride standard was published shortly after the cancer risk of this substance was established, and after asbestos manufacturers began to suffer multimillion-dollar liability losses shortly after the 1972 asbestos standard was issued. Both of these nonregulatory factors could have accounted for the observed reduction in exposures.

Even though each of the cited studies has its deficiencies, taken together, they present a convincing story. OSHA has not come close to the expectations of one of its early sponsors, Congressman William A. Steiger, who expected a 50% reduction of injury rates as a consequence of the Act's passage.[7] OSHA has been criticized for weaknesses in its standards, inadequate expertise, poor management, and deficient enforcement policies. Although there is certainly room for improvement in its current policies, even an expert agency with a well-managed inspection program would probably have little impact on workplace conditions.

OSHA's FUNDAMENTAL LIMITATIONS

OSHA's safety and health inspectors periodically pay unannounced visits to America's workplaces. If inspectors find a violation of the regulations, they issue a citation and impose a penalty, which is supposed to reflect the seriousness of the danger to workers' health and safety. Employers may contest the citation, but in most instances they must pay the penalty and correct the hazard by a given date.

The basic reason for OSHA's ineffectiveness is its excessive reliance on enforcement of health and safety standards. OSHA operates on the theory that the thread of sanctions will lead most employers to comply with its regulations and that the occasional recalcitrant employer will be caught and compelled to come into compliance as well. A brief look at the Agency's task and its resources suggests why it cannot achieve a substantial reduction in workplace hazards by simply enforcing standards. OSHA's 1,100 inspectors are responsible for protecting the health and safety of 50 million workers at 2 million workplaces. (The rest are covered by state programs.) In fiscal 1987, the agency conducted about 60,000 inspections. In other words, OSHA inspected 3% of covered workplaces. Even if we disregard the less hazardous sectors of the economy (retail, personal, and business services) and put aside consideration of the problematic agricultural sector, OSHA inspects fewer than 20% of all manufacturing plants and construction sites each year.

Because firms can expect to see an inspector less than once every 5 years, the impact of enforcement activity is necessarily limited. Most firms will not fear imminent discovery of hazardous conditions. Moreover, health and safety conditions change from day to day as a result of random events, changes in production processes, and the presence or absence of adequate maintenance. These factors mean that an OSHA inspection every 5 years can be expected to uncover only highly visible and persistent health and safety hazards. Even if the inspection corrects all apparent problems, changing practices and inadequate maintenance may soon erase the benefits.[8]

Although hazard reduction in inspected workplaces is constrained by the necessity of continual vigilance, OSHA's deterrent effect is even more limited. Even for serious violations (those that may result in death or serious physical harm), OSHA's average penalty has hovered around $200 in recent years. Given that manufacturing and construction sites have less than a 20% chance of being inspected, the average employer would anticipate paying that $200 amount over a 5-year period. For violations that cost more than $40 per year to correct, employers would save money doing nothing until after they were inspected.

How could the impact of OSHA's enforcement activities on "voluntary" compliance be significantly increased? There are two obvious ways: either penalties could be raised substantially or inspection activities could be stepped up. Neither alternative is realistic. Consider a serious violation of the asbestos standard that costs $5,000 a year to correct. To convince an employer with a 20% chance of being inspected in any given year that he should voluntarily comply, the employer would have to expect at least a $25,000 fine—and this assumes that the violation would be detected by the inspector. Such penalties are not permitted under the OSHA legislation.

Neither are more frequent inspections the answer. The Occupational Safety and Health Act sets a maximum penalty of $1,000 per serious violation. Employers with a serious violation costing $5,000 a year to correct would therefore have to expect more than five inspections (and thus more than $5,000 in fines) a year before they would comply voluntarily. OSHA inspection operations capable of deterring such violations would have to exceed 25 times their current level. The resources necessary to inspect at such a level, even if the most hazardous workplaces were carefully targeted, are certainly not consistent with a balanced Federal budget.

INVOLVING WORKERS IN INSPECTION

To increase its impact, OSHA needs allies to monitor workplace conditions and to provide employers with additional incentives to reduce hazards. Occupational safety and health professionals can help in this effort, but they are not present in every workplace. When they are, they often face a conflict between their obligation to protect worker health and their employers' needs to increase profits.[9,10] OSHA's logical allies are the workers who are at risk. Workers are always present at the work site, and, because they are the prime beneficiaries of efforts to improve workplace safety, it seems reasonable that they have a substantial role in achieving that objective.

When it designed the Occupational Safety and Health Act of 1970, Congress was aware of the importance of worker involvement. The Act requires OSHA to inspect a workplace when there is a formal (written) worker complaint about hazardous conditions. During an inspection of a unionized workplace, a worker representative accompanies the OSHA compliance officer; when there is no union, the compliance officer consults several workers. After the inspection, proposed citations, penalties, and abatement dates must be posted where employees can read them. Finally, the Act forbids employer discrimination against any worker participating in legal health and safety activities. As a matter of policy, OSHA had extended some of these rights in the late 1970s. At that time, OSHA promulgated a rule that required workers accompanying an inspector to be paid. OSHA also had a policy that all post-inspection conferences with employers were to be open to workers and their representatives. Both of these policies were rescinded during the Reagan years. Currently, OSHA can meet alone with an employer and agree to reduce penalties substantially. The workers' only right is to have the agreement explained to them.

If workers are to act as a citizen occupational safety and health inspection force, these rights must be extended. First, they must be trained in the recognition of occupational hazards and given information about the hazards in their place of employment. The OSHA Hazard Communication Standard has traveled a short distance toward the goal of adequate training and information. OSHA has provided funding for private-sector training and education through the New Directions Program, but this program was extremely limited in scope. A more recent effort funded by the National Institute of Environmental Health Sciences is confined to hazardous waste workers. Most worker-oriented occupational health and safety training programs have been developed by unions or by local grassroots coalitions, COSH groups (Committees for Occupational Safety and Health).[11,12]

A worker inspection program also requires arrangements to facilitate consultation between workers and their employers about reducing hazards. A natural setting for this is the joint labor-management health and safety committee. If joint committees are to act as a vehicle for worker inspection, every workplace over a minimum size should have such a committee. Committee members must be trained. They must have access to all information about current workplace hazards and should be able to personally observe any area of the workplace. They should also be informed in advance about the impact of planned changes in plant, equipment, processes, and chemicals. They should be paid for all committee work and have the right to bring expert consultants into the workplace. Worker members of the committee should be elected or appointed by their union or, if not represented by a union, elected by nonmanagement employees.

Knowledge about workplace conditions is not of itself sufficient for the committee to have a substantial impact on management's decisions. When management refuses to eliminate very hazardous conditions, committee members must be able to take action. The most simple and effective step is to shut down the operation until agreement can be reached or until OSHA can be called in to determine suitable remedial action. This creates an incentive for the firm to act quickly so that production can begin again. A related action that would both create extra safety incentives and remove workers from risk is to broaden the limited right to refuse unusually hazardous work currently available to workers.[13-15]

Some employers may be tempted to discipline workers who use these new rights to take part in health and safety decisions. Nothing will chill worker participation as effectively as the threat of job loss. As a consequence, vigorous enforcement of rules protecting workers from discrimination for health and safety activities is critical to the success of such a program. This would require a substantial new commitment by OSHA, because its record of investigating alleged discrimination and protecting workers' rights has been woefully inadequate.[16,17]

Some of these rights have already been obtained in labor-management contracts. For example, in many of the plants it represents, the United Automobile Workers Union has, among other rights, safety representatives and safety training paid for by the employer. The United Steelworkers of America, through many of its contracts, has established paid safety committee work and walkaround rights, as well as an internal procedure that links the right to refuse hazardous work with the safety committees. Such gains in only a few of the strongest and most committed unions are not adequate to address the problems we are discussing. There must be broader statutory rights for all workers. Greater worker authority in occupational safety and health is not an untried or impractical idea. Other countries have had considerable experience in this area. Two well-known examples are Sweden and Canada.

SOME FOREIGN MODELS

Sweden

Sweden has had a system of worker participation in occupational safety and health for decades. Currently, every workplace with five or more workers is required to have a safety steward, whereas those with at least 50 workers must have a joint labor-management safety committee. There are currently 110,000 safety stewards in Sweden.[18] Both safety stewards and safety committees are charged with providing safety information and training. They receive full pay while discharging their safety duties and receive special training. About 650,000 Swedish workers (more than 1 in 10) have received a basic work environment course, while an advanced course is given to 30,000 to 40,000 workers every year.[19]

In 1974, the Worker Protection Act gave union safety stewards the right to suspend an operation that is an "imminent and serious danger for employee life or health" until a government inspector arrives.[20] This right has been exercised an average of about 100 times per year over the last 15 years, but with declining frequency since 1979. Because Sweden's labor force is less than 5% that of the United States, this is equivalent to over 2,000 such actions annually in this country.

Canada

In Canada, occupational safety and health regulation is primarily provincial in nature. All of Canada's provinces have provided for mandatory joint health and safety committees, and four (Ontario, Manitoba, Newfoundland, and Quebec) also have provisions for worker health and safety representatives. Provincial regulations require at least half the members of health and safety committees to be workers either elected by their fellow employees or appointed by their union. Committee members and health and safety representatives are paid for time spent performing their duties. In Saskatchewan, Manitoba, and Quebec, the employer must pay as well for attendance at approved training courses. Although committee powers vary by province, there are some common themes. Members of joint committees and health and safety representatives are typically entitled to receive information on worksite hazards, to receive and respond to worker complaints, to investigate serious accidents and hazardous conditions, to accompany a government inspector, to participate in the resolution of problems arising out of refusal to perform hazardous work, and to consult with experts. With the exception of the province of Quebec, committees can act only in an advisory capacity. In Quebec, joint health and safety committees have additional powers, giving them a central role in occupational safety and health planning. These include the right to choose the company physician, to approve the company occupational health and safety program, to develop health and safety training, and to select personal protective equipment.

In several Canadian provinces, workers receive substantially greater protection against discrimination for health and safety activity than in the United States. For example, a worker who has been engaged in occupational safety and health activities and is disciplined or fired is presumed to have suffered from illegal discrimination. The employer has the choice of proving otherwise or providing the worker with full compensation for lost wages.[21]

Finally, Canadian workers who refuse hazardous work are provided with a dispute-resolution procedure that is superior to that in the United States. When a Canadian worker refuses work and does not reach agreement with management that the job is sufficiently safe to warrant return, the worker or employer can call a government inspector. The inspector will either require the employer to correct the hazard or will determine that there is no unusual hazard and order the worker to return to the job. Thus, when the employer and worker disagree, the inspector acts as an impartial and expert arbitrator.[21] Our procedures are much slower and generally do not involve an independent examination of the disputed conditions by a government inspector.[13]

RECENT ACTIVITY IN THE UNITED STATES

These ideas have received considerable attention in the United States over the past several years. The COSH groups have provided early leadership in this area. For example, in 1984, the Philadelphia Area Project on Occupational Safety and Health (PHILAPOSH), published *A Job Safety and Health Bill of Rights*.[22] Among the rights enumerated are: access to all health and safety information, payment for union-sponsored training, and the right to shut down dangerous operations. In some states, legislation has been drafted to attain greater worker involvement in abating hazards. The Pennsylvania Public Employee Occupational

Safety and Health Bill would require the establishment of joint health and safety committees with the right to investigate accidents and regularly inspect the workplace. Elsewhere, groups are considering submitting legislation that would require all but the smallest workplaces to have labor-management health and safety committees. Committee members would have access to health and safety information, annual training at the employer's expense, and the right to investigate work and hazards, to bring in outside consultants, to advance notice of any new processes, equipment, or chemicals to be introduced, to shut down hazardous operations until corrected or checked by OSHA, and to participate in meetings or agreements between government agencies and management. Attendees at a 1987 AFL-CIO national conference discussed mandatory joint health and safety committees, obligatory health and safety training for workers, and a strengthened right to refuse hazardous work.[23]

CONCLUSION

Studies of the effectiveness of the Occupational Safety and Health Administration have uniformly shown little or no reduction in workplace injury rates. Although there is certainly room for improvement in its current policies, even an extremely well-managed agency would have limited impact. In the past, OSHA has used its small field staff to ensure that inspected employers are in compliance with health and safety standards. It has had a limited role in educating workers and employers and in supporting hazard surveillance and control activities by workers and their unions. If OSHA is to transcend its limitations, it must have a broader vision of its mandate. More effective regulation is possible if workers understand workplace hazards and supplement OSHA's inspection efforts.

OSHA can provide support for worker training, more stringent requirements for informing workers under existing right-to-know regulations, incentives for employers to involve workers and their unions in hazard reduction, greater opportunity for workers to participate in the inspection and hazard abatement process, and increased protection against discrimination for health and safety activities.

In addition, new laws and regulations could support increased worker involvement in workplace health and safety, using workers as a volunteer inspection force. Models exist in other countries, notably Canada and Sweden. Examples include statutory labor-management health and safety committees and the right of workers and their representatives to shut down hazardous processes and to refuse hazardous work.

Last and most important, the Federal government must take steps to reestablish workers' faith that OSHA will keep safety and health as its first priority. This good faith is necessary if OSHA is to receive the input from workers that it needs to be effective.

REFERENCES

1. SMITH, R. S. 1979. The impact of OSHA inspections on manufacturing injury rates. J. Human Resources **14:** 145–170.
2. VISCUSI, W. K. 1979. The impact of occupational safety and health regulation. Bell J. Economics **10:** 117–140.
3. MENDELOFF, J. 1979. Regulating Safety: An Economic and Political Analysis of Occupational Safety and Health Policy. MIT Press. Cambridge, MA.

4. SMITH, R. S. 1979. The impact of OSHA inspections on manufacturing injury rates. J. Human Resources **14(2):** 145–170.
5. MCCAFFREY, D. P. 1983. An assessment of OSHA's recent effects on injury rates. J. Human Resources **18:** 131–145.
6. U.S. CONGRESS, OFFICE OF TECHNOLOGY ASSESSMENT. 1985. Preventing Illness and Injury in the Workplace. :268. U.S. Government Printing Office, Washington, DC.
7. ZECKHAUSER, R. & A. NICHOLS. 1978. The Occupational Safety and Health Administration—An overview. *In* Study on Federal Regulation, Appendix to Vol. VI. U.S. Congress, Senate Committee on Governmental Affairs. :163–248. U.S. Government Printing Office. Washington, DC.
8. BODEN, L. E. & D. H. WEGMAN. 1978. Increasing OSHA's clout: Sixty million new inspectors. Working Papers **7:** 43–49.
9. WALTERS, V. 1982. Company doctors' perceptions of and responses to conflicting pressures from labor and management. Social Problems **30:** 1–12.
10. WALSH, D. C. 1987. Corporate Physicians: Between Medicine and Management. Yale University Press. New Haven, CT.
11. BERMAN, D. 1981. Grassroots coalitions in health and safety: The COSH groups. Labor Studies J. **6(1):** 104–113.
12. LEVENSTEIN, C., L. I. BODEN & D. H. WEGMAN. 1984. COSH: A grass-roots public health movement. Am. J. Public Health **74:** 964–965.
13. ASHFORD, N. A. & J. KATZ. 1977. Unsafe working conditions: Employee rights under the Labor Management Relations Act and the Occupational Safety & Health Act. Notre Dame Lawyer **52:** 802–836.
14. GROSS, J. A. & P. A. GREENFIELD. 1985. Arbitral value judgments in health and safety disputes: Management rights over workers rights. Buffalo Law Rev. **34:** 645–691.
15. BACOW, L. S. 1980. Bargaining for Job Safety and Health. The MIT Press. Cambridge, MA.
16. MINTZ, B. W. 1984. OSHA: History, Law, and Policy. :606–607. Bureau of National Affairs. Washington, DC.
17. MCMANUS, J. M. 1987. Deadly Dilemma. Wisconsin Committee on Occupational Safety & Health. Milwaukee, WI.
18. SODERLUND, S. 1987. Working Environment in Sweden. The Swedish Work Environment Fund, Stockholm.
19. 1987. Occupational Safety and Health in Sweden. The Swedish Institute, Stockholm.
20. KELMAN, S. 1981. Regulating America, Regulating Sweden. M.I.T Press. Cambridge, MA.
21. NASH, M. I. 1983. Canadian Occupational Health & Safety Law Handbook. CCH Canadian Ltd. Don Mills, Ontario.
22. ENGLER, R. 1984. A Job Safety and Health Bill of Rights. Philadelphia Area Project on Occupational Safety and Health. Philadelphia, PA.
23. WRIGHT, M. 1987. Discussion paper on New Laws and Worker Rights. AFL-CIO National Health and Safety Conference, Nashville, TN.

An Invitation to Act

MARGARET SEMINARIO

Director of Health and Safety
AFL-CIO
815 16th Street, N.W.
Washington, D.C. 20006

I have been in Washington for almost eleven years now. I came in under a friendly administration and have been one of the few to stay through a not-so-friendly administration. Every four years, just before the next election, people come in to Washington to decide what they should do. What is the platform? What is the program? Where are we going in the future? This is all very nice and it is good to see old friends and to talk about ideas. But talk is cheap.

Those of us in the labor movement have been struggling for the last eight years to make gains in this area of occupational health. And we have made gains despite the history of the last eight years and the obstacles we have had to overcome, both with respect to an administration that was deeply committed to deregulation and an economy that was going rapidly downhill. Things looked very bleak. Nevertheless, we have been able to make some gains, to learn some lessons, and even to establish new ground.

In the late 1960s, when the issues leading us to the Occupational Safety and Health Act were being discussed, an important basic issue was to change the relationship between workers and employers under the structure of the Act. A great deal of hope surrounded this effort. However, what resulted was a piece of legislation that did not address the employer–employee relationship, but which, rather, gave the government primary responsibility and a great deal of discretion to act. Unfortunately, too much hope and too much power were vested in government. If the government wants to enforce the law, it will enforce; if it does not, it will not. And there is very little that anybody can do about it.

In the years since passage of the OSHAct, we have had some limited success in the area of standard-setting. When it comes to enforcement, though, there is very little that workers or the unions can do if the government does not want to do its job.

In short, we have come to realize that there is a basic inadequacy in the program established under the Occupational Safety and Health Act. Too much trust was placed in government. Now when we look at things that have to be changed, we see that that aspect has to be changed. We now know that we cannot always depend upon the government to do its job.

Even if we had the best of all worlds and a government that was committed to enforcement, we would still have problems with enforcement. The size of the inspection staff has never gone above 1,400 to 1,500 inspectors nationwide. Thus the government does not even have the ability to provide the necessary coverage in even the most hazardous of workplaces.

Clearly then, there is a need for a change in emphasis and a change in focus. I am not saying that we should abandon a strong enforcement scheme. The cause of occupational health and safety will only progress in this country if we have strong regulations and the strong backup of federal enforcement. However, the experience of the past decade has taught us that we must look at ways in which we can develop better programs for health and safety in workplaces across this country on a more uniform basis. The big companies with the big unions are doing a pretty good job in this area. We must study mechanisms by which we can expand that activity to smaller shops with weak unions or no unions at all.

In our view, the only way to accomplish this goal is to empower the workers and the unions to have the power in workplaces to deal one-on-one directly with management on health and safety problems. Structures must be established in workplaces across the nation in the form of committees. Those committees, those worker representatives, must be given the right and the responsibility to deal with health and safety problems. The basic issue is to create joint labor–management committees in workplaces across the United States which will have the power to do routine inspections of the workplace.

All of these structures exist in other countries; this is not a radical idea, but one that makes sense in dealing with health and safety problems in workplaces in this country. Further, I think we have heard a consensus from the other participants at this workshop that empowerment of workers is needed if we are truly to achieve health and safety in the workplace in this country.

The next problem is how this empowerment of workers will be brought about. How will these provisions find their way into law? Laws and protections are not automatically granted, but must be won, and they are won through struggle. Those of us in the labor movement are looking to the next three- to five-year strategy for major reforms in the occupational safety and health laws in this country.

We may not be able to do everything initially at a federal level. We may have to go out and test the waters in the states or communities where people are willing to listen and where there is more receptivity to these kinds of issues. But we must act rather than sit around and rehash the same ideas, and we have to develop a plan for action.

The AFL-CIO had a big conference on health and safety in November 1987 in Nashville. It was attended by some 900 to 1000 trade unionists from across the country coming to Nashville to deal with issues of health and safety. These people were elected by their local unions and paid by local treasuries, yet the level of discussion and the sophistication of that audience was ten times higher than it has been here. People got down to business. What were the problems? What were the issues? What needed to be done?

Here I have heard that there is a general agreement about the problems that exist and where we need to go. But we have not had any discussion of how we are going to get there. By contrast, those of us in the labor movement are getting our act together. We are sitting down to figure out strategically what we need to do in this area.

I am told that some challenges were made to the unions at this workshop. We were criticized for not being here in record numbers. To answer that I will tell you that attendance at a workshop like this is a luxury for union members. But we have been attempting to do our job, however imperfectly. When we have gone to OSHA for the standard-setting hearings and to the Hill to deal with new legislation, we have not seen many of the groups represented at this workshop. So I would put the challenge to you to join forces with us to advance the cause of occupational safety and health programs in this country. There is major work to be done. We in the labor movement are engaged in that work and we invite you to join us in the work. For the first time in a long time, we are able to agree upon the direction in which we should go. Now we need colleagues to become involved in the struggle to develop the kind of enforcement schemes that we must have for protection of workers in this country.

Round Table 6: Discussion

DAVID H. WEGMAN (*University of Lowell, Lowell, Mass.*): Margaret Seminario has presented an important challenge to us. As physicians, we, for the most part, are not representative of workers. Indeed, few of us have had experience with physical labor. We need to be more active than we have been.

We cannot afford to buy into the current thinking of the Reagan administration; rather we must work to change that agenda.

RICHARD RAVEN (*Massachusetts Division of Occupational Hygiene, Boston, Mass.*): Ms. Seminario, you referred to strategies that need to be developed to expand workers' rights under the Occupational Safety and Health Act. What are some of them?

MARGARET SEMINARIO (*AFL–CIO, Washington, D.C.*): We are in the process of developing the kinds of changes, specifically legislative changes, affecting the basic protections that need to be reformed under the Occupational Safety and Health Act. They are quite easily identified. One problem is that the OSHAct did not establish clear rights for participation by workers and unions. That is one thing that has to be changed. And both the whole standard-setting process and the whole enforcement process need to be corrected. Those are three key identifiable areas.

We need to develop legislative proposals that respond to these issues and build the activity. We need to educate the public, scientists, and politicians that these are the problems. That is why conferences like this are good, because they provide an opportunity for us to compare notes, think together, talk together, and thus to educate one another.

As far as developing strategies for implementation, the basic issue is to have a political atmosphere where you can move to have these kinds of legislative changes adopted. I hope that we will soon have a Congress that is receptive to these kinds of proposals. But that will not happen by simply drafting proposals and visiting staff people on Capitol Hill. It requires a lot of organization, and a lot of education; it is a political activity which has to start with the elections in 1988.

In a sense, it is easier for us in the labor movement to engage in this frank political process, because we *are* political organizations and that is what we do. For someone who is a state employee or working at a university, it is more difficult because his or her involvement and activities may not necessarily match the institution's position. However, it is very helpful for those persons who cannot get involved politically to have access to the basic information, the analysis, the experience, and the basic documentation concerning the problems that exist.

In summary, I do not expect everyone here to pick up a banner and to have their state or university join in. However, the kind of work you do day in and day out, the identification and the analysis of problems are going to be critical in developing the kinds of reforms that are needed.

JAMES WEEKS (*United Mine Workers of America, Washington, D.C.*): This is an important discussion, because it is examining the cultural gap that exists between scientists and labor, a gap that we must try to bridge. One of the ways in which labor functions to achieve rights is through collective bargaining. This is foreign territory for most scientists.

Also, at the United Mine Workers of America, we are discovering a number of provisions in the OSHAct that have never been enforced. One of them is a petition for modification of standards; under OSHA it is called the petition for variances. It has been used extensively by management. We have been in the process of filing dozens of petitions for modifications, and I think we are driving the coal operators and MSHA crazy, because it is entirely within our legal rights to do so. We have been doing it for substantial matters.

In dealing with our members on a regular basis, I have found that there are dozens of creative ways of making a difference.

WEGMAN: Tony Robbins used to say that we do not need more Acts, we need new *actions*. I think we may need both.

LINDA RUDOLPH (*California Department of Health Services, Los Angeles, Calif.*): As we have talked about ways to improve the standard-setting process, ways to improve compliance with standards, and ways to increase enforcement, it occurred to me that a parallel debate has been going on in the environmental protection community. Barry Commoner's article in the *New Yorker* has stimulated much reflection as to why our society has failed to deal adequately with environmental protection, to set adequate standards, to regulate environmental pollution, and to achieve effective enforcement. Out of that discussion, a consensus is emerging that alternative strategies should be tried as an extension of previous activities in environmental enforcement. In particular, the environmentalists are beginning to focus more on actions that work to ban outright the bad technologies, thus forcing research on new technologies that are alternatives to the toxic technologies that we keep trying unsuccessfully to regulate. I wonder whether this toxic-reduction strategy that is emerging in the environmental community is applicable in the workplace setting.

LESLIE BODEN (*Boston University School of Public Health, Boston, Mass.*): There are quite a large number of goals that could be accomplished without any new legislation at all, not only within collective bargaining, but, also with an OSHA that had the will to act.

One obvious example is OSHA's terrible record in enforcing the antidiscrimination section of the OSHAct. The fact is that OSHA basically discourages workers from bringing these claims. It takes from four months to more than a year for OSHA to decide what to do, basically invalidating the kinds of protection that workplaces ought to have.

Let me give you another example: OSHA decided some years ago to encourage employers to take responsibility themselves by telling them that they did not have to be inspected any more if they did a couple of not very useful kinds of things. But OSHA could have encouraged employers in a much more constructive way, urging them to get together with workers and unions to set up real joint–management co-determination arrangements without any new legislation at all. They can do that through the rule-making process.

ANTHONY MAZZOCCHI (*The Institute for Labor Studies, New York, N.Y.*): As a public health advocate, I think we ought to redefine what advocacy means. At this stage of development persons ought really to decide whether they are advocates or neutralists. Advocacy means standing for something, defining, having a discussion among ourselves as to what the blueprint should be. There are two ways this can be done. First, we in the labor movement must assign some vitality to ourselves, we must reexamine where we are and work on a new quest to assume power. The second is by co-determination. Co-determination only comes about when people have equal power. The history of the labor movement in this country in the last five or six years has been a history of concessions. This history has to be seriously examined. We are weaker than we have been. By contrast look at the situation in Canada. The Canadian Labour Congress took the position that there would be no concession. The former OCAW union in Canada, which is now the Energy and Chemical Workers Union, doubled their membership under this policy, dealing with the same companies we confront in the United States. They have not lost a worker through decertification. They confront the employer with an elevated level of consciousness. They also have a political party with which they can operate. So do the Swedes. We do not.

The question is one of power. Collective bargaining is fine if you have power. I have not seen anybody sit behind collective bargaining tables these days with enough power even to hold what they have. I have been looking at what is happening to workers on a local level for the last five years. I have been at plant gates twice a week, because 42 years ago, when I was a younger guy, people had confidence in your ability to struggle and win. That confidence no longer exists.

I have been on plant floors and I am telling you that I have never seen a situation involving health and safety as bad as I see it today, with some notable exceptions. You saw what happened with the mine workers who are empowered. Jim Weeks' data show it. Where you have inspectors and the union has power, mortality diminishes. When you have the same number of inspectors with no union and no worker empowerment, you have no improvement. The fact of the matter is that no matter how many new regulations you get, there is a large gulf between what happens in Washington and what happens on the shop floor. Workers are disillusioned, cynical, and skeptical because they feel entirely powerless. The public health community must therefore enter into new debates over the question of power and rights. These rights ought to be sharply defined, and that is going to call for confrontation.

At our next meeting there ought to be a reality session. We have to let the people who are on the shop floors describe exactly the realities of the shop floors. Any of you can walk into any workplace and understand the problem, either by observing it or working in it for a short time, in the context of the existing rules. That will give us a better understanding of the realities of the American power relationship.

Linda Rudolph mentioned Barry Commoner's article. As Barry Commoner said candidly, with all the laws and with all of the movements, we are further behind now than we were twenty years ago. We have to do some real soul-searching and define ourselves as advocates and we have to create arenas where the advocates can come together as advocates and not as neutralists.

WEGMAN: Tony, I appreciate those comments. Many of us began work in this field by participating in the hearings that you prepared from the workforce and from OCAW in preparation for the passage of the OSHAct.

I am reminded of Irving Selikoff's lecture in which he recounted some history in which public health workers were activists who took risks and made judgements. We have become much too self-centered and oriented toward technological answers; we have turned away from political answers.

Tony Mazzocchi's charge that those of us in the public health community return to advocacy is an appropriate one, and one that we had better attend to.

PART V. WORKERS' COMPENSATION, LITIGATION, AND THE
PREVENTION OF OCCUPATIONAL DISEASE

Workers' Health, Safety, and Compensation in Historical and Cross-National Perspective

An Overview

RAY H. ELLING

Department of Community Medicine and Health Care
University of Connecticut Health Center
Farmington, Connecticut 06032

This paper suggests a framework of struggle for improvement of workers' health and safety (WHS) and workers' compensation (WC) and briefly surveys the historical experiences of several countries in order to provide a basis for suggested changes in the United States in the 1990s and beyond.

A FRAMEWORK FOR WORKERS' HEALTH AND SAFETY

As late as 1972 the International Labour Organization's (ILO) *Encyclopedia of Occupational Health and Safety* titled its article on the subject of this paper, "Workmen's Compensation."[1] Only at the close of the 1970s did the Connecticut State Legislature amend "the Workmen's Compensation Act" to "Worker's Compensation Act" effective October 1, 1979.[2] The women's movement and the increasing participation of women in paid labor outside the home had finally forced the change. This recent development reflects, as does the whole history of WHS and WC, its growth and change through struggle. The struggles of gender have been joined with those of class in this recent development. Perhaps class struggles have been primary in the development of WC:

> Underlying the political process involved in the passage of compensation laws was a fundamental clash of interest between employers and workers. Workers wanted to use the financial club of compensation benefits to both succor the injured and to maximize the financial incentive employers had to act to *prevent* accidents. Employers were not opposed to accident prevention or the relief of the injured as abstract or moral propositions; but business owners and managers were guided by a second set of considerations—their desire to maximize revenues (subject, of course, to some constraints) to both increase their own gain and to avoid giving competitors an edge that might eventually endanger the very survival of the enterprise itself. The basic contradiction between the imperatives of business-owners and the objectives of the employed created an antagonism that existed long before compensation laws were first considered by legislatures. Indeed, the extent and bitterness of the class conflict engendered by contention between labor and capital over unsafe working conditions and by the legal and direct personal clashes between injured workers and employers over the level of financial relief to be given to accident victims was an important consideration to many employers, who were willing to accept a small increase in the cost of doing business if this friction could be mitigated.[3]

Although this is not the forum in which to develop sociologic frameworks, it should be noted that others may disagree with class and gender struggle as an explanatory framework for WC and other social welfare measures. Orloff and Skocpol[4] survey and dismiss several explanations in a very scholarly contribution: (1) the logic of industrial development which requires social insurance at a certain point; (2) the relative greater strength of liberalism and laissez-faire ideology in the United States, prohibiting WC from developing as soon and as completely as in Europe, particularly Britain; and (3) comparative working class strength and strength of the labor union movement in particular. They offer the idea of a relatively autonomous state bureaucracy (such as the British civil service), doing technocratic things on its own to better the lot of working people. Although there is much to be learned from their work, including their tracing of U.S. WC and other social legislation to the Civil War veterans' benefits, I find the struggle model more convincing. Certainly Asher[3] and others[5] find the class struggle model most clarifying. Indeed, my own historical and current comparison of general provisions for workers' health and safety leads me in this direction, for I found more adequate protection in Sweden, Finland, and the German Democratic Republic, where workers' movements are comparatively strong, than in the Federal Republic of Germany and the United Kingdom where workers' movements are not as strong. The United States offers the least adequate WHS system and has the weakest workers' movement among those of the six study countries.[6]

Before going into WC, I will briefly describe a few of the most striking provisions for WHS in Sweden, East Germany (GDR), and Finland and contrast these with those same aspects in the United States to suggest what remarkable achievements can flow out of comparatively strong workers' movements. A workers' movement is stronger when it:

- has followed with deliberation and pride a class-based strategy of struggle in clear recognition of the labor theory of value;
- has oriented itself with a broad philosophy of social well-being, including socioeconomic justice, education, health, housing, self-realization, and human dignity for all—not just wages and hours and conditions of work (such breadth makes coalition building more feasible);
- works through, supports, and is supported by a credible labor party;
- through the labor party has held and currently holds state power;
- continues to organize on the basis of laws favorable to labor unions (closed shops, sympathy strikes permitted, etc.);
- has pursued gender and ethnic solidarity and avoided splinterism;
- has a high percentage of the paid workforce organized (perhaps better than 85% of Swedish workers are union members, including high proportions of clerical, technical, professional, and scientific workers, whereas today in the United States it is falling toward 15%); and
- enjoys high employment and low exposure to loss of jobs to other countries in the capitalist political-economic world-system.

Although all these elements have not been perfectly realized in any of the six countries I studied, perhaps Sweden offers the best example of a strong workers' movement, the GDR (though of a different form) is about on a par with Sweden, and Finland follows closely.[7]

Some selected examples of WHS achievements from these countries with comparatively strong workers' movements follow:

Sweden: Sweden can be characterized as having a worker-based system in which more than 110,000 union health and safety representatives have been trained in WHS for 40 hours or more; these "reps" have a majority on joint union-management health and safety committees which have the power to hire and fire WHS personnel (thus the mistrust of "company quacks," so prevalent in the United States, is disappearing); these reps also have the power to stop the production process when they perceive a hazard, even a long-acting hazard; and all workers have the right to refuse hazardous work without fear of retribution; finally, there generally is no problem with the right to know as the Law of Codetermination brings union and management together to plan all aspects of production, including the chemicals and other materials to be used. In the United States workers are still struggling for the right to know and have not yet seriously raised the right to refuse or the right to stop hazardous production.

German Democratic Republic: The GDR in 1981 began vigorously implementing a law requiring a complete hazard survey for every workplace in the country, with continuous follow-up health exams for workers exposed and a time-ordered plan for removal or control of hazards according to priority based on severity of risk. Today in the United States OSHA has been so weakened that it cannot inspect more than 2% of workplaces each year, and neither NIOSH nor OSHA or any other agency has a working program of hazard surveillance for the workplaces of this country.

On the important (though all too often ignored) matter of adequate links between first-line general health care and WHS, although the United States has many medical schools with hardly any required study of WHS (my own school, the UConn Medical School, is one of those that only offer an elective course)[8]; medical schools in the GDR require 36 hours of WHS.

Finland: Finland has vigorously implemented a law requiring coverage of every workplace in the country with adequate occupational health services. The United States, by contrast, has hundreds of thousands of workplaces with nothing more than first-aid kits and fire extinguishers.

Many more contrasts could be described, but I must move on to the focus of workers' compensation.

WORKERS' COMPENSATION

As early as 1849, in reaction to the widespread but abortive revolutionary attempts in Europe in 1848, Otto von Bismarck, the "Iron Chancellor" of Prussia, said, "The social insecurity of the worker is the real cause of their being a peril to the state."[9] Later it was his anticipatory action in the form of the first national health insurance and first WC adopted in 1883 that helped take the wind out of the sails of the strengthening socialist workers' movement.[10] In Bismarck's words, these acts were passed "to cut the legs off" the socialist workers' movement.[11] At the same time that he was fighting the revolutionary movement with such sophisticated means, members of his own party were calling him, Bismarck of all people, a "socialist," for they saw these beginnings of the welfare state as threatening the then sacred principles of early capitalist development—individualism and laissez-faire. (Today, of course, these words are anachronistic in the age of neoimperialist monopoly capitalism, because the gigantic projects of mammoth transnational corporations, in competition with others, require a partnership with government and its access to capital through taxes and control of competition through legislation and regulation.) Of course, passage of the first WC law did not mean that it offered adequate compensation. In fact, it was quite minimal, and years of struggle lay ahead before the very interesting system found today in West Germany (FRG) evolved. I will come back to this system.

The earlier phases of capitalist development were very rough indeed on working men, women, and, yes, children.

> Many, many thousands of these little, hopeless creatures were sent down into the north, being from the age of seven to the age of thirteen or fourteen years old—overseers were appointed to see to the works, whose interest it was to work the children to the utmost, because their pay was in proportion to the quantity of work that they could exact . . . cruelties the most heart-rendering [were] practiced upon the unoffending and friendless creatures who were thus consigned to the charge of master manufacturers; they were harassed to the brink of death by excess of labor . . . were flogged, fettered and tortured in the most exquisite refinement of cruelty; . . . they were in many cases starved to the bone while flogged to their work and . . . even in some instances were driven to commit suicide. . . . The profits of manufacturers were enormous; but this only whetted the appetite that it should have satisfied, and therefore the manufacturers had recourse to an expedient that seemed to secure to them those profits without possibility of limit; they began the practice of what is termed "night working," that is, having tired one set of hands, by working throughout the night, the day-set getting into the beds that the night-set had just quitted, and in their turn again, the night-set getting into the beds that the day-set quitted in the morning. It is a common tradition in Lancashire that *the beds never get cold*.[12]

In the United States the struggle for the 10-hour day dated back to at least 1835. Later the struggle for an 8-hour day centered in the national strike of 1886 which ended with the Haymarket Massacre. Both these efforts were tied to the hazards of work.

Accident rates, especially in steel, mining, and railroads, reached astronomic proportions around the turn of the century and afterward. In the single year of 1907, there were 3,242 deaths in the coal mines and 4,534 workers were killed on the railroads.[13] It was said of the brakeman, who had to put his hands between cars to uncouple them, "A brakeman with both hands and all his fingers was either remarkably skilled, incredibly lucky or new on the job."[14]

Workers and their families were at great risk. Their only recourse was to sue their employers. But the employer had several common legal defenses that made success in such suits unlikely. First, the worker had to prove that the employer was at fault in the accident. In addition, employers often used their other defenses with success:

(1) Contributory Negligence. The worker could not recover any damages if the worker had been negligent in *any* degree, regardless of the extent of the employer's negligence.

(2) The Fellow Servant Doctrine. The employee could not recover any damages if it could be shown that the injury had resulted to any degree from the negligence of a fellow worker.

(3) Assumption of Risk. The injured worker could not recover any damages if the injury was due to an inherent hazard of the job of which he had, or should have had, advanced knowledge.

As Downey concluded, "By this concatenation of judge-made doctrines . . . some seven-eighths of all work injuries were left without legal relief."[15] Somers and Somers point out that the use of the fellow-servant doctrine in this way did not follow precedent for in the early part of the nineteenth century it had been clearly established that a master *was* responsible to third parties for injuries inflicted upon them by one of his servants in the course of his or her employment.

They highlight the class bias involved by quoting Dodd's explanation: "the desire of the judges to encourage large industrial undertakings by making the burdens on them as light as possible."[16]

In addition, work-related diseases were almost totally uncompensated at the time for a variety of reasons[17] and still remain highly problematic today even within WC laws. As Barth[18] notes, the German law of 1883 and the Austrian law of 1897 recognized occupational diseases as compensable, but there were many problems in their being identified in an agreed-upon way. (Later presumptive lists were developed as a partial solution.) The British statute of 1897 took no note of work-related disease, but was amended less than a decade later.

> That the British quickly amended their law of 1897 to cover occupational disease might suggest that the American states, many of which shortly thereafter passed their own compensation laws, would specifically incorporate provisions for diseases. The states, however, excluded any mention of diseases in their earliest statutes; but there is evidence that the issue was not simply overlooked in their haste to pass these first laws. The Wainright Commission, which resulted from pressures to pass a workers' compensation statute in New York, reported that occupational disease probably fell outside its purview and that it would report later on the subject. However, later reports made no mention of the issue.[18]

Going back to the period in the United States just before WC laws began to be adopted by the individual states, several sources note that although employers were able to avail themselves of the common law defenses against tort liability suits by workers, several factors led to increasing success and larger awards in such suits.

First, the workers' movement was growing in strength and becoming more militant. For example, the "one big union," the Industrial Workers of the World (IWW or "Wobblies"), won the important "bread and roses" strike at the Lawrence textile mills in 1912. Solidarity had been achieved across gender and ethnic lines against vicious repressive measures of the bosses and police. As Big Bill Haywood put it in his speech celebrating the victory, "The women won the strike."[19]

Second, public outrage over working conditions also played a role. In the Bread and Roses Strike, the case of Camella Teoli made national headlines and caught the attention of President Taft's wife. "Two weeks after she'd started work [at age thirteen] at the Washington Mills, Camella Teoli was scalped: her hair got caught in a machine for twisting cotton. She was hospitalized for the next seven months. The company paid her doctors' bills, but not her lost wages."[20]

Third, the ground for this public outrage had been prepared in part by the Muckrakers—Upton Sinclair (*The Jungle*, 1906, on work in the meatpacking industry) and Crystal Eastman (*Work Accidents and the Law*, 1910). These and other works "were effective in arousing public awareness of horrible working conditions of the times, with temperatures freezing in the winter and boiling in summer, child labor common (as young as five years old), long hours, and no ventilation."[21]

These several sources of pressure brought about the passage of more protective employer liability laws, first for railroad workers. These were extended to miners and industrial workers in only a few jurisdictions before 1910.

> But in the first decade of the twentieth century, as labor union membership increased, as labor became better organized for legislative lobbying and as the Socialist Party of America increased its representation in legislatures, several states—most notably Oregon, Ohio and Colorado—began to remove the common law defenses that had

protected negligent employers against successful tort suits by injured workers. Concurrently, state judges, especially in Minnesota and Wisconsin, began to alter their interpretation of the common law of industrial torts in a manner that allowed injured workers higher rates of recovery of damages. Immediately, employers felt the financial pressure of these developments, as liability insurance companies, in the insurance business to make a profit, quickly raised their premiums for accident insurance. By 1909, when several states established investigative commissions to draft workmen's compensation laws, very drastic employers' liability bills were pending in the legislatures of most industrial states. Pressure for the enactment of these laws was mounting; in Ohio labor broke through with the 1910 Norris law, which left negligent employers virtually defenseless against tort litigation. In Oregon, the legislature passed an equally drastic liability statute. Everywhere business spokesmen, representing large and small establishments, sounded the alarm: additional "radical" liability legislation had to be blocked.[22]

Thus, in the face of increasing numbers and size of injury awards, disturbing to capitalists not only for their effect on profits, but also for their unpredictability and consequent inability to properly plan for the cost of doing business, the owners began to accept, even push for, the passage of WC laws. Asher assesses this development this way:

But business spokesmen drove a hard bargain: they insisted that a definite limit be placed on the increased outlays for injured workers and strove to attain a level of predictability of costs for accident compensation which could be achieved only by making injured workers sacrifice almost completely their right to sue negligent employers, a right that workers regarded as essential to making employers obey safety legislation and avoid gross negligence. The political weakness of both organized and unorganized labor during the years of the enactment of pioneering compensation legislation, and—I would add—in the years that followed, led lawmakers to accede to most of the terms requested by business spokesmen who wanted to be assured that state-mandated welfare capitalism would substantially reduce class conflict but would not substantially reduce profits.[23]

For a time the U.S. systems (enacted by the states; no federal legislation was passed) reflected a mix of so-called voluntary and compulsory approaches. This had been an issue with all social insurance—health, unemployment, disability, WC, and the like—in Europe as well, employers generally favoring a voluntary approach. Much of this debate occurred in the meetings of the International Congress of Insurance against Industrial Accidents (later the Congress of Social Insurance). This association

which was organized in Paris in connection with the World Exposition in 1889 and which met at frequent intervals until the eve of the World War, witnessed a recurrent battle between the adherents of the principle of compulsion and those who advocated subsidized voluntary insurance. At its session of 1908, however, the victory of the former at least in theory was virtually conceded.[24]

In the United States this struggle went on until 1917.

There was at first considerable doubt on constitutional grounds that the European type of compulsory law would be permissible in the United States. As a result the "elective" compensation law was devised. This gave both the worker and his employer the right to choose between the newly created compensation system and the old damage suit arrangement. Pressure was exerted, however, to prevent rejection of compensation by the employer by providing that such a choice would deprive him of his three defense doctrines of assumption of risk, fellow servant and contributory negligence. Conversely, the worker who chose to adhere to his damage suit rights was handicapped by restoration of the defenses to his employer. As the Supreme

Court of the United States upheld the legal propriety of the compulsory type of compensation law in 1917 (*N.Y. Central Ry. Co.* v. *White,* 243 U.S. 188), there was no longer any reason for the elective type of measure.[25]

There were many more problematic aspects to WC laws. In 1934, Armstrong summarized the U.S. situation this way:

> Most of the American acts started with an undue number of the worst features of the various continental laws . . . [and] the great majority of American laws still contain a marked number of clauses which make them far less satisfactory compensation measures than the current laws of the important foreign industrial countries.[26]

The death benefits for surviving family members were not adequate and only in the case of six states—Arizona, Nevada, Oregon, New York, Washington, and West Virginia—and the Federal Employees Compensation Act did these benefits carry through the period of family dependency. Another problem, taken over from the British system, was that workers were usually left to their own devices to avail themselves of the law, there being no administrative or assistance machinery to facilitate the worker's filing and pursuit of his or her case. This lack of support for workers to pursue their cases coupled with another major failing of these laws—that workers might be charged with total or partial responsibility for their accident (something Berman develops in detail, as "blaming the victim," even in the educational approaches to WHS in which "the careless worker" was invented)[27]—meant all too low a rate of success in deserving cases. Also, insurance companies that entered this field for profit were likely to deny and fight all claims.

> Other major shortcomings of many American compensation measures are the following. First, certain codes contain penalty clauses which exclude from benefits or reduce benefits in situations where a variety of types of misconduct or "gross negligence" contributes to the injury. These clauses are to be criticized in that they lead to litigation and also because they shut out from compensation benefits thousands of workers who are injured at their work. Second, in order that the cost of compensation may be kept down, total compensation for all types of injury is limited to an arbitrary sum, regardless of the particular requirements of individual cases. Moreover specific permanent injuries are scheduled with corresponding compensation amounts, which are not adjusted with reference to the age and occupation of the worker. Third, weekly benefits, although usually stated as a percentage of the wage earned, are scaled down, by the inclusion of a low maximum benefit figure, to an amount inadequate to maintain the workers' family even at the lowest current standard of living. Fourth, occupational disease is not compensated as an industrial injury; even in the minority of states which do make provision, compensation only for listed diseases is allowed. Fifth, no provision for a state insurance carrier is made in thirty-one of the acts, so that the "poor risk" employer, whose business is rejected by the commercial companies, is left without any practicable opportunity to protect his workers.[28]

Whatever the failings of WC laws and their surrounding systems (for the United States Berman[29] terms it the "compensation-safety apparatus") and the failings are many, though faults vary greatly across nations, by 1932 Armstrong[30] found in her comprehensive survey of social insurance (WC, health, old age, disability, and unemployment) that WC was the most ubiquitous, with 119 systems in 62 countries. It was "well nigh universal."

Because Britain's law loaned many of its features to so many others, in large part because the United Kingdom was then the dominant center of the core capitalist nations in the political-economic world-system, and the cultural hegemony emanating from this center influenced colonies, former colonies, and

others,[31] it is worth noting that its cumbersomeness and many unsatisfactory aspects eventually led, under a strong Labour government just post WWII, to its replacement with the Industrial Injuries Act of 1946. In addition to all the aforementioned problems, the British system, contrary to many initial expectations and predictions, was incredibly litigenous. In being restricted initially to "the dangerous trades," disputes developed as to which jobs in what industries were included. With its definition as a factory-related act, disputes of an amazingly complex variety developed. As one observer put it, "Although we know generally what a 'factory' is I defy the Factory Inspectors themselves to say, what may or may not be a factory for the purposes of the Workmen's Compensation Act."[32] The exquisite character of the many disputes is suggested by the following:

> Many legal cases were generated by the wording of section 7(1) which applied the Act to "any building which exceeds thirty feet in height, and is either being constructed or repaired by means of scaffolding." Did scaffolding include a board resting on chairs, or the chair itself? Could the branch of a tree constitute scaffolding in particular circumstances? In *Veasey* v. *Chattle* (1902) the Court of Appeal held that a crawling board resting on a roof was scaffolding. Did the thirty feet rule include buildings which had been or would be over the height limit? This question was not settled until 1899 when the Court of Appeal ruled against such an interpretation. But there remained the difficult question of how a building was to be measured—should footings and chimneys be included, how should buildings on sloping ground be treated, what was the position when underground constructions, such as wells or subterranean railways were involved?[33]

By contrast, the German law had many advantages over the British law:

> Although there were some basic similarities (e.g., no-fault, finance provided wholly by employers—though in Germany this was so only after thirteen weeks—and earnings-related benefits), the German system of work accident insurance was very different, both in its principles and its administration, from that of Britain. Unlike the British scheme it was closely linked to the rest of the social insurance system; it provided for accident prevention, medical treatment and rehabilitation, whereas the British scheme did none of these things; in Germany insurance was compulsory and private companies played no role, whereas in Britain insurance was voluntary with proprietory companies possessing an important share of the market. A full list of contrasts would be extensive. Much closer to the German system were, *inter alia*, those of Austria (1887), Norway (1894), Greece (1901), Russia (1903), Switzerland (1906) and Hungary (1907). No official examination of continental experience preceded the British Act of 1897. According to Wilson and Levy, Britain lagged behind most other countries in terms of the level of cash benefits, provisions of medical expenses, surgical appliances and rehabilitation.[34]

In his brief overview of foreign experience for protection of WHS, including brief attention to WC, Ashford[35] surveyed eight European countries. Although it is unsure whether the United States does any better or worse in job safety and its compensation because "all statistics on occupational injury and disease represent gross underreporting [and thus] statistical comparisons between countries are not very revealing," it seems certain that most European systems do a better job of recognizing and compensating occupational disease.

> The programs for reporting, controlling, and compensating occupational disease are all far superior to those of the United States. In Sweden, occupational illness has been compensable for twenty years, and a steadily increasing number of diseases has been reportable and compensable since 1939, with an updated list provided in 1967. Under the German BGS insurance scheme, 47 occupational diseases are compensable. In France, there are 48 compensable occupational diseases, and if a disease is not

included as compensable, an employee can sue at common law. In France and Britain, a physician is required by law to report and diagnose properly all cases of occupational disease. In Britain, disease caused by twenty chemical substances or their derivatives as well as pneumoconiosis and byssinosis must be reported to the Factory Inspectorate. In Italy, control of 47 hazardous substances has been required by law since 1952 (amended 1967). In many cases, an illness may be classified as occupational if a hazardous substance which can cause a variety of illnesses is found in the work environment, even if no direct connection is known.

The point about linkages between WC and prevention deserves special emphasis. Initially, labor leaders had looked to employ liability acts and later WC not only as a way of relieving some of the misery workers and their families suffered because of the slaughter and maiming going on through work; they had hoped that if the employers had to pay, they would clean up their acts. As Harry D. Thomas, secretary of the Ohio State Federation of Labor, put it in 1910:

> . . . our object has been at all times not to get compensation or collect damages, but . . . to prevent accidents; and when safety laws have been made and deliberately violated and accidents continue to occur with as much frequency as before, we have come to the conclusion that the only way in which the employer will eliminate accidents in his plant as far as possible is to make him liable for all that occurs; and then he will find it cheaper to buy safety devices than to pay damages.[36]

But it hasn't worked out this way for many reasons. The levels of compensation—sometimes only 50% of wages in some U.S. states (whereas several European countries provide 100%)—and the ease of avoiding any payment through contesting cases are among the many reasons. Probably the most important factor is the comparative overall weakness of the workers' movement in the United States. But just with regard to the way premiums are collected without motivating either employers or insurers to clean up, Ashford observes:

> Workmen's compensation insurance, while mandatory in many of the countries studied, varies in the form it takes and the extent to which it affects accident and illness prevention. In France, Finland, and Germany, premiums (which are paid by the employers) are based on a percentage of the total wage bill, risk level, and firm performance record. In France, the threat of rate increases serves as an important economic lever in controlling accident and illness, particularly since the Regional Caisses have an inspection role. The British system utilizes a flat-rate premium and offsets the lack of individual firm incentive (caused by spreading the risk) by enabling employees to sue their employers for negligence to cover any damages not paid for by workmen's compensation insurance.[37]

My own comparison of provisions for WHS in six industrial countries does not highlight the overall strength of the West German system, but for the concerns of this paper, this oldest WC system in the world has evolved into one of the greatest interest.[38] Whereas in the United States it is hard to discern any important impact of the insurance industry and WC laws on prevention in the overall WHS system, in West Germany the WC system has evolved to become the very center of the system for protecting workers. Legal mandates come from two sources: the laws or ordinances of the national state and regulations issued by the three types of Mutual Accident Insurance Associations (the *Berufsgenossenschaften*). The latter began as self-help insurance-advisory agencies of the employers. Today these organizations are legally mandated public nonprofit corporations to cover work accidents and sickness in industry groupings—steel, shipbuilding, mining, and the like. They are grouped under three categories: industry (36), agriculture (19), and a number for public service. There is a 50–50 representation of employers and unions on the controlling boards of the *Berufsgenossenschaften*.[39] Thus, they are a major channel through which the workers' movement can have an influence on WHS. Generally, these laws, regulations, and the like from these different sources are said to be nonoverlapping. They proceed from more general to more specific measures as shown in TABLE 1.

Thus, the insurers are involved in every aspect of WHS in West Germany—setting of standards and regulations; inspection; training of WHS personnel and of employers and workers; and reimbursement for medical and rehabilitation expenses as well as compensation. Possibly the key characteristic of the system is its functioning more or less like a set of state-regulated public utilities with equal representation in the control structures of the potential or actual adversaries—organized labor and management.

TABLE 1. Parallel Structure for WHS Laws and Regulations in FGR

From the State	From the Insurers
Laws	Reich's insurance codes
Ordinances	Accident prevention regulations
General implementing ordinances	Rules for application of the accident prevention regulation
Generally acknowledged safety engineering and occupational health rules	Generally acknowledged safety engineering and occupational health rules
DIN[a] standards	DIN standards
VDE[b] regulations	VDE regulations
Directives, etc.	Directives, etc.

[a] DIN = German Industrial Standard.
[b] VDE = Association of German Electrotechnicians.

NEW DIRECTIONS

What lessons can we suggest from this all too cursory historical and cross-national overview of WHS and WC? One certainly is that considerably more in-depth work of this sort should be supported. It is high time for an update of the kind of cross-national survey Armstrong[30] did back in the 1930s. Such work, it is hoped, would not simply assemble a catalogue of provisions in different systems, but would also look into the dynamics of class and gender struggles and other political-economic contextual forces shaping systems in particular ways.

Two rather different strategies of reform can be envisioned. The first, tied more directly to the WC system, is piecemeal in approach. The second envisions more encompassing changes in the health system. I will not prejudge here the political-economic chances of either approach, although I personally favor the more encompassing strategy.

With respect to the WC system, it is a bit presumptuous of me to make suggestions from this brief overview. I am not as expert on the subject as are others who have given much more attention to the matter. A recent set of conference papers is of some help in this regard.[40] A good start would be made in improving the U.S. system if the ILO model was followed.[41] Although I am hesitant in making them, a distillation of my recommendations follows:

- It is high time for a national law to be adopted that would smooth out some of the hodge-podge variations of multiple state laws and assure minimal standards.
- Such a law should establish WC as a public nonprofit utility with equal representation of organized labor and management.
- Such a law should inject strong motivational forces into the WC system so as to bring about real preventive efforts.
- In this connection, no-fault compensation, which provides 100% of lost wages or income and benefits, should be provided.
- Work-related compensable diseases should be included on a presumptive list (I believe the Federal Republic of Germany uses a list of 55), and additions should be made as epidemiologic and other research establishes reasonable grounds for supposing a work connection.
- Tort liability of employers should be reestablished in cases of employer negligence or violation of strengthened OSHA standards and regulations to guard a punitive element in the system so as to cut down on company concealment, dishonesty, and wrongdoing and generally to enhance the preventive aspect of the system.
- An independent WHS service should be set up through a network of independent state-supervised clinics to cover all workplaces (as is required in Finland) so as to bring work-related disease fully into the picture and properly compensate injured workers as well as lead to prevention of such illness.[42]
- First-line general health care providers should be trained in WHS and linked into a clinic network as just suggested for continuing education.[43]

Alternatively, a more comprehensive approach would establish a fully regionalized national health service,[44] one that would explicitly take WHS adequately into account, especially as regards necessary links between first-line general health care and WHS. The Dellums Bill offered each year in Congress for more than a decade would go a long way toward meeting what is intended here. Compensation adequate for the maintenance of a decent life-style should be given to every citizen with a disability regardless of source (work-related or not). Such a social security disability system would simply remove the strife and confusion from the worker compensation system. Countries like Sweden today provide 90% of usual income during sickness and shift to such a system as I intend here when disability is permanent, either partial or total. Whether compensation should be related to earning power above an adequate floor is one of those points on which I feel others are more expert and able to advise.

Finally, for reasons indicated herein, this more encompassing approach should still provide for tort liability when damage from work has occurred because of employer negligence or wrongdoing.

Of course, in line with the framework suggested at the outset of this paper, I am not optimistic that any of this will happen in the United States in the near future. The struggle for workers' health and safety is long and hard because its improvement lies at the heart of the production process, and there is nothing more jealously guarded by the capitalist than control over the means and processes of production and there is nothing more important to the class-conscious worker than to claim her or his full due from a process organized to expropriate the surplus value produced by the workers' labor. The primary need is for the workers' movement to rejuvenate and spread, keeping such goals in mind as have been suggested in this specific sphere of concern, as it gathers strength for a much needed transformation of our society in a more humane direction.

NOTES AND REFERENCES

1. QUINN, A. E., 1972. Workmen's Compensation. Encyclopedia of Occupational Health and Safety. Vol. **L-Z**: 1515–1518. International Labor Organization. Geneva, Switzerland.
2. Bulletin No. 34 "Workers' Compensation," The Workers' Compensation Act as amended in 1979. Issued by The Board of Commissioners. October 1, 1979, Hamden, CT. Quote from p. 4. Note that the quote gives a singular possessive, "worker's," whereas the bulletin's title and text otherwise uses the collective "workers'," the practice I follow in this paper.
3. ASHER, R. A. 1986. A Flawed Precedent: The Legacy of the Original Workmen's Compensation Laws. Paper prepared for the annual meeting of the Organization of American Historians, April 12. I owe a special debt to Robert Asher, Professor of History at the University of Connecticut, Storrs, for this paper and some of his other works, notably: 1969. Business and Workers' Welfare in the Progressive Era: Workmen's Compensation Reform in Massachusetts, 1880–1911. Business History Rev. **43**: 452–475. Workmen's Compensation in the United States, 1880–1935. Unpublished Ph.D. dissertation, University of Minnesota. 1973. Radicalism and Reform: Workmen's Compensation in Minnesota 1910–1933. Labor History **14**(Winter): 19–23. I also benefitted from Robert Asher's reading and critique of an early draft of this paper.
4. ORLOFF, A. S. & T. SKOCPOL. 1984. Explaining the politics of public social spending. Am. Soc. Rev. **49**(December): 726–750.
5. QUADAGNO, J. S. 1984. Welfare Capitalism and the Social Security Act of 1935. Am. Soc. Rev. **49**(October): 632–647. Social welfare legislation in general in U.S.A. is seen as waxing and waning in relation to the ferment or heat in the system. *See* Regulating the Poor. 1971. F. F. Piven & R. A. Cloward, Eds. Pantheon. New York; see also Morse.
6. ELLING, R. H. 1986. The Struggle for Workers' Health. Baywood. Amityville, NY.
7. More discussion of these criteria or elements of a strong workers' movement is offered in my book (ref. 6). The comparatively weak situation for the United States is highlighted *in* Working Class Modernization and American Exceptionalism. Economic and Industrial Democracy Series, 1980. Shalev, M. & W. Korpi, Eds. Vol. **1**: 31–61. Sage. Beverly Hills, CA. The capitalist world-system is examined in the works of Wallerstein and many others. See, for example, Goldfrank, W. L. 1979. The World-System of Capitalism: Past and Present. Vol. 2 of Political Economy of the World-System Annuals. Sage. Beverly Hills, CA.
8. About half of U.S. medical schools require some WHS; the average is 4 hours. The others offer only elective work or have nothing. Levy, B. S. 1980. The Teaching of Occupational Health in American Medical Schools. J. Med. Ed. **55**: 18–22.
9. As quoted by Sigerist, H. E. 1943. From Bismarck to Beveridge: Developments and trends in social security legislation. Bull. Hist. Med. **13**: 365–388; quote and source p. 376.
10. All observers I consulted begin the story of WC with the German law of 1884: Quinn, *op. cit.*[1]; Asher, *op. cit.*[3]; Sigerist, *op. cit.*[9]; Orloff and Skocpol, *op. cit.*[4]; also the important cross-national comparative article by Armstrong, B.N. 1934. Workmen's Compensation. Encyclopedia of the Social Sciences. E. R. A. Seligman, Ed. Vol. **XV**: 488–492. Macmillan. New York; and Barth[18] whose work is cited below. However, Rubinow, I. M. 1934. Social Insurance. Encyclopedia of the Social Sciences. E. R. A. Seligman, Ed. Vol. **XIV**: 134–138. Macmillan. New York, says: "Although it is usual to ascribe the beginnings of the movement to the first compulsory accident insurance act of 1883 in Germany, which was rapidly followed by others covering sickness and old age, its sources derive from earlier periods. . . . A step toward the development of state insurance along somewhat different lines was made by France in 1850 and Italy in 1883 in their establishment of state insurance funds in which participation was voluntary and individual but which offered to the workman assurance of security on a non-profit basis, the state at times even contributing to the insured workman's premium." (pp. 134–135).

11. "um die Beine abzuschneiden," Sigerist, *op. cit.*[9]; p. 380.
12. Marx's quote from Fielden in Vol. I of *Capital* first published in 1867 as cited in Edwards, R. C. *et al.* Eds. 1972. The Capitalist System, Prentice-Hall. Englewood Cliffs, NJ, quote from p. 66, some deletions (. . .) added.
13. PAGE, J. A. & M. W. O'BRIEN. 1973. Bitter Wages. :47. Grossman. New York.
14. Bruce, as cited in MORSE, T. 1987. Dying to Know: The Workers' Struggle for the Right to Know. Unpublished Ph.D. dissertation, Ph.D. Program in Social Science and Health Care, University of Connecticut :15. I would like to acknowledge Tim Morse's special contribution to this paper. His suggestion of sources and critique of an early draft were most helpful.
15. DOWNEY, E. H. 1924. Workmen's Compensation. :144. Macmillan, New York. As cited in Morse, *op.cit.*,[14] p. 16.
16. DODD, W. F. 1936. Administration of Workmen's Compensation. :5. Commonwealth Fund. New York.[5] as cited by Somers, H. M. & A. R. Somers. 1954. Workmen's Compensation. John Wiley. New York.
17. MORSE, op. cit.,[14] makes the important point that workers' knowing the hazards could turn against them if employers used the "assumption of risk" defense. Thus, there were few motivating supports for the right to know in this early period.
18. BARTH, P. S. with H. A. Hunt. 1980. Workers' Compensation and Work-Related Illnesses and Diseases. MIT. Cambridge. MA; quote from p. 2. Also Fuchs, S. 1972. Compensation of Occupational Diseases. Encyclopedia of Occupational Health and Safety. Vol. **L-Z:** 1518–1521. ILO. Geneva.
19. CAHN. W. 1980. Lawrence 1912, The Bread and Roses Strike. Pilgrim. New York.
20. COWAN, PAUL. Introduction to Cahn, *op. cit.*[9]
21. MORSE, p. 18.
22. ASHER, *op. cit.*,[3] pp. 4–5.
23. *Ibid.,* pp. 2–3.
24. RUBINOW, *op. cit.*,[10] p. 135.
25. ARMSTRONG, *op. cit.*,[10] p. 490.
26. *Ibid.,* p. 490.
27. BERMAN, D. M. 1978. Death on the Job. Monthly Review Press, New York.
28. *Ibid.,* pp. 490–491.
29. BERMAN, *op. cit.*[27] Part of the extent of business domination of this apparatus in the United States is given by the following quote (pp. 74–75). "A half-dozen organizations have for decades had an important role in defining the business response to the problems created by dangerous working conditions, but a description of the activities and financing of such groups is hardly adequate to characterize the scope of the business role in occupational safety and health. In fact, every insurance claims representative, every corporate industrial hygienist, safety engineer, and medical director functions as part of the compensation-safety apparatus. In order to understand the workings of this system it is necessary to look at a number of topics: the ideas which guide management safety practice; the activities of the National Council on Compensation Insurance in setting insurance rates; the changes in the business role as standards-setting moves from private to public arenas and from an emphasis on safety to an emphasis on health; and the training, attitudes, and practices in the principal occupational health specialties. . . ."
30. ARMSTRONG, B. N. 1932. Insuring the Essentials. Macmillan. New York.
31. For a consideration of world-systems theory (work by Immanuel Wallerstein, Andre Gunder Frank, and others) in relation to workers' health and safety see Elling, *op. cit.*,[6] especially chapter 5, "Framework."
32. RUEGG, A. H. 1905. The Laws Regulating the Relations of Employers and Workmen in England. London: 149, as cited in Bartrip, P. W. J. 1987. Workmen's Compensation in Twentieth Century Britain. :26. Aveburg, Aldershot, U.K.
33. BARTRIP, *op. cit.*,[32] pp. 25–26.
34. *Ibid.,* pp. 148–149.
35. ASHFORD, N. A. 1976. Crisis in the Workplace, Occupational Disease and Injury, A Report to the Ford Foundation. :506. MIT. Cambridge, MA.
36. As quoted in Asher, *op. cit.*,[3] p. 3.

37. ASHFORD, op. cit.,[35] p. 507.
38. For more detail, see Elling, op. cit.[6]
39. "Berufsgenossenschaften," pp. 165–167, in Woerterbuch zur Humanisierung der Arbeit. Bundesanstalt fuer Arbeitsschutz. Bremerhaven, 1983.
40. CHELINS, J. (ed.). 1986. Current Issues in Workers' Compensation. W. E. Upjohn Institute for Employment Research. Kalamazoo, MI.
41. For detailed references and a summary of ILO recommendations see Quinn, op. cit.[1]
42. LANDRIGAN, P. J. & S. B. MARKOWITZ. 1987. Occupational Disease in New York State. Proposal for a Statewide Network of Occupational Disease Diagnosis and Prevention Centers. Report to the New York State Legislature, February 1987. Environmental and Occupational Medicine, Department of Community Medicine, Mount Sinai School of Medicine of the City University of New York. A very significant report which details the need for and recommendations concerning such a network of WHS clinics in New York State.
43. ELLING, R. H. & K. GREENLUND. 1988. First-line General Health Care Providers and Environmental and Workers' Health. A report based on an exploratory research. Department of Community Medicine, University of Connecticut (reproduced).
44. The concept of regionalization as used here includes such elements as involvement of citizens at all levels of the health service in determining its priorities and assessing its achievements, closed-ended financing, etc. A schema of 10 interwoven elements of regionalization is developed in Elling, R. H. 1980. The Cross National Study of Health Systems, Political Economies and Health. Transaction Books. New Brunswick, NJ, esp. pp. 100–101.

DISCUSSION OF THE PAPER

MITCHELL ZAVON: I learned some years ago, on a visit to Switzerland after a visit to Spain, that things were not always what they seemed to be. I had been told by a French physician in Madrid, as he looked down his nose at me because we did not have a physician for every plant, that in France they had a physician for every plant.

When I was visiting in Switzerland, we looked at some plants of the Geigy Corporation. They pointed to a plant in Germany, one in France, and one in Switzerland and described how the physicians in the Swiss and the German plants interchanged when they had to cover for each other. I asked about the physician in the French plant? They looked at me and said: "Oh yes, but he is in 300 other plants as well." The question is: How does it really work in Sweden and in the other countries you have cited?

ELLING: You are right to ask about variation and how fully coverage is being implemented. Although the question was directed toward Switzerland, the country that is actually attempting to cover all workplaces is Finland. An amazing effort is being made to bring in physicians for short-term courses and to certify them. Companies have to sign up either with a local municipal service or with a private polyclinic, like an HMO, to make arrangements for workers' health.

I was at a conference in October in Finland to learn more about this system. The evidence presented seemed quite convincing that the Finnish had in fact moved a long way toward implementing this law. This is not to say that the private clinics are going to function in just the same way as the public ones; there are variations still within the country.

ERIC JANNERFELDT, (*Swedish Embassy, Washington, D.C.*): After hearing Ray Elling, I should say that I am proud to be Swedish. As with so many other things, however, it is important to remember that things may look better in the laws and on the books than they are in reality and that also applies to Sweden. We have come further than you have in the United States, but the background is a bit different. Sweden has a long history of political stability and excellent industrial growth. We survived two world wars and did not have to enter them.

These issues are important to remember when it comes to realizing why we are where we are. It is not a simple situation in which the United States and Sweden started at equal points with equal resources and equal commitment to safety. I should mention that the Swedes have an almost excessive interest in safety, perhaps due to the proximity of our powerful neighbor, the Russians. But whatever the cause, that sense of the importance of safety has carried over also into the workplace.

Of course, all of this has been done at a cost. We have the highest taxes in the world. We have a very large and, in a sense, an unproductive governmental sector, and we have been criticized for going too far in our regulatory efforts. I think that even in Sweden, we are seeing the limits of what can be done with regulation, and right now we are in the midst of trying different approaches.

When it comes to learning from Sweden, you have to realize the difference, but there are some lessons too. There has been a lot of talk about regulation; yet there are limits to what it can achieve.

If the regulation is to be effective, there has to be effective enforcement. We do not have that in Sweden. There also must be an acceptance of regulation, and I do not mean acceptance only in the political sense. I mean an overall broad acceptance in society that the regulation is something that has merit, that is good, and that really justifies the increased costs and complications. It is not enough to write something into law; there also must be consensus and acceptance.

If there is one major lesson to be learned from the Swedish occupational health and safety system, it is to characterize it as a worker-based system. The action is in the plant, in the health and safety committees, and in the wide net of well-informed people, including local study circles.

I do not mean to pretend that everybody is always enthusiastic and actively involved in reading the latest pamphlets from the Work Environment Fund. However, the structure at the local level and the degree of involvement are amazingly high and admirable. It strikes me that the control really rests there, and that the awareness of the hazards and doing something about them indeed rests much more with the workers than it does in any other system.

TEE L. GUIDOTTI (*University of Alberta*): I share the common view that Europe is an exceedingly valuable source of new concepts and innovative ideas in occupational health. The Swedish, Finnish, and German systems are very useful in introducing new ideas. Whether these ideas will actually work on a demonstration basis in the more pluralistic and expansive societies of North America is an open question. Dr. Jannerfeldt from Sweden pointed this out very nicely.

What is needed is a laboratory to demonstrate whether or not these ideas work. There are 10 such laboratories in the provinces of Canada in which various models are being applied. Among the most interesting is in the Province of Québec where there exists not only a provincial equivalent to NIOSH, which is doing very good research in safety-related behavior, but also a very innovative system of community occupational health clinics, similar to what is being proposed for New York State. This is a network that is now relatively well implemented, and data exist to permit its evaluation.

The point I am making is that a great deal is going on north of this border, ranging from a highly sophisticated infrastructure along the lines of those of

Québec and Alberta, to a less sophisticated structure on both coasts. Careful evaluation of that experience can teach us as much in the United States as the study of the National Health Insurance schemes in Britain and Canada taught us about health care financing.

DOROTHY WIGMORE: Another important lesson to be learned from Québec, and perhaps from Manitoba, is the involvement of the workers. You speak about the need to have workers trust their doctors. In Québec, the joint worker-management safety committee has the right to hire and fire the doctors. They also have the right to decide on the nature of the training programs and to choose protective equipment.

There are many problems with the workers' compensation systems in the various provinces, but in some places where more worker-oriented political parties have been in power, attempts have been made to improve that situation. Improvement certainly is taking place in Manitoba at the moment. We are looking at developing an occupational health service that would function along the lines of the WHO definition of the occupational health services, and that uses the Québec model to a certain extent. We also looked at countries such as Sweden for help and guidance.

The other place that people ought to be aware of is New Zealand, which has a very interesting workers' compensation system that is linked to their health care system. Because they have universal health coverage, that connection makes life a little simpler when it comes to dealing with some of the workers' compensation issues with which everyone here is familiar.

ELLING: I agree that it is very important to look at other experiences, because it is high time that we were more systematic, not just in a cross-sectional way, but in a dynamic historical way. I certainly support the recommendations to look further at other experiences.

New Developments in Workers' Compensation Law

T. FORREST FISHER[a]

Campbell Soup Company
Camden, New Jersey 08101-0391

The basic purpose of workers' compensation legislation is to provide the prompt payment of specified benefits to an injured worker, regardless of the question of fault. The workers' compensation laws of the individual states vary considerably in content and scope, especially as they apply to occupational diseases.

The Occupational Safety and Health Act of 1970 established the National Commission on State Workmen's Compensation Laws. The Commission was directed "to undertake a comprehensive study and evaluation of state workers' compensation laws to determine if such laws provide an adequate, prompt, and equitable system of compensation." The Commission presented its report to the President in July 1972. The Commission's report called for liberalization and some degree of uniformity of the state acts.[1]

In the years since the Commission's report several changes have been made in the individual states' workers' compensation acts; however, a lack of uniformity in the individual state acts persists. The greatest difference between state acts exists in the area of occupational disease, which is usually defined as an industrial disease contracted independent of an accidental injury and arising out of employment. The occupational disease discrepancy in the state acts is complicated by the fact that the occupational disease may be delayed in onset; in fact, the development of occupational disease may be spread over many years and over several employers.[2] The compensability of the occupational disease is further complicated by the additive or synergistic effect of the environment external to the workplace and individual lifestyle, as well as genetic factors.

The report of the National Commission on State Workmen's Compensation Laws served as a stimulus for the revision and improvement of several state acts. It was, however, not the first attempt at reforming state workers' compensation acts, as substantial reform had taken place in New York, California, Oregon, Maryland, Idaho, and Pennsylvania prior to the Commission's Report.[3]

The differences in the workers' compensation acts of the individual states were increased with the publication in 1983 of the "Suggested List of Ten Leading Work-Related Disease and Injuries" by the National Institute for Occupational Safety and Health. This list included: (1) occupational lung diseases, (2) musculoskeletal injuries, (3) occupational cancers, (4) severe occupational traumatic injuries, (5) occupational cardiovascular diseases, (6) disorders of reproduction, (7) neurotoxic disorders, (8) noise-induced loss of hearing, (9) dermatologic conditions, and (10) psychologic disorders.[4]

Many of the state workers' compensation acts do not have provisions that accommodate these conditions. Since 1983, we have observed a movement of reform by some states to accommodate these conditions. For example, effective

---

[a] Past President of the American College of Occupational Medicine, S.S.W. Seegers Road, Arlington Heights, Illinois 60005.

July 1, 1987, amendments were made to the state workers' compensation law in Montana. These changes included the following:

(a) exclude from coverage injuries from emotional or mental stress and disease not caused by an accident;

(b) make heart attacks compensable only if they are the primary cause of physical harm; and

(c) change the definition of occupational disease to exclude physical or mental harm arising from emotional or mental stress or from a nonphysical stimulus or activity.[5]

Political, social, and economic pressures are constantly increasing benefits to keep pace with the rising cost of living. We note activity in some states to implement reform that would accommodate health care cost containment and case management. The most consistent thing about the individual state workers' compensation act is change.

I propose that there is a need, more than ever before, for a national scheme, built from the ground up, to deal with workers' compensation. The present individual state laws handle occupational disease poorly, at best. There is a need for a formula determining disability based on impairment, environmental influence, lifestyle influence, hereditary influence, and workplace exposure. There is a need for a formula to prorate the liability among contributing employers.[2] I feel that physicians and attorneys have not performed well in the current system. Much of the data to support the reward is based on subjective, as opposed to objective data, and once the reward is determined, not enough of it reaches the worker. There is a definite need for more scientific objectivity and less adversarial negotiation. There is a need for more documented exposure, as opposed to assumed exposure.

I propose that it is time to consider the development of a national board (please note, I did not say a federal board but a national board [not under federal control]) with equal representation from labor and industry that would: (1) develop and control rules and regulations of workers' compensation for the nation, (2) oversee regional boards, and (3) accept or reject appeals for evaluation of regional board decisions.

The regional boards would accept or reject a request for an evaluation of a claim submitted by the worker. The regional boards would also have equal representation from labor and industry.

Regional medical centers should be identified to evaluate each case for which a claim is submitted to the board. Where possible, these evaluation centers could be located in the educational resource centers. Testing would be performed by specialists to develop objective data. Work hardening centers could be used to evaluate rehabilitation data and assist in preparing the claimant for return to the worksite. Funding of the board could be made on the basis of cost-plus for claims settled. The employers could continue with the current system of insurance to support the payment of their claims either through private insurance carriers, self-insurance, or a special fund provided by the regional board. The settlement of compensation claims could still be handled through four basic methods[1]: (1) the formal agreement method, (2) the direct settlement, (3) formal claim petition, and (4) the hearing method.

The payment for temporary total disability, permanent total disability, permanent partial disability, and death could continue as it is at the present time; however, there would be one uniform scale throughout the nation. Individual employers would be required to maintain a list of panel physicians for selection by the injured for treatment. The national board would be advised to establish and maintain minimal requirements for claim submission and the regional boards would be advised to accommodate those who need help with reading, writing, and claim preparation. Serious effort would be made to provide easy access to the system and to accommodate scientific data submitted by the treating physician, the evaluating panel physician, claimant, and employer. Flexibility of the system would be maintained to accommodate changes in the scientific literature.

I feel that such a system would provide fair and uniform compensation with maximum reward for the claimant on a national scale.

REFERENCES

1. U.S. CHAMBER OF COMMERCE. 1986. Analysis of Workers' Compensation Laws. Washington, D.C.
2. DANZON, P. M. 1987. Compensation for occupational disease: Evaluating the options. J. Risk & Insurance **54**: 264–280.
3. The Report of The National Commission on State Workmen's Compensation Laws, July 1972. Washington, D.C.
4. NATIONAL INSTITUTE FOR OCCUPATIONAL SAFETY AND HEALTH. 1983. Suggested List of Ten (10) Leading Work-Related Diseases and Injuries. National Institute for Occupational Safety and Health. Atlanta, GA.
5. Comp. News in Occupational Hazards. December 1987: 20. Penton Publishers. Cleveland, Ohio.

DISCUSSION OF THE PAPER

JOHN CHONG (*McMaster University, Hamilton, Ontario, Canada*): I am concerned about the recognition of occupational disease. This is a central issue in any health care or public health system or workers' compensation system throughout the world. Without a category of health professionals trained in occupational health, it is not possible to recognize the work-related disease. Underreporting is a frequent result. The key issue you have identified is that of training all health professionals at the undergraduate, postgraduate, and continuing educational levels.

At McMaster University, we have tried very hard to target our educational reforms at all levels. Undergraduates are trained in occupational health, as well as in a specific area. But many barriers need to be overcome to implement this program. Some problems stem from underrecognition of the importance of occupational and environmental causes of disease.

I would like to ask how we can succeed in getting students' attention early. How can we transform the very constrained medical model, the diagnosis and treatment model, which is already ingrained in a high proportion of students when they enter medical school, to a more prevention-oriented effort? Without that change in orientation, many of the concepts that we have discussed will never reach fruition.

FISHER: You have made a good point. As occupational physicians, we must be represented on medical schools' curriculum committees because that is where the decisions are made. Medical schools are not preparing physicians for dealing with cost-containment or with quality-of-care issues. They are not developing physicians who are prepared to think about preventive medicine.

Another thing you can do is to encourage local industries and medical schools to collaborate to bring their students into industrial facilities. I just spoke at the medical school of the University of Medicine and Dentistry of New Jersey in Stratford, New Jersey addressing the students and the residents in the field of occupational medicine. They need exposure to the concept of preventive medicine; it is foreign to them.

If we are going to get good data and good scientific programs, physicians have to be the bottom line in the system. No matter what you do within the plant, that patient has contact with the physician outside the plant, and that physician has to recognize occupational disease.

You are right: There is a big job ahead of us. There are not enough of us to do it, but we can try.

ALAN ENGELBERG (*American Medical Association, Chicago, Ill.*): Many medical specialty groups from orthopedists to emergency physicians are tripping over each other trying to get into occupational medicine. Internists tried to say they were the only ones who could do it. In this context, I would like to ask you, Dr. Fisher, whether, when you were President of the American Occupational Medical Association, you tried to bring in some of these specialty groups to meet with your Board of Directors. Did you broach the idea of anything like specialty centers in occupational medicine? If you did, how was that accepted by these other specialties who are now trying to get into the practice of occupational medicine?

FISHER: I did broach it, and they were not keen on it. I have no problem with the internists or the orthopedists or anyone else wanting to practice occupational medicine. The more the better. My problem is that most of them tend to look only at the acute case, but do not follow up. When a doctor treats a patient, he does not look at the cause of the exposure. He does not come down on the employer or go into the worksite.

That is the problem. The occupational physician cannot practice occupational medicine in the closet. He must go into the workplace to see the exposures. That is where the patient is located, and it is there that you have got to stop the future exposures.

Treating the acute case of carbon monoxide poisoning today does not stop the process. You have got to get to the source. That is my concern with this business of every doctor wanting to practice occupational medicine, while wanting to stay in his white coat and office. You cannot do it.

JAMES CONE (*University of California, San Francisco, Calif.*): Our problem has been in dealing with the American Board of Preventive Medicine in regard to occupational medicine. We need to examine the performance of the Board in the field. Is it advancing or retarding the field?

Our experience suggests it may be retarding the interests of occupational medicine. Therefore, we should examine the original rationale for founding the Board, which was to raise the performance and standards in the field and to promote the education of physicians in occupational medicine. Too often the Board seems to create obstacles.

FISHER: From the standpoint of the American Occupational Medical Association, we would like very much to establish an independent board in occupational medicine. The problem now is that such a proposal has to be voted upon by all the other existing board representatives. The American Board of Preventive Medicine covers general public health, aerospace medicine, and occupational medicine. I think that there is a need for an independent occupational medicine board separate from the other two. Occupational medicine is a specialized area, and the lack of a separate board is a shortcoming.

VALERIE WILK (*Farmworkers' Justice Fund, Washington, D.C.*): I would like to call your attention to the fact that when we are talking about reform of workers' compensation, we should remember that agricultural workers are not even covered by workmens' compensation laws in half of the states. When you are talking about only 1200 board-certified occupational medicine physicians in the U.S., how many of those are based in the cities as opposed to rural areas? I was pleased to hear Dr. El Batawi acknowledge earlier the agricultural component of the workforce.

FISHER: One of the amendments to the Gaydos Bill on the House floor was to exempt agricultural facilities that have seasonal workers who work fewer than six months a year from notification. That is a real problem.

TEE L. GUIDOTTI (*University of Alberta, Faculty of Medicine, Edmonton, Alberta*): In Canada a free-standing board was, in fact, established—the Canadian Board of Occupational Medicine. It has had a wonderfully salutary effect on the primary certification agency, the Royal College of Physicians and Surgeons, leading eventually to breaking up the logjam and to the establishment of occupational medicine as an independent specialty apart from what had previously been the general area of community medicine. Now, there are, in effect, two pathways to certification in Canada—a direct path, and an indirect path, which is eminently suitable for the lateral transfer of specialists from other areas into occupational medicine. This is a very interesting development, but one of the major benefits of the alternate pathway was its effect on the primary board specialization pathway.

FISHER: Similarly, in this country, most of the practicing occupational physicians and many of those who are board-certified are the result of mid-career conversions.

MITCHELL R. ZAVON (*Agatha Corp., Lewiston, N.Y.*): As someone certified in everything including industrial hygiene, I agree with virtually everything you have said, but one huge area has been overlooked: Most workers are not seen by doctors. They are seen by nurses. Most plants are not visited by doctors. If the workers are lucky, they are visited by a qualified, competent industrial hygienist.

We live in an age of specialization. Although I have taught that the physician should get out in the plant so that he knows what the worker is exposed to, a busy physician in private practice has to be extremely dedicated to do that.

We depend on the specialist, the industrial hygienist, or the safety engineer, to describe the situation to a physician or to a nurse who is knowledgeable. We should not ignore the fact that the nursing component of the occupational health team is more critical than is the physician, and that the industrial hygienist is more important in cleaning up the work environment than is the physician.

We need the concept of the team to be reinstated. During the 38 years I have practiced occupational medicine, I have seen the team sundered by one specialty area after another opting to get out from under the umbrella. In some industries these specialists do not even report to the same people.

One last comment on workers' compensation laws. Having spent many years in Ohio, I am not at all sure that that state-run model is one that we should emulate. I was not successful within that system in inculcating the notion of prevention. My advice fell on deaf ears in a state-run "nonprofit" system, which has been profitable for the politicians and the political process within the state.

FISHER: A major problem I see is that many facilities do not have a full-time hygienist. They use an insurance carrier to provide hygiene services. A related problem is that the plant manager or production manager, both of whom are lay persons, are typically given the responsibility for knowing when the hygienist has to be called in. In the last year I have visited 39 of our facilities with that very purpose in mind—to sensitize the nurses to finding the exposures and to knowing when to call the hygienist.

Tort Litigation

A Goal, a Source of Polarization, and a Possible Tool for Prevention

RONALD SIMON

Connerton, Ray & Simon
1920 L Street, N.W.
Washington, D.C. 20036-5004

I shall begin by describing the workers' compensation system, because I have been working in it for fifteen years. Then I'll talk about the tort liability system. Specifically, I shall give an example of a particular chemical about which I am preparing a trial, and shall use this example to explain why the tort system is effective. Finally, I shall conclude with a few comments about lawyers. There appeared to be some lawyer-bashing at this workshop, and while much of that is well deserved, I believe that the role of lawyers in protecting injured workers is crucially important.

First, the workers' compensation system. I'm sure I was placed on the program because I disagree with most of the things the last speaker, Dr. Fisher, said. The goal of the tort litigation system is one that leads to prevention, to deterrence, and in fact to more polarization. There will be more polarization from the tort system, but that's not necessarily bad.

A workers' compensation system, particularly one with a national board, will tend to move away from polarization. Such a system will also tend to produce results that are drastically tilted against the worker and other persons whose position of relative power in society is small. A national board will mirror the orientation of the persons on those boards and the persons and interests opposing compensation for workers.

The workers' compensation system was instituted at the turn of the century. On a state-by-state basis, people are said to have given away their tort rights with regard to workplace injuries in exchange for the right to be compensated without regard to fault. This trade-off was effected merely by passing a law implementing this system. In 1900 tort rights weren't worth very much. That the system included the provision of medical benefits for injured people was significant in 1900, but is hardly so in our era when most workers have health insurance. Finally, anyone who has experience in the Workers' Compensation system knows that it is hardly nonadversarial.

I was a law professor for many years, and I had my students try cases in a workers' compensation system, including in the largest and some would say most infamous workers' compensation system, the Veterans Administration.

The Veterans Administration is nonadversarial by statute. The standard of proof is that every reasonable doubt must be resolved on behalf of the claimant. The Veterans Administration's highest administrative body has allowed 13% of cases that come before it each and every year. If someone from the Veterans Administration were here, they would explain to you that this isn't a quota; it just happens that for many years in a row, 13% of the people win.

The 13% win rate is very small. By contrast, in jury trials the rate is about 50%. In most compensation systems it's much higher than 13%. As a person who has made a study of the Veterans Administration, I can testify that the 13% quota is inflated.

For example, once one of my students missed a deadline. That's the worst thing a lawyer can do. I was terrified for the student and went to someone in authority in the agency, musing aloud about a way to deal with this problem, how I could have the veteran's case tried even though the deadline had been missed. I was told there would be no problem at all. One could appeal the missing of a deadline, and one would always win.

I was puzzled. How could that be? The person from the government explained it to me. They have a 13% quota of cases that they have to grant. If they grant your case and say that you didn't miss the deadline, it counts as one of the 13% granted cases. However, the case still has to be sent down and tried on the merits. They can grant a case, include it in the 13%, and still never give the claimant a nickel, because the claimant will later lose on the merits.

Those who have been in a workers' compensation system know how stringently the worker is questioned by the "nonadversarial" judge even if there's no party on the other side. The judge is typically more inquisitorial than any jury would ever be. The notion that we can pass a law and create a nonadversarial system just doesn't fit the facts.

Typically in these "informal" systems, paid counsel is on the other side, and will raise every imaginable technical, nontechnical, and foolish objection to the victim's claim. Even when there is no opposing counsel, one finds that the industrial boards or whoever is deciding these cases looks at them in a very adversarial way. This is worse when you get the kind of system that was suggested by Dr. Fisher. The national board he proposed would function like the Veterans Administration.

The Veterans Administration testifies about its actions on a regular basis to the Congress. It says that it cannot allow a claim for a disease that is caused by a chemical unless there is a *consensus in the scientific community*. It claims that just because I could find an expert who would affirm that a particular bladder cancer is caused by a dye or a particular leukemia by benzene, that is not enough to prevail, because the company would have doctors that would say the opposite. The Veterans Administration says that as long as there's no consensus, the national board will not allow compensation.

This is why I prefer trial by jury. As a lawyer who has worked for years on litigation concerning toxic chemicals, I can assert that there's never going to be a consensus, but that there will always be somebody on every side of a question. Furthermore, a national board is necessarily going to be extremely conservative. Both logic and our experience tell us this. A compensation system based on supposed scientific expertise will drift drastically towards conservatism.

The conservative drift has two different causes. The first is that those who have the money and power to fund and control scientific studies are the manufacturers of chemicals, who have good reason to deny their dangers. The second is the skepticism that is inherent in scientific pursuit. Scientists require a high level of proof to conclude something is proved scientifically. The way that scientists approach uncertainty will cause a national compensation system controlled by them to be very difficult for claimants.

Regarding regulatory decisions, it was also suggested by Dr. Fisher that we need more regulation from the Occupational Safety and Health Act (OSHA) and other federal regulatory schemes to protect worker health. This is one subject on which I agree with the current President of the United States, namely, that the regulatory system has not been successful in protecting the public.

My typical clients and audiences are trade unionists, workers, veterans, and community groups who are the victims of toxic chemicals. In addressing these groups, as well as lawyers who represent them, I point out that we don't know of any other substances like asbestos. There are many factors that make asbestos unique: the exposure of so many people; mesothelioma, the unique marker disease; the ability to find the fibers when a person is dead; and the unique X-ray findings. Tracing the injuries caused by another chemical is much more difficult. If you try a case of a person now who is dying of disease caused by asbestos, there's very likely not to have been any warning on the product. The workers who were in shipyards or in the construction trades received no warnings about the asbestos. In the trial of these cases we blow up reproductions of letters to show what the companies knew and concealed and compare this to what the workers were not told. However, the current regulatory process leads to an environment in which there generally are some warnings. For most of the dangerous chemicals that people are now exposed to in the workplace, there is a material safety data sheet (MSDS). There is a regulatory process under OSHA. Pesticides are regulated under the Federal Insecticide, Fungicide, and Rodenticide Act (FIFRA).

The regulations have created a system that is better. There's lots of information. There can be no doubt that warnings and information are very beneficial. However, the regulatory environment also poses grave threats to public health.

This can be seen from the example of chlordane and heptachlor. This chemical, which has been produced as a pesticide since 1948, has been under intense regulatory scrutiny for at least fifteen years. It is regulated under FIFRA, and at this moment it cannot be manufactured for sale in the United States. What had been manufactured can be sold and applied in the United States. Of course, it can be manufactured and sold in a lot of other countries, though most of the countries of Western Europe have banned its use.

The regulatory history reveals claims by its manufacturer that it is safe. The company has epidemiologic studies that claim to prove it does not hurt anybody, and there was a government policy that allowed it to be used. The company claimed that workers in its plants had been checked and were showing no adverse health effects.

Because persons came to us who were sick, lawyers began to challenge the claims of safety. We found out something that most of you have already learned. If you look at the studies that said the chemicals were safe, you will find this conclusion in the executive summary and the conclusion of these studies. However, if you sit down and look at the data in those studies, you will not find that the chemical was safe. You will find that there were statistically significant increases in a variety of diseases that were never reported in the conclusion. We found that almost every study that was done on this chemical was done by the company that manufactured it, and that these studies had a unique set of qualities.

Number one, many studies were never reported in the scientific literature, nor were they ever peer reviewed. These studies were conducted in-house or by paid contractors. Because they were never reported in the literature, the conclusions were never reviewed by independent experts. The second thing we found was that the conclusions in these studies were rarely, if ever, supported by the data in the studies themselves.

As far back as the 1950s, we found studies that claimed to show that the chemical did not enter houses if it was properly applied to the exterior. That's what the introduction to the study said, that's what the conclusion to the study said, and that's what all the reports of the study said. That's what all the company literature said; that's what all the government reports said. But if you actually go and look at the raw data, if you actually reexamine the gas chromatographs, you will see the chemical in the houses. It was consistently there even though reports said it was not.

Another problem with the regulatory process is that as a product moves through it, all of the actions are controlled by lawyers. Only in protracted tort litigation do these studies come to light. The way in which a lawyer gets these documents in litigation is in itself instructive. First, the lawyer asks the company for its studies. Even though they are required by law to produce the studies, the companies rarely give them to you. The second step is to go to the judge repeatedly to force the company to produce the studies. After you have spent time and money to force the company to follow its legal obligation to produce its studies, the company tells the judge that they will provide the studies if you sign a piece of paper that you won't show them to anybody else. (Heaven forbid that someone else should see the studies and realize that they don't support the reported conclusions!) After you get these studies, you analyze them and try to compare the data in the studies with the conclusions that have been drawn.

In a workers' compensation system, it's very difficult to get the studies the company has done, because the question of what the company knew is not relevant. In a tort suit what the company knew is relevant for two reasons. What the company knew is compared to what they told you in order to determine whether they provided adequate warnings. The consideration of fault is irrelevant in a workers' compensation system.

What a company knew is also important in terms of punitive damages. Punitive damages is an award of damages based on moral fault and an expression of punishment to deter reckless and outrageous conduct. There is an opportunity to judge a company who knew about a chemical and compare this with what it did and said. Punitive damage considerations are based not on science but on moral principles such as retribution and punishment. These concepts are very important and have absolutely nothing to do with a workers' compensation system.

I have clients who, when a machine exploded and a 2000-pound door was shot across a room and through a 14-inch brick wall, were killed or maimed. In the plant there was a lot of wrongdoing that caused that tragedy. But if the wrongdoing was by the employer in the state of Virginia and in most states, the only remedy is workmen's compensation. Workers' lives aren't worth very much under that system. If I could take their case to a jury and I could show that their injury was caused by the wrongdoing of their employer, a jury would find their lives and injuries to be worth much more. A jury could evaluate both the suffering and the wrongdoing. But under a workers' compensation system neither of these is considered, and my clients' lives are not worth much. Retribution and deterrence are human values that the workers' compensation system has taken away.

The tort system has ways of getting a lot of this information that the regulatory and Compensation systems lack. The government does not have the will to look at these chemicals themselves; neither does it have the resources to go through each study and to reevaluate it.

As you know, the tort system is under attack. People in corporate America and the insurance industry have tried to persuade the public to move tort liability toward a workers' compensation system. People in the trade union movement, who have tried to make the compensation system better, are often attracted by that line of reasoning. What you need to ask yourself is why big business is trying to take away the tort system and make it into a workers' compensation system. You don't need much imagination to come up with the answer. The workers' compensation system is to their advantage because it limits the liability of companies who injure people. The company enjoys limited financial exposure and the focus of their wrongdoing is removed. The burden of proving causation is still there, but there is a severe limit on damages. At the same time all the issues that go with corporate wrongdoing are taken away. If the question of liability and wrongdoing is eliminated and damages are severely capped, the element in the system that could encourage companies to behave disappears.

By severely limiting damages and eliminating all aspects of blame, the workers' compensation system institutionalizes the relative position of power of the participants. By taking away any possibility of redress, the injured worker is rendered powerless. By limiting the damages that the injured person can recover, the system in effect removes the incentive to uncover the wrongdoing, because it will go unpunished. The company has the resources to defend the compensation case to whatever extent it chooses on limited grounds or causation. With a compensation system, where the damages are very limited, there's very little reason for the case to be aggressively pursued, since there's very little that can be accomplished in doing it. The maximum exposure of the company is very slim, no matter what it has done. Given the limit on liability imposed by the compensation system, it is truly remarkable that companies so vigorously contest compensation claims, and administrative tribunals are so reluctant to grant compensation.

I can offer further elucidation as to why big business wants a compensation system. Next week I'm going to attend a meeting of corporate counsel called by the Bureau of National Affairs to discuss legal issues that threaten the existence of corporations. One topic addresses "events that can put a corporation into play." I have been asked to speak about product liability and toxic torts because corporations are now aware that if they make decisions that seriously injure many people, the entire existence of the corporation can be threatened.

Some corporations have been found by juries to have caused so much devastation that they are seeking refuge in the bankruptcy courts. These bankruptcies by solvent companies are efforts to shield the company against the wrath of juries who hear the sordid facts of corporate wrongdoings. The extreme efforts companies make to escape juries cannot be ignored. A major corporation's existence can be put into play only because these cases of wrongdoing can be taken to court. If a workers' compensation system in which damages are severely limited is implemented, you can be confident that no matter how many people a company murders, it will never be put into play. Its existence will not be threatened and the deterrent effects will be eliminated. The cherished moral values that create justice will disappear.

We need the tort system because it provides the necessary incentives for both the worker to get significant compensation and the companies in terms of some risks and deterrence. I want to quote from Robert Sherrill, who reviewed books about the Dalkon Shield and the asbestos industry. These books detail how lawyers played a role in the Dalkon Shield and in the asbestos litigation in uncovering and demonstrating what the companies did wrong. The lawyers had the incentive to uncover the examples of conscious deception practiced by the sellers of these products. These discoveries would never have been made in a compensation system in which the issues of wrongdoing, and concealment of the known dangers of the products, are irrelevant. Sherrill's remark is taken from a publication called *Grand Street*, which is a literary review. His opening paragraph expresses better than I can why we need the tort system and what its role is in the American system of justice.

> There is something over 1500 men and women on the death rows of America. Given the social context in which they operated, one might reasonably assume that they

were sentenced to be executed, not because they are murderers but because they were truly inefficient. Using guns, knives, the usual foot paraphernalia, they dispatched only a few more than their own numbers. Had they used asbestos, mislabeled pharmaceutical drugs, devices, defective autos, illegally used and illegally disposed chemicals, they could have killed, crippled and tortured many thousands of workers and other people and they could have done it without much fuss at all.

We need the tort system because it raises the moral issue of wrongdoing. If we go back to the Old Testament, we see that the notion of responsibility—and irresponsibility, or wrongdoing—is an essential part of our values. A workers' compensation system that places no fault is truly a system without a crucial element of justice.

DISCUSSION OF THE PAPER

SCOTT JACOBS (*Office of Management and Budget, Washington, D.C.*): I work in the Office of Information for Regulatory Affairs in the Office of Management and Budget.

I appreciate the value of your comments. Your statement that regulation has not worked and cannot work does not seem well supported, however; you said that regulation makes it more difficult to sue later on. It seems to me, though, that you must consider that regulation may make it *unnecessary* to sue later on, and no worker wants to preserve the right to sue if that means incurring a disease.

Second, you said that tort increases the risk for employers. It also increases the risk for employees who go through the system. I would like you to address the capriciousness of the tort system and talk a little bit about the equity considerations.

SIMON: First, on the issue of regulation, there is no question that if regulation worked, conditions in the workplace would be better. Similarly, if my kids behaved, I would not have to punish them. It is that simple. Unfortunately, history is against us. History indicates that the nonadversarial system does not work in our society.

As for capriciousness, that issue does not trouble me at all. To be sure, our system is capricious. However, we live in a democratic society and the risk of having different outcomes is one of the consequences of living in this society. One definite risk of a situation in which plaintiffs go to different juries is different results; that reflects the fact that we have different states, that is, federalism. Indeed, if you go back to *The Federalist* papers, on which our nation is based, you have to realize that a conscious decision was made by the Founding Fathers to accept a risk of different results rather than run the risk of uniform results which might be far skewed to one direction or the other; capriciousness is a small price to pay for freedom. It is a trade-off that I am willing to accept.

MICHAEL GOCHFELD (*New Jersey Medical School, University of Medicine and Dentistry, Newark, N.J.*): I would like to switch attention away from the macro level which you have been covering and toward an issue on the micro level. Peter Schuck, in a review of the Agent Orange tort litigation, was commenting on some of Judge Weinstein's decisions and formulas, that is, his algorithms, two of which had to do with assigning proportional responsibility based on the manufacturer's share and on the proportion of excess damage to which a particular case was attributed. I think that Schuck was questioning whether we were ready for such fine-tuned algorithms in the tort system. What is the current stage of evolution? If, for example, we keep the tort system, what is our stage of evolution in actually making it work for very complicated cases such as class action suits?

SIMON: A lot of questions are implicit here. Judge Weinstein's famous decision in the Agent Orange case has spawned some literature, in which you will find an article by Len Schroeder entitled "Demystifying Judge Weinstein." Weinstein's view, in essence, is that you cannot prove anything without human epidemiology. Making limitations like that is hardly rational. In terms of the difficulty of cases, there is no doubt that cases can become very complex.

With regard to the specific issue of proportional responsibility, generally in most states we have what is called joint and several liability; this term means that any of the proportional parties can be assessed for all of the damages. Some states have passed other laws; California now has proportional responsibility.

Complexity is an issue that is generally raised along with equity. The best authority on the issue of complexity is the Rand Corporation. Rand is hardly a liberal institution. It is biased against trade unions, plaintiffs' lawyers, and any other people who are on our side of the political fence. Rand has found that a large percentage of the money goes to the lawyers. However, they have also found that the majority of it goes to the defense firms, not to the plaintiffs' lawyers, who get contingencies. Rand has further found that almost all of the complexity is due to procedural maneuvers made by the insurance companies in their own defense. The complexity is not inherently there; it is something that people are paid by the insurance companies to do in order to stonewall cases.

DON ELISBURG: (*Occupational Health Foundation, Washington, D.C.*): Given all you say about the defects of the workers' compensation system, it is no more nonadversarial than a jury trial. Its ability to handle occupational disease is clearly almost nonexistent. The administrative and regulatory efforts that have gone into the system are dismal and well documented.

Is it not true, though, that if you throw this system into some kind of court action (jury trials), in the blink of an eye, the courts are going to have to create the equivalent of a workers' compensation system to handle the volume of cases? In other words, when you consider loading a million or more cases a year onto the court system, as has happened with asbestos litigation, which has basically bypassed the workers' compensation system, the courts have, in district after district, set up a judge-run administrative tribunal equivalent to that of workers' compensation to evaluate and settle cases.

SIMON: Don Rand has looked at this question specifically. He found that the overcrowding of the courts and their complexity did not suggest a workers' compensation system in any of these subjects except with the potential question of asbestos. Let me point out what the situation is with asbestos. I believe that there are 30,000 pending claims in court now. Rand suggested that even with 30,000 pending claims, we are not even near the point where an administrative system is needed.

Further, the courts have not set up an administrative system. All they have set up is a system to deal with the litigation. Previously, there was the Wellington proposal, which allegedly would have speeded settlements; then, however, the defense came up with a plan for paying people less than five cents on the dollar. They were going to kill a man for less than you would get under workers' compensation laws. As a result, a mesothelioma victim who is dying of a painful cancer would be getting paid less than $10,000.

It may turn out that ultimately there will be some kind of administrative system. I think, however, that there will be a crucial distinction, and that such a system will tip over once we are into a Manville situation, which results when the victims and their families come to control the corporation. In that situation, those people and those interests can decide where the money will go once the company has set it aside. Then, and only then, is some kind of administrative system logical. Until that point, all an administrative system does is create another barrier.

I suggest that an administrative system would function much like the malpractice law that doctors want in various states. In that proposed law, before a patient can sue for malpractice he must go before a panel of seven doctors. A person has to spend three years reaching that panel, and only if he can survive that system does he have a right to sue.

An administrative system might ultimately be reasonable if a corporation has set aside enough money to pay damages. Until that happens, however, I would say not.

ELISBERG: This same discussion took place with all of the federal judges at the American Bar Association last summer, a discussion in which massive toxic torts and asbestos were the focal points. Judge Lambrose, who has some thousands of cases in Cleveland, described the way in which he handles the cases. He uses special masters, medical review teams, with 150 lawyers in the courtroom working on some settlement negotiations. The question then arose: when do you get to the jury trial that really makes the difference? The judge was basically saying that in the way his system operates, a person wanting a jury trial would get it about 1997.

SIMON: It is true that the federal courts are involved in a variety of experiments. There are, for example, procedures called summary jury trials. Some people allow the lawyers to speak for one hour to a jury and then see what happens. In Philadelphia, judges are involved in trying the damages first, and then the liability. The courts are experimenting with various ways of handling these problems. Each one has to be studied as to its individual benefit.

Making the court system work better is a good goal, as is improving the compensation system. I did not say we should abolish the workers' compensation system, but rather that it is not a panacea. The court system is also having great problems in finding ways to speed up the process.

The court system works best in Philadelphia, but there nothing more has been done than making the jury trials go faster. There are no special settlement arrangements; the cases just move faster.

BILL HIRZY (*NFFE, Washington, D.C.*): Our union represents the professional workers at the Environmental Protection Agency (EPA), including those who do the reviews on chemicals like chlordane.

I would like to address the point that was raised by the representative of the Office of Management and Budget (OMB), Mr. Scott Jacobs, but with a somewhat different conclusion. It is important to distinguish between the policy makers in the government and the professional civil service. Those of us who are in the professional civil service take a lot of heat because of decisions that are made by the political leadership. When you say that the government does not have the will to do a good job in an area such as reviewing pesticides, this distinction becomes very important. One must understand why it is difficult to get accurate reviews of pesticide data. Right now we are fighting a very antiprofessional performance management system in the pesticides program which very few people understand and about which there is going to be a lot of publicity quite soon. Our people— professionals, toxicologists, chemists and others—are given a certain number of points for reviewing a study. A review of an LD 50 is worth so many points; a review of a two-year cancer bioassay is worth so many points. It makes no difference how complex a study is, how complete a study is, or what types of animals the study uses, you get X points for reviewing that kind of study. You have to accumulate a certain number of points in order to get a successful performance evaluation. It does not take a genius to figure out that this system encourages quick processing of paper and that it discourages the thoughtful, professional review of data. We have had people in our bargaining unit blasted and downgraded by their management because they do too good a job of reviewing the data. It is a terrible situation. We are fighting that.

You need to get ready for the time when much better reviews come out of the EPA. Our union is not going to sit still and allow the ethics of our various professions to continue to be subverted by political management. It goes without saying, as the representative from the OMB said, that it is much better not to have damaged workers. It is a terrible shame that the OMB did not take that attitude when, for instance, they tried to torpedo the asbestos rules and to ban the phasedown rules for lead in gasoline. Fortunately, our union played a large role in rescuing those regulations from the black hole into which the OMB tried to force them.

SIMON: I could not agree more with that. However, it is important to remember that corporations are not bad guys nor are other people. There are many dedicated, competent, reliable and moral people who work in corporations. It is not a question of people being good and bad. It is a question of how decisions are made.

In my presentation about the regulatory posture, I made the point that the regulatory process is almost entirely controlled by lawyers from the moment a firm tries to put a product on the market. The whole city of Washington is dominated by law firms who do nothing but conduct products through the regulatory system. When a lawyer is involved in this process, he or she is necessarily guarding the lawyer's ethics, that corporation's interest, that corporation's desire to have things come out a certain way. Necessarily, then, he or she is not being all that careful about disclosing data about the chemical that might be damaging. So the regulatory process, in drawing in lawyers, tends to politicize the process in a way that is not always very useful.

What happened in my chlordane litigation was that the company had been dominated by lawyers since 1973. The company had done such a bad job that lawyers were essentially making every decision. Consequently, the lawyers did not turn over damaging information to the government. That is exactly what you expect a lawyer to do. That is a lawyer's obligation to his client. In essence, then, politicalization is not unique to the government. It holds true in corporations also. We have to look at everybody's role in it.

LINDA RUDOLPH (*California Department of Health Services, Los Angeles, Calif.*): Yesterday, and for the past several years, people in the occupational and environmental health communities have spent a lot of time discussing their concept of right to know, notification of workers regarding risk, and notification regarding hazards. In California, Proposition 65 mandates that companies issue a warning prior to releasing a chemical with a substantial listing of carcinogenic or reproductive hazards. Proposition 65 requires "clear and reasonable" warning (which has yet to be defined). Ironically, the California Manufacturers' Association is threatening to petition for exemption from "clear and reasonable" warning for any company that complies with the hazard communications standard. I would like you to expand on your point about the implications for the tort liability system of providing material safety data sheets (MSDS). Particularly, I would like your views in light of the recent rulings that have favored the tobacco companies because they printed the government-required warnings on cigarette packages.

SIMON: That is a good question. The regulatory system is going to be in the position of defending these large companies who comply by issuing government-approved warnings. This is what happened with chlordane and is the same defense manufacturers have developed for the three-wheel vehicles that roll over and kill people. The government said that they could sell them; the fact that they kill people is tough luck.

What I learned, though, in my litigation experience, is that these government warnings are the products of negotiation between a government agency, which is understaffed and often dominated at the top by people with varying political interests, and lawyers who are defending the company. What happens in that unbalanced sort of negotiation is that warnings do not include many important factors. For instance, in the case of chlordane, there are 57 components in technical chlordane, none of which is even disclosed on the label. Under the Federal Insecticide, Fungicide, and Rodenticide Act (FIFRA), there is a list of insecticides. However, the label tells you only the name of the pesticide itself and not all of its other ingredients. These other ingredients are called "inert ingredients," by statute, a term which implies that they are nontoxic to insects. However, they may be toxic to humans, but the label is not required to say anything about that. These so-called "inert ingredients" include propylene oxide, which is a known carcinogen, and carbon tetrachloride. The regulatory system creates a situation which at first blush is going to bolster the company's defense. In the end, however, tort litigation will be required to get at the bottom of what really is in these chemicals and what is not being disclosed.

Round Table Papers: 7. Restructuring Workers' Compensation to Prevent Occupational Disease

Workers' Compensation and the Prevention of Occupational Disease

DAVID L. MALLINO
*Industrial Union Department
AFL-CIO
815 16th Street, N. W.
Washington, D.C. 20006*

After some 17 years of experience in addressing the issue of occupational disease prevention and its relationship to the OSHA regulatory system, it can safely be concluded that regulation alone cannot adequately address or resolve the problem. Indeed, the sheer number and extent of workplace toxic exposures are such that OSHA regulation alone is simply inadequate to effectively reduce exposures to the point where disease can be prevented. Even if the policy difficulties of setting effective OSHA standards on the thousands of toxic substances in the workplace could be overcome, which is highly doubtful, the necessary enforcement and compliance mechanisms to implement the standards are not available. In these times of staggering budget deficits it is unrealistic to expect any Administration or Congress to make the kinds of budgetary commitments required to field an army of compliance officers and attendant legal, technical, and other personnel necessary for effective enforcement and implementation.

This is not to suggest, however, that the regulatory approach should be abandoned, for it is the front-line defense in reducing toxic exposures. Neither is it suggested that the current regulatory system cannot and should not be improved. Indeed, after nearly 8 years of summary neglect by the Reagan Administration, the OSHA/NIOSH regulatory regime is in shambles and in desperate need of rebuilding and restructuring. It needs more effective policy direction as well as an increased commitment of resources. Moreover, the Occupational Safety and Health Act itself probably needs to be revisited and undoubtedly changed to take into account all that has been learned about workplace health and safety since it was enacted in 1970. Even a casual survey of the technical, scientific, medical, economic, legal, and policy factors that have surfaced since passage of the Act inevitably leads to the conclusion that the statute should be reviewed and changed where necessary to take into consideration the experience of the last 17 years. Many of the assumptions on which the Act was initially based either are not valid today or do not fit the realities of the 1990s. I believe that it is time to review and reevaluate those assumptions and modernize the statute as necessary.

However, even if major positive changes can be made in the OSHA regulatory scheme, at least two additional policy tools need to be created to effectively deal with occupational disease prevention. The first is occupational disease risk notification, medical monitoring, and health promotion. Workers who have already been exposed to high levels of toxic substances and who are at high risk of latent occupational diseases need a federal program to identify, notify, and counsel them so as to either prevent the disease from occurring in the first place or diagnose it early enough for successful treatment. The regulatory system alone cannot help these workers, because it is predicated on prospective protection.

Because these previously exposed workers are already at high risk and may currently be carrying the latent disease "time bomb" in their bodies, it does them little good to confront a future workplace where the regulatory system has resulted in lower exposures. Although reduced exposures can have a positive effect in reducing the cumulative risk burden, what these high risk workers really need is the scientific and medical information necessary to protect themselves from disease through medical surveillance and health promotion. What is needed is the program mandated by the High Risk Occupational Disease Notification and Prevention Act of 1987 which has passed the U.S. House of Representatives and is currently pending before the U.S. Senate. The positive aspects of such a program are recognized not only by the labor movement and the public health community, but also by major segments of the business community such as the chemical, electronics, paint and coatings, and parts of the insurance and asbestos industries, all of whom are actively supporting passage of the legislation.

The second policy tool required as a critical supplement to the OSHA regulatory system is basic workers' compensation reform that allocates the total costs of occupational disease where it rightfully belongs—on the production of goods and services. For a whole host of reasons, some of which are outlined herein, employers, through the workers' compensation system, have not had to bear the costs of occupational disease and therefore have had no economic incentive to clean-up the workplace and reduce or eliminate toxic exposures. For all practical purposes the workers' compensation system simply does not compensate for occupational disease and never has.

Currently, the workers' compensation system compensates less than 10% of all occupational disease cases and most of these are relatively minor illnesses such as dermatitis. Of the 10% involving serious diseases, nearly all that are ultimately compensated must first be litigated over the basic question of compensability.

As originally conceived in the early 1900s, workers' compensation was to be a "no-fault" insurance program by which employers assumed financial responsibility for injuries to workers due to "personal injury by accident arising out of and in the course of employment." The idea was to move away from the legal problems of attempting to determine negligence and to simply provide certain benefits to workers and their families to overcome the economic hardships of work-related injuries and death. For the most part, the system was designed to compensate for traumatic injuries and death resulting from workplace accidents. Occupational disease, which theoretically is covered by workers' compensation programs, has, however, been effectively excluded from the system.

Part of the problem is that a number of state workers' compensation laws include what have been called "artificial barriers" to occupational disease compensation. These barriers include requirements that a compensable disease be "peculiar" to the workplace, or not an "ordinary disease of life;" or to be compensable a disease must first be listed on a specific schedule of diseases; or not be an infectious disease; or that disease claims must be filed within a restricted time period from the time of exposure rather than the onset of disease.[1]

Most of these artificial barriers have little or no relation to modern medical science which has concluded that most occupational diseases are multicausal in nature and have relatively long latency periods from the time of initial exposure to the actual manifestation of disease. Some asbestos-related diseases, for example, have latency periods as long as 25–30 years.

Even more basic than the artificial barriers, however, is what I have termed the "iron rule" of workers' compensation which I believe is the single, most important legal factor barring compensation for occupational diseases.[2] As just indicated, the original no-fault concept was predicated on the qualifying notion that a worker must demonstrate that his injury/illness/death was due to a "personal injury by accident arising out of and in the course of employment." Although the "personal injury by accident" test has largely been removed from most state and federal compensation laws, the iron rule of workers' compensation remains "arising out of and in the course of employment."

For the most part, the "arising out of and in the course of employment" test has required the demonstration of a direct cause and effect relation between the injury/illness/death and the job before a worker can qualify for benefits. In most cases of traumatic injury or death, the cause and effect relation is clear; a worker loses a hand in a stamping machine, falls from a scaffold, or is killed in a grain elevator explosion. In each case the injury or death clearly arose out of and in the course of employment, and the worker is awarded workers' compensation benefits no matter who was at fault.

The matter becomes much more complicated, however, when the iron rule is juxtaposed against serious occupational diseases. For many of these diseases, such as work-related cancers, it is often difficult, if not impossible, to determine a specific cause and then link it specifically to a particular workplace exposure or set of exposures. Unlike traumatic injuries that are direct and immediate, many occupational diseases have long latency periods and are often multicausal in nature; therefore, it is often impossible to link a specific toxic exposure to a specific industrial substance and prove that it was the sole determining cause of the disease exclusive of any other factor or factors. As a result, most occupational diseases cannot meet the direct causal test and therefore fail the "arising out of and in the course of employment" requirement.

Over the years, the artificial barriers and the iron rule have combined to effectively deny workers access to benefits under workers' compensation, even when they are aware of the relation between toxic workplace exposures and their disease, which in many cases they are not.

This lack of information is another major obstacle to occupational disease compensation. Indeed, the overwhelming number of occupational disease cases never enter the workers' compensation system. In the first place, many workers are simply ignorant of the toxic exposure-disease relationship and therefore die believing that their lung, bladder, or brain cancer was an "act of God" or just plain bad luck. Moreover, even when they are aware of the linkage, workers do not have access to all the information they might need to make a case, especially the highly technical data on the toxicity of the substance, its known health effects, or their past exposure levels. Very often they do not even know the true chemical name of the substance to which they were exposed.

Although some of this information gap should be overcome through the recent OSHA Hazard Communication Standard as well as the High-Risk Notification legislation should it become law, progress under the best of circumstances will be slow. However, even with all the available data and information, workers are still confronted with worker compensation laws that make it difficult, if not impossible, to successfully pursue a workers' compensation claim. As stated earlier, nearly all workers' compensation claims for occupational disease must first be litigated over the basic question of compensability.

The first hurdle, of course, is the presence of artificial barriers included in many state laws. Thus, for example, if the worker has lung cancer—which is an "ordinary disease of life"—he has no claim in those states that bar compensation for such diseases no matter how much data he can muster to demonstrate a link between the workplace and lung cancer. If the state has overly restrictive time limitations on filing disease claims, which a number of states do, then the worker is disqualified if his latent disease does not become manifest until after the filing deadline. In those states that bar compensation for infectious diseases, any health care worker that contracted AIDS because of contact with infected blood would be unable to qualify for compensation.

Even without the artificial barriers to compensation, which some states are beginning to eliminate, the iron rule of "arising out of and in the course of employment" remains the key issue. Because the multicausal nature of most occupational diseases makes it very difficult to prove an exclusive workplace cause and effect relationship, the burden of proof on the worker becomes overwhelming.

As a result, most lawyers are reluctant to accept workers' compensation disease cases on a contingency basis, because they get paid only if they win the case. Workers, therefore, are left with the unenviable option of paying a lawyer on a retainer to persue a claim that under the best of circumstances is difficult to win. This, plus the fact that most workers' compensation benefits are traditionally low and inadequate, places the worker in a very disadvantageous position. Indeed, most workers, given all these hurdles, simply do not bother with the workers' compensation option, thereby relieving the employer of any costs.

Rather than pursuing the workers' compensation route, many, if not most, diseased workers have turned to the public welfare system for a measure of economic relief, most notably the Social Security system including Social Security Disability, Supplemental Security Income, Medicaid, and Medicare. The House Committee on Education and Labor recently estimated that the cost of occupational disease to the Social Security system alone is some $5.4 billion annually. To this must be added another $1.7 to $4.3 billion in annual wage loss and other medical costs.[3] Thus, without counting such additional public costs as lost tax revenues, the direct costs of occupational disease to the federal government and workers are about $7.1 to $9.7 billion a year, which is nothing more than a direct public subsidy to American industry.

More recently, workers have begun turning to another source, the tort system, in an effort to obtain a measure of economic justice. Although the workers' compensation laws have traditionally barred workers from suing their employers for workplace injuries and illnesses by application of the so-called "exclusive remedy rule," workers have always been able to sue third parties who may have contributed to the injury or illness. More often than not, these "third parties" are product manufacturers who introduce a product into the workplace that caused or contributed to the harm. Most such product liability suits have been aimed at the manufacturer of industrial equipment that causes traumatic injuries or death, but recently workers have been successfully pursuing toxic torts directed at the manufacturer of toxic chemicals and other hazardous substances. Perhaps the most dramatic and successful toxic torts have involved asbestos and asbestos-related diseases, but as more becomes known of the relation between other toxic chemicals and diseases, these too are becoming the focus of work-related toxic torts.

For well over 15 years, ever since the report of the National Commission on State Workmens' Compensation Laws concluded that workers' compensation was "generally inadequate and inequitable," the labor movement has been seeking federal reform of workers' compensation.[4] Although a number of reform bills have been introduced in the United States Congress over this period, none has ever gone beyond the public hearing stage. Although the reform issue remains very complicated, involving a host of economic, legal, medical, scientific, and public policy questions, the bottom line involves three basic and fundamental reforms: increased benefits, elimination of artificial barriers to disease compensation, and expansion of the iron rule of compensation, especially for occupational disease claims.

Traditionally, workers' compensation has provided three types of benefits: weekly wage replacement, medical care, and rehabilitation benefits. Of these, the weekly wage replacement benefits are by far the largest cost item and therefore present the greatest problem in terms of reform. Although workers' compensation is supposed to replace two thirds of an injured worker's weekly wage, every state has placed a maximum cap on what a worker can collect, which in most cases does not approximate the two-third level. Indeed, on average the weekly wage replacement benefits have traditionally been inadequate to meet the economic requirements of injured workers and their families. Moreover, wide disparities exist in the maximum benefits workers are entitled to, from a high of $1,108 a week in Alaska to a low of $140 a week in Mississippi, not including Puerto Rico which pays a weekly maximum of $31. At the beginning of 1987, 37 states (including the District of Columbia and Puerto Rico) paid maximum weekly benefits of less than $350 and only eight states paid over $400 a week.

To put all this into some perspective, at $350 a week, a totally disabled worker with a family to support can only collect $18,200 a year. In 14 states, the maximum benefit is $250 or less, or $13,000 a year, and of these 14 states, six pay a maximum of $200 a week or less, which is $10,400 a year. In Mississippi, a totally disabled worker can collect a maximum of $7,280 a year for himself and his family whether he needs it or not, and in Puerto Rico he can collect $1,612.[5]

There is simply no question that in the overwhelming number of cases, weekly wage replacement benefits are far too low to afford injured workers and their families anything approaching economic security or equity. Thus, we believe that at a minimum there should be a national standard that requires all states to pay wage replacement benefits at two thirds of the worker's weekly wage subject to a maximum of 200% of the average national weekly wage in manufacturing which last year was about $692 a week or $36,000 a year. This, of course, would apply only to the highest paid workers in the country. For the lowest paid, no matter what their actual weekly wage, we believe that economic justice demands a minimum payment of 50% of the average national weekly wage, which would be about $173 a week or about $9,000 a year. Most workers, of course, would fall somewhere in between.

In terms of artificial barriers to occupational disease compensation, the reform issue is simple. These barriers, which have little relation to modern medical science, need to be eliminated. It makes no sense to deny benefits to workers because their lung cancer, for example, is an "ordinary disease of life" whether or not it is related to the workplace. At a minimum, workers exposed to carcinogens that have been linked to lung and other common cancers should have the opportunity to demonstrate the linkage and be paid benefits if the relation can be proved. The same is true for other work-related diseases. The test should be work-relatedness, not some arbitrary determination that may or may not be related to the workplace.

With respect to reforming the iron rule of compensation, what is required is an expansion of the concept of "arising out of and in the course of employment." Rather than requiring workers to prove a direct cause and effect relation between exposure and disease, which is very difficult if not impossible, the test should be a demonstration of whether the exposure was a contributing "factor" to the disease. Thus, the question should not be "did the workplace *cause* the disease" but rather "was the workplace a *factor in causing* the disease." In other words, rather than applying the Newtonian concepts of cause and effect to occupational disease compensation, what the modern industrial situation requires is the adoption of factor analysis for compensation purposes.

There is nothing new in the approach. As a matter of fact, it was incorporated into the first two workers' compensation reform bills introduced by then Senators Jacob Javits (R.-N.Y.) and Harrison Williams (D.-N.J.) in 1973 and 1975. The 1973 bill proposed to expand the iron rule by providing that "an injury (illness) shall be deemed to have arisen out or in the course of employment if *work-related factors were a contributing cause* of the injury (illness)." Although somewhat different, the 1975 bill held that "an injury (illness) shall be deemed to have arisen out of and in the course of employment if *work-related factors were a significant cause* of the injury (illness)."[6] Under either approach, all a worker would have to prove was that he was, in fact, exposed to the toxic substance, that the substance in question had been scientifically linked to the disease, and that the cumulative exposure was a contributing or significant factor in causing the disease.

To make this factor analysis concept fully operational, any reform must also include certain presumptions concerning exposure and disease. Working with Drs. Irving Selikoff, Philip Landrigan, and William Nicholson of Mt. Sinai Medical Center in New York, we have developed a set of worker population-based presumptions for occupational disease that can be characterized as the "30% rule."

Essentially the 30% rule states that a compensable occupational disease is one in which, through the use of epidemiologic and clinical studies, it can be demonstrated that a given worker population exposed to the substance in question exhibits at least a 30% increased incidence of the disease compared to a nonexposed population. In other words, when it can be scientifically shown that an exposed population of workers has a disease rate 30% greater than that of a nonexposed population, the disease in question would be deemed to be work related. The individual worker with the disease in question would then have to prove that he was a part of the exposed population and that his individual exposure was sufficient to have been a factor in causing his disease.[7]

To finally complete the reform of the iron rule, a third ingredient must be added to the factor analysis and 30% rule, which is a set of time-based exposure presumptions. In this respect, we believe any reform should include a formula that links a presumption of disease to a defined period of individual exposure. Thus, for example, using Selikoff's data for asbestos, it might be that a worker, depending on his job, would have to have had at least 5 years of asbestos exposure in a chemical plant in order to qualify for a presumption of lung cancer, or 15 years of exposure for a presumption of asbestos-related cancer of the larynx.[8] Each time-based exposure presumption for a specific disease could be established by regulations promulgated by the Department of Labor.

Should the traditional iron rule governing workers' compensation be reformed to include factor analysis, the 30% rule, and time-based exposure presumptions, it would dramatically expand what heretofore has been a very limited workers' compensation approach to occupational disease. Indeed, if properly formulated and institutionalized, such an expansion would go far in finally providing social and economic justice to the tens of thousands of occupational disease victims who have been effectively excluded from the workers' compensation system.

Moreover, by increasing workers' compensation benefits and eliminating the artificial barriers to occupational disease compensation, such reforms, by placing the entire burden on the production process to pay for occupational disease compensation, would provide a powerful economic incentive to employers to reduce exposures and clean-up the workplace. As it is now, employers for all practical purposes are paying little or nothing for occupational disease and, in fact, are being subsidized by the public welfare system and workers themselves. The only current incentive for employers is the OSHA regulatory program which, after 17 years, has only been able to produce a relatively small handful of health standards governing some 20–25 toxic substances. In addition, at least for the last 8 years, the enforcement of these standards has been nearly nonexistent. I believe that without a properly reformed workers' compensation system that bears the full economic burden for work-related diseases, the ultimate prevention of these diseases will largely remain an unmet public goal.

NOTES AND REFERENCES

1. The artificial barriers to occupational compensation were first raised as a reform issue by Senator Harrison Williams when he introduced his 1975 Workers Compensation reform bill. They were also identified and analyzed in the *Report of the Interdepartmental Workers Compensation Task Force*, U.S. Department of Labor, 1977.
2. MALLINO, D. L. 1979. Policy Dimensions of Workers Compensation. A report prepared for the United Steelworkers of America and published as part of the "Hearings of the National Workers Compensation Standards Act of 1978," U.S. Senate, Committee on Labor and Human Resources, March–April, pp. 483–573.
3. U.S. House of Representatives, Committee on Education and Labor, Report on the High Risk Occupational Disease Notification and Prevention Act of 1987, pp. 7–8.
4. National Commission on State Workmens' Compensation Laws, Report of the National Commission on State Workmens' Compensation Laws, U.S. Department of Labor, 1972.
5. These data were compiled from annual AFL-CIO analysis of workers' compensation and unemployment insurance state laws. See AFL-CIO, "Workers Compensation and Unemployment Insurance Under State Laws January 1, 1987."
6. U.S. Senate, S. 2008 (1973) and S. 2018 (1975).
7. The 30% rule was incorporated into the "Occupational Disease Compensation Act of 1985" (H.R. 3090), introduced by Representative Pat Williams (D.-Montana), Section 15(b)(7).
8. The time-based presumptions were also incorporated into H.R. 3090, along with specific presumptions based on the Selikoff *et al.* data. See H.R. 3090, Section 6(c).

Workers' Compensation and the Prevention of Occupational Disease

PETER S. BARTH

Department of Economics
The University of Connecticut
Storrs, Connecticut 06268

One of the core goals of workers' compensation insurance in the United States is to reduce the incidence of injuries and diseases arising from the workplace. The system seeks to accomplish this by using financial incentives both to reward those employers who operate safe and healthful establishments and to punish those with poor performance records. In a general sense, the method of experience rating is quite simple. When a business has a poor track record in terms of injuries and diseases, its workers' compensation insurance premiums will be raised, thereby increasing the firm's costs. This will tend to undermine the firm's competitive position and could even force the firm to shut down. From a more positive perspective, the employer with an exemplary record derives competitive advantages, earning both greater profits and virtue as rewards.

Economists as well as social activists appear to favor such experience rating. The former are attracted because of the efficiency that springs from assigning costs to their source. For them, proper resource allocation dictates that unsafe establishments sell their output at prices that reflect the full economic costs of producing them. Such costs would include the indemnity and medical payments of workers' compensation. If the firm can no longer compete because of its high compensation costs, let it leave the industry if it cannot improve its record.

Aside from economists, many others appear to support experience rating, apparently believing that some sort of justice is served by it. They perceive this as a punishment of reckless employers where few or no other sanctions exist.

Does the workers' compensation system actually deliver on its goal of encouraging health and safety at the workplace? If not, could the system be made to work so as to assure the achievement of this goal? Without an unequivocal response to the first question, answering the second one is especially speculative. Regrettably, even though workers' compensation is more than 75 years old, at least in several of the states, the evidence is only shaky that the system does induce employers to operate as the theory suggests. If the data do show such a relation, the link appears to be weak. Yet the argument here is not to suggest that workers' compensation insurance is irrelevant as an inducement for employers to behave. Instead, the point is that although injuries due to accidents represent the best possible case for loss control measures by employers, *occupational diseases*, especially the long latent ones, offer no such payoffs for businesses. The following represent several reasons why the compensation system cannot be counted upon to deliver a healthful workplace:

 1. The problem in the case of certain diseases is especially great because of the long time lag between the exposure and the first manifestation of illness. In a society in which business is often accused of thinking only for the short run—and

that may mean no longer than the time till the issuance of the next quarter's earnings statement—does one expect an employer to worry about an increase in workers' compensation premiums 10 or 20 years down the road?

Preoccupation with the short run may be perfectly rational from a managerial or an economic point of view, although hardly desirable from a public health perspective. For example, a dollar spent on reducing a workplace health risk today must save the firm $4.66 in compensation costs 20 years down the road with a discount rate of 8%. If the latency period is 30 years, unless an investment of $1.00 today saves $10.06 in 30 years, it is not worth the expenditure, with a discount rate of 8%.

As imposing as the force is of such discounting, an even stronger argument exists against the likelihood of a socially responsible outcome. Suppose a decision to invest in a healthier workplace would yield a positive payoff to the firm in 10 or 20 years. What is the probability that the persons deciding on the expenditure today will be able to derive credit for the decision a decade or two in the future? Clearly, that probability must be very low, because those individuals may be retired or deceased, working in some other part of the firm, or working for another employer. Thus, they can expect little or no chance for reward in the future for their current decision to make an expenditure. An alternative way to express this is that employees who, from a social perspective, make poor decisions for the firm today are not likely to be identified and held responsible when the consequences come home to roost.

2. One way for a business to keep compensation costs down for occupational illnesses is to provide a less hazardous workplace. However, that is not the only method. Instead, employers, or their insurers, may find that a cheaper approach is simply to defend themselves vigorously against any such workers' compensation claims. By doing so, the employer or insurer will often settle the claim with the worker, resulting in a lower indemnity payment than the statute mandates. Combining this with the probability that no claim will be filed for the disease, the compensation costs to the employer for occupational disease will be relatively low, thereby providing little incentive to clean up the workplace. Why is it that no claim may result? When the worker (or survivor) does not know the cause of the disease or where and when the hazard was encountered or what his or her rights to compensation are, claims for compensation simply do not materialize.

3. Many employers appear to have little confidence in state workers' compensation agencies, viewing them as lacking in sophistication and as making capricious decisions in difficult or complex cases. Hence, these employers feel that they may still have to pay for compensation when the worker was not made ill due to exposure at their establishment. Possibly, the hazardous exposure occurred in some other employer's establishment. In any case the employer will perceive that the economic reward, in the form of lower compensation costs, will not materialize from the decision to clean up the workplace.

An expression of this attitude is heard often in the cases of three categories of disease claims. First, many employers are paying for temporary and permanent disability claims for back problems when there was little the employer could have done to prevent them. In some states, the costs of back cases exceed 25% of the costs of all workers' compensation. Secondly, some of the heart cases being paid for by employers were undoubtedly beyond the control of the employer. Third, many of the stress claims (other than heart) that are beginning to emerge in some states are also seen as basically uncontrollable by employers. With all three of these categories of cases becoming more important, it is hardly surprising that employers believe that compensation costs are generally unavoidable. As such, a subtle message is communicated to employers, that is, their own actions are unrelated to their compensation costs.

4. Thus far, all the arguments have dealt with diseases. A more general issue, however, is that most employers do not face a dollar-for-dollar saving when they reduce compensation costs. Many (smaller) employers are not experience rated at all. Although their premiums will vary from those of other employers depending on their industrial classification and level of payroll, they simply are not experience rated. And though larger employers are experience rated, their rates are not entirely a function of their experience. The closest we come to pure experience rating occurs under self-insurance programs, which are limited, typically, to the few, largest employers in the jurisdiction.

5. The final argument also applies as much to issues of injury as to disease. Workers' compensation costs vary considerably across states, industries, and employers. Although some businesses face very high workers' compensation costs, such as longshore work, timber, and mining, the average employer pays about 1.5% of payroll for workers' compensation insurance covering both injuries and illnesses. One must wonder about the importance given to this rate of expenditure in many businesses. Even a 50% reduction in one's insurance costs will save a firm less than three quarters of a percentage point of payroll. Serious efforts (and expenditures) to clean up the workplace can hardly be expected to result, regularly, where the potential future savings are so relatively minimal.

A primary, but not exclusive, area of difficulty in assuring healthful workplaces is in the long latent diseases. At least three other areas exist where workers' compensation does not assure socially sound employer practices. First, it is most unlikely that any American jurisdiction would award indemnity benefits under workers' compensation for reproductive disorders resulting from hazardous workplace exposures. (It is possible, however, that medical treatment costs could be paid by workers' compensation.) Second, hazards transmitted by workers to others which result in disease for the latter are not covered by workers' compensation. For example, children sickened by lead carried home from the workplace are simply not a part of the workers' compensation system. It must be noted, however, that because such third parties are uncovered by workers' compensation, they do have access to the tort system.

A third area of special difficulty occurs in cases of infectious diseases. Workers frequently encounter obstacles in any quest for compensation in which they are victims of "ordinary diseases of life." Again, my point simply is to demonstrate that the workers' compensation system cannot be counted on to deliver a healthful workplace.

If workers' compensation is ineffective currently at providing adequate safety and health for workers, can it be made tougher or stricter? To do so would satisfy those who seek retribution against employers whose workplaces have caused disease. I am persuaded that such a strategy is a mistake, however, at least in cases involving long latent illnesses.

It seems anomalous that members of organized labor would seek "justice" in such form, whereas some in their ranks have been working to eliminate experience rating in the unemployment insurance area. For those encouraging this type of change, experience rating has served too well, encouraging some employers to vigorously and regularly fight claims for unemployment compensation. Perhaps correctly, they perceive experience rating not as a spur to employment retention, but instead as a reason for employers both to limit employment creation and to challenge applications for compensation by unemployed workers. The analogy in workers' compensation is that employers are induced by experience rating to stonewall claims, and not necessarily to make the workplace more healthful.

By eliminating experience rating in cases of long latent disease, the employer has less of a stake in fighting claims. Indeed, the employer would then have no disincentive to alert workers and the public heath community that a hazard may have existed at the workplace. It could open the door to the possibility of greater employer-worker cooperation in the entire disease prevention process. It also would serve to eliminate a source of employer discrimination in the hiring and retention of workers previously exposed to hazards.

Finally, it must be noted that the single most significant difficulty in workers' compensation for industrial diseases is the underutilization of the system. The core problem is one of ignorance, that is, regarding etiology, source of exposure, and rights to benefits by workers and their survivors. To ameliorate those is an immense responsibility of government, the public health community, and organized labor. The latter is especially limited in carrying this out when well below 20% of the American labor force is organized.

Restructuring Workers' Compensation to Prevent Occupational Disease

EDWARD J. BURGER, JR.

Institute for Health Policy Analysis
Georgetown University Medical Center
Washington, DC 20007

I will take the liberty of rephrasing the issue put to us in this roundtable session and word it as a question. Should the workers' compensation system be structured or restructured to prevent occupational disease? It is my conviction that, indeed, although prevention of disease and disability should be paramount social goals, one should perhaps not look to the financial compensation system as the vehicle for reaching that goal. Indeed, it is more than just conceivable that our traditional pattern of seeking to serve multiple goals through both workers' compensation and tort law processes—punishment, deterrence, and financial compensation—has contributed to the frustrations in these instruments of social accommodation and to their failure to deliver relative to their expected promise.

In a strict sense, the title given to this session, restructuring workers' compensation to prevent occupational disease, concerns the potential of the financial incentives to operate on the employer to offer a nonharmful workplace. The conventional wisdom has been that such incentives are effective and that one has only to increase the financial penalty to the employer for not providing for safety (that is, not preventing disease) sufficiently in order to reach an optimum level of safety and prevention.

Richard Victor, then at the Rand Corporation, indicated that the theoretic conventional wisdom is not necessarily borne out in practice. The relationship is much more complex than the simple statement would support. Financial incentives for injury prevention exceed those for disease prevention. Furthermore, as Victor has suggested, when high workers' compensation benefits do tend to be found in association with higher injury rates, it is not clear which is the independent variable. He has proposed that the high injury rates may cause high compensation benefits, rather than the reverse.[1] In a complementary study, Victor cautioned that generalizations about the size (or existence) of workers' compensation financial incentives should be made with the greatest of care.[2]

Another examination of this issue of incentives and prevention can be seen in a relatively recent study of the asbestos industry. An empirical study of that industry sought to determine what economically motivated behavior for controlling asbestos exposure among workers might have been expected if the employer, in 1948, had possessed the knowledge about the asbestos hazard and about the technology for controlling exposures that was available in later years. The conclusion reached in this inquiry was that such a hypothetical employer would have acted exactly as the real asbestos industry did.[3]

Our own inquiries, particularly for product liability and tort law suits, have indicated that deterrence as a function of threat of liability is a much less predictable outcome than may be generally believed. Furthermore, the end result may even be perverse.[4]

I would like to offer the following proposals:

1. A system of financial compensation for disease and disability or premature mortality should concentrate exclusively on the goal of financial compensation. That is, it should comprehend the combined desires of wage replacement, direct costs of medical care, plus, perhaps, certain important intangibles of loss of enjoyment due to incapacitation.

2. A system of financial compensation for injuries and disease associated with conditions in the workplace should be integrated with other social compensatory schemes. A distinction between that component of lung cancer which is due to underground mining and that arising from unknown cause or from cigarette smoking is one that is essentially impossible to make. To attempt to do so will inevitably lead to argument, disagreement, and tensions and in the long run will, in part, be arbitrary. I note with interest that the Canadians are moving in the direction of more general integration of their several schemes of compensation.

3. An important question arises as to whether we should continue to rely on the findings of causal association in deciding whether to compensate or in choosing the particular instrument for compensation. Again, particularly for disease, Canada has been moving away from a strict cleaving to cause for compensation decisions.

It is my conviction that if one is to preserve a test of causation, that test should be performed rigorously, observing all of the traditional tests of validity and quality of medical-scientific factual information. Otherwise, I would strongly urge that we not parade behind the fiction of observing cause as a test.

4. Finally, I would like to open up a new relation between practicing medicine and the functions of occupational medicine. Here, I return specifically to the issues of prevention. Traditionally, those professionals who have provided occupational health services to industry have been divorced from clinical practice and from the general care of employees and their families as patients. This situation has essentially been an economically dictated pattern of division of labor within the medical profession. It makes no sense. Furthermore, it detracts from efficient prevention endeavors in industry. I would urge some new and creative thinking about how to recombine these two functions. I would propose that a more integrated scheme could, indeed, bring benefits ultimately to the health of workers, including the prevention of disease and disability.

REFERENCES

1. VICTOR, R. B., L. R. COHEN & C. D. PHELPS. 1982. Workers' Compensation and Workplace Safety: Some Lessons from Economic Theory. The Institute for Civil Justice, Rand Corporation, Santa Monica, California.
2. VICTOR, R. D. 1982. Workers' Compensation and Workplace Safety: The Nature of Employee Financial Incentives. The Institute for Civil Justice, Rand Corporation, Santa Monica, California.
3. DEWEER, D. H. 1986. Economic incentives for controlling industrial disease: The asbestos case. J. Legal Studies **15**: 289–319.
4. Causation and Financial Compensation for Claims of Personal Injury from Toxic Chemical Exposures. 1986. Institute for Health Policy Analysis, Georgetown University Medical Center, Washington, DC.

Making the Law Responsive

ROBERT STEINGUT[a]

Bear Stearns & Co., Inc.
New York, New York 10004

As one who has left state government on a day-to-day basis, I am honored to be here. Previously, I had the opportunity of participating in New York State government with Governor Cuomo and with the members of the legislature in trying to make some very modest changes in the New York State workers' compensation system.

A central point permeating the remarks of Drs. Barth and Burger, as well as those of many other contributors to this workshop, is the fact that, in many ways, the workers' compensation system is somewhat perverse and schizophrenic since it does not do what it was originally designed to do.

The system was designed to remove controversies between workers and their employers from traditional court settings. It was supposed to be a system that would fairly compensate individuals who were injured or became ill through no fault of their own, and a system that would decently compensate them.

Obviously, that is not the state of affairs today in New York State or in most other states in this country. We have a system that is litigious and adversarial. Its most perverse aspect, in my opinion, is the fact that it is motivated by profit.

The exclusive state fund is one experiment tried by a number of jurisdictions in this country in an effort to rectify the problems of the system. In this regard, I disagree with Dr. Barth's approach to occupational disease and experience rating.

One basic characteristic that all business people respond to is the profit motive. The degree, therefore, to which we, as a society, reward corporations for improving their safety standards and preventing disease and injuries is the degree to which we can help to prevent the future onslaught of new diseases.

One of the key problems that we face is developing a heightened social and societal awareness of the problems of occupational disease. It took us too long a time to change a very basic problem that we had in New York State regarding the statute of limitations in the Workers' Compensation system for the long-latency occupational diseases. Until just a year and a half ago, people who suffered from meselthelioma, for instance, were precluded from even filing a Workers' Compensation claim in New York State because the law, until then, demanded that benefits claims be filed within a year of initial exposure to the injurious substance. Clearly, that situation was wrong and took much too long to rectify.

Workshops such as this one and exchanges of information are important. Even more important is the desire of those of us here and those in the trade union movement to embark on an educational and informational campaign, a political campaign, to heighten society's awareness of the problems of occupational disease and illness. Such a campaign is necessary to heighten our government leaders' sensitivity to these problems and to act as catalyst for progressive change in the system. But remember that all of the meetings in the world of the already committed will mean very little unless we encourage changes in the law and changes in public awareness.

---

[a] Present address: 245 Park Avenue, New York, N.Y. 10167.

From my experience in New York State, I know that the method of some legislators is a piecemeal one: they will take care of benefits one year and the statute of limitations in another year, but they are not interested in revising the system.

Our job, and I can speak to this because I was an elected official in New York City for nine and a half years before joining the state administration in New York State, is to heighten the community's awareness of the problems that all of us face in our workplaces. We must make occupational disease a high national priority and a high local priority. We must insist that our local representatives and elected officials take some positive action or at least begin discussion as to how we, as a society, ought to be insuring that the workplace is safe for everyone.

Restructuring Workers' Compensation to Prevent Occupational Disease

DOMINICK J. TUMINARO
Counsel to the Chair, Committee on Labor
New York State Assembly
Albany, New York 12248

More than 15 years ago the Report of the National Commission on State Workmen's Compensation Laws identified prevention of injuries and illness as a second principal objective of the workers' compensation systems. But the goal of preventing occupational disease has yet to be realized. The workers' compensation systems are replete with structural impediments which undermine effective contributions toward the prevention of occupational disease. Barth and Hunt[1] have identified most of these problems and have made recommendations that might have a salutary impact.

In New York, a new focus on preventing occupational disease has emerged even as a recent estimate of its magnitude has added visibility to the issue in the public policy sphere and stimulated action by a coalition of the labor and public health communities.[2]

This paper discusses some of the presently existing barriers to the linking of the compensation system to the prevention of occupational disease as well as some promising recent efforts to link the state workers' compensation system to the prevention of occupational disease in New York State. The prospects for progress, while promising, are yet uncertain. The commitment of legislators and government policymakers to this hitherto neglected area of workers' compensation will only be sustained if a vigorous coalition campaign can be continued in the years ahead.

DIMENSIONS OF THE PROBLEM

The gap between estimates of the incidence of occupational disease and the number of occupational disease cases being compensated reflects the fact that the costs of occupational disease are presently being borne by society rather than by employers, who have control over workplace conditions that produce illness. Thus, despite some assertions to the contrary, Barth and Hunt clearly are correct in their observation that, "[w]orkers' compensation creates no adequate incentive for improving health at the workplace to prevent long latent diseases" (Barth,[1] p. 260).

The recognition that the system, historically designed around "no fault" principles, has broken down in relation to occupational diseases is widely shared by diverse observers who have examined it.[3]

In New York, which is not atypical of what prevails nationally, of 112,828 compensated cases closed in 1979, only 1,391 or 1% were occupational disease cases; of this number, 29% were for hearing loss. Only 3% of all compensation awarded was for occupational disease.[4]

The cases that are being handled account for an inordinate amount of time and expense associated with the litigation of a range of issues about which varying degrees of medical and scientific uncertainty may exist. Indeed, the rate of controversions throughout the nation's states is markedly higher for occupational disease claims than for accidental injuries.

CONTROVERSIONS AND DELAY: IDENTIFYING CAUSES AND FASHIONING REMEDIES

Until controversions and delays are effectively addressed, claims for occupational disease will continue to remain largely outside the workers' compensation system or will continue to be grossly undercompensated through the use of inadequate lump-sum payments often agreed to by financially hard-pressed workers facing medical costs without wage income.

As Shor[5] has pointed out, "the root of the problem is that the employer (or his insurer), and not a financially disinterested factfinder, makes the first determination of whether the claimant has sufficiently proven the exposure-disease link. . . . If a neutral party, neither the claimant nor defendant, were making the determination based on fact rather than on personal interest in the case, the burden of proof could be put on the party contesting the determination. Currently, the burden is one-sided."

As the Interim Report put it, "individual employer liability appears to provide a strong incentive for employers (or their agents) to adopt a defensive litigation strategy which results in extensive litigation within a no-fault system." That report made four important recommendations addressed to the state workers' compensation system's treatment of occupational disease claims (pp. 99–100):

1. Establish legal presumptions to reduce the difficulty of proving the cause of occupational disease.
2. Establish an employer- and/or producer-financed trust fund to pay benefits.
3. Eliminate artificial barriers to occupational disease claims in the law.
4. Establish a neutral administrative body to administer the compensation of occupational disease claims.

To these I would add the following provision: payment of medical expenses for controverted claims. To achieve a more equitable and expeditious payment of medical expenses incurred by individuals filing for worker's compensation benefits, a system should be developed in which health insurers are required initially to pay the cost of medical care for individuals seeking care for a suspected work-related illness or injury. If an individual's claim is sustained by the worker's compensation system, the health care insurer would be reimbursed at the time of settlement or award. If no award is made and the worker is not financially responsible, the insurer could be reimbursed through a special fund. This system would remedy the present situation in which often neither medical insurance nor worker's compensation coverage is available to pay the cost of health care for individuals. As a result of this lack of coverage, individuals often defer a much-needed medical evaluation, and secondary prevention interventions are often foregone.

In sum, steps must be taken to remove barriers to compensation that presently result in the failure to impose the real costs of occupational disease on employers who control workplace conditions. Increased costs may provide an incentive for the employer to clean up the workplace and eliminate hazards that cause disease. Providing knowledge to workers so that they and their unions may press for safer working conditions may also contribute to prevention.

OCCUPATIONAL HEALTH AND EDUCATION TRAINING OF WORKERS FUNDED BY ASSESSMENTS ON WORKERS' COMPENSATION PREMIUMS

Barth and Hunt[6] recommended the dissemination of information on workplace hazards to both workers and employers as a means to contribute to the prevention of occupational disease. In New York, the state legislature, responding to an initiative of the New York Committee for Occupational Safety and Health (NYCOSH), established a $5 million grant program, funded by an assessment on workers' compensation premiums, to train workers concerning occupational hazards, right to know, and workers' compensation in 1985. NYCOSH led a coalition effort in which labor unions, COSH groups, and occupational health professionals strongly lobbied for the program.

Now in its third year, the program in its first year elicited worker-training proposals totaling more than $11 million, attesting to both the need for such training and the strong interest on the part of unions, COSH groups, employers, and health professionals in the academic sphere.

Training courses and curricula, films, and other resource materials specifically targeted to worker populations at risk of occupational disease have been produced and disseminated. Such programs constitute an approach to the prevention of occupational disease that follows up on the right-to-know movement of the early 1980s.

A mere legal "right to know" can hardly make a substantial contribution to preventing workplace exposures and illnesses, without the training that educates workers to the hazards they face and the means to protect themselves. The program is likely also to have an important educational impact on employers, particularly smaller employers, who as Barth points out, "[i]n some instances . . . know little more than their employees about the hazards to which they are exposed."

OCCUPATIONAL DISEASE DIAGNOSIS AND PREVENTION CENTERS FUNDED IN PART BY WORKERS' COMPENSATION REIMBURSEMENT FOR OCCUPATIONAL DISEASE SCREENINGS

According to a recent estimate by Landrigan[7] of Mount Sinai Medical Center in New York, "[o]ccupational exposures are responsible each year for more than 35,000 new cases of disease and for an estimated 5,000–7,000 deaths in New York State. The majority of these cases are not recognized as work related by physicians in conventional medical settings. Consequently, diagnoses of occupational disease are frequently not made, and appropriate specific medical intervention is typically not undertaken. Although total cost of occupational diseases in New York State is not known, a partial estimate of only five occupational diseases is placed conservatively at $600 million (in 1985 dollars) per annum.[8] Because of the widespread underdiagnosis of occupational disease, these costs are generally not borne by the workers' compensation system, but instead are transferred to workers and their families, to third-party payers, and to social programs funded by general revenue sources.

Landrigan went on to state that a "new agenda for occupational health is urgently needed in New York State." A central element of this agenda, more fully delineated in the report, is the establishment of a statewide network of fixed and mobile occupational clinics staffed by doctors, nurses, industrial hygienists, and other professionals trained to evaluate the connection between work and disease. Such a clinic network will permit early diagnosis and rapid intervention, and ultimately will contribute to the prevention of occupational illness in New York State.

Under New York law, however, the workers' compensation system does not pay the medical costs of occupational disease screenings unless such screening results in a positive diagnosis of an occupational illness. Even if an individual or group of workers has clearly been exposed to dangerous levels of toxic substances in the workplace and a screening is medically indicated, no compensation for the costs of such evaluations will be made.

The clinic network is seen as a promising effort toward the prevention of occupational illness, and it seems eminently reasonable that the law be amended to require that the workers' compensation system contribute toward the cost of such efforts through payment for occupational disease screenings for workplace exposures associated with disease.

INTEGRATING WORKERS' COMPENSATION CLAIMS INFORMATION INTO HAZARD SURVEILLANCE AND PREVENTION EFFORTS

An ancillary and closely related element in New York's approach to preventing occupational illness will be the development of a statewide data collection system incorporating workers' compensation claims' information to identify hazardous occupational exposures and diseases and thereby target enforcement and preventive efforts toward hazardous industries with worker populations at high risk.

CONCLUSION

Barth has observed that as we implement reforms that have the effect of really compensating workers with occupational diseases, we are likely to see, in the short term, some substantial increases in the costs of compensating occupational disease. But he also observes that "[t]he costs to society, and to employers, of occupational diseases are already being borne even if they are not being compensated."

Accordingly, it seems reasonable to infer that increases in compensation costs will provide real visibility to the problem and provide a stimulus to employers and society to undertake serious efforts at improving health and safety in the workplace. To suggest that we cannot afford reforms of the system fails to consider that we already bear the losses associated with occupational exposures and illness, and the real issue, as Barth notes, is "who will suffer the direct and immediate burden for them." It is unjust for workers and their families to suffer the twin failures of our present legal regime either to prevent illness or to compensate sick workers.

NOTES AND REFERENCES

1. BARTH, P. & H. HUNT 1980. Workers' Compensation and Work-Related Illnesses and Diseases: 257–274. M.I.T. Press. at Cambridge, MA.
2. LANDRIGAN, P., S. MARKOWITZ, *et al.* Occupational Disease in New York State, Report to the New York State Legislature, February 1987. Unpublished.

3. See, "An Interim Report to Congress on Occupational Diseases," submitted to Congress by the U.S. Dept. of Labor, 1980: 54–78; Barth and Hunt, *ibid;* APHA Policy Statement No. 8329 (PP): Compensation for and Prevention of Occupational Disease. APHA Public Policy Statements 1948–present, cumulative. Washington D.C. APHA, current volume; reprinted in Am. J. Public Health (March 1984) **74** (3) 292; see also the report of the Crum & Forster Insurance Company's Task Force on Occupational Disease, released in June, 1983; reported on by S. Tarnoff in *Business Insurance* (August 1983).
4. Compensated Cases Closed in 1979. Research & Statistics Bulletin No. 40 (March 1983).
5. SHOR, G. 1980. Workers' compensation: Subsidies for occupational disease. J. Public Health Policy: 333.
6. BARTH & HUNT, *ibid.*: 262, 265.
7. LANDRIGAN, *ibid*: 6.
8. *Idem*: 38–51.

Round Table 7: Discussion

LESLIE BODEN (*Boston University School of Public Health, Boston, Mass.*): Yesterday I criticized OSHA. Today, I would like to agree with what Peter Barth and other panelists have said, namely, that the workers' compensation system is generally not where we ought to invest time and energy to prevent occupational disease. I would also like to add two items to Peter Barth's excellent list of reasons why we should not invest heavily in workers' compensation. Where there is a successful tort suit, the employer ends up paying virtually nothing because the employer's insurance company is allowed to recoup workers' compensation payments from the manufacturers, say, of the asbestos. Secondly, even in occupational injury cases, where studies have been done to identify the preventive impact of workers' compensation, no impact has been found. If in the case of occupational injury no impact is detectable, then, given all the problems of compensating occupational diseases, you really cannot expect, and maybe should not expect workers' compensation to do more than what its name says: to compensate workers and if we can get it to do even that, we probably will have accomplished a great deal.

One final point is that both workers' compensation and the tort system are private remedies. By contrast, one of the great strengths of OSHA regulation is that it is public. Thus it has brought issues of occupational disease and injury into the public eye much more than has tort litigation. To the extent that it has had a tremendous educational effect in the United States, OSHA regulation has been very effective. When I see episodes on occupational health on *60 Minutes* or even fictionalized episodes concerning the problem in various weekly or monthly TV shows I realize that OSHA has at least been successful in its ability to alert and to make public the problems of occupational disease.

PHILIP LANDRIGAN (*Mt. Sinai School of Medicine, New York, N.Y.*): I agree; in the introduction to this workshop we said that one of the great successes of the Occupational Safety and Health Act is that it has created an ineradicably high level of expectation—a phrase I borrow from Eula Bingham—in regard to occupational health. It is very important—intangible, but very real.

DAVID L. MALLINO (*AFL–CIO, Washington, D.C.*): On the question of whether workers' compensation can help to prevent occupational disease, I believe that if benefits increase dramatically and the basic rules on causation are changed, it will be possible through workers' compensation to lay costs where they properly belong, that is, on the production process. With such changes, you may be talking about a big economic incentive that employers currently do not have. Right now, the only incentive for an employer to clean up the workplace is the OSHA regulatory system, and after seventeen years of experience with that system, we still only have 24 health standards.

BODEN: I am concerned that trying to make those changes may cause some ill effects on the compensation part of the system, effects that we may live to regret. What insurance companies worry about is not disease prevention. If they can achieve loss prevention by contesting a claim or by screening out of employment those workers whom they think are at high risk, they are going to do that. As a result, disease may increase and compensation may suffer. Those are issues to worry about before changing the system.

NICHOLAS ASHFORD (*Center for Policy Alternatives, M.I.T., Cambridge, Mass.*): Peter Barth has said it and Les Boden has said it. The lack of economic incentive to prevent occupational disease is best described by the following example: the economically rational owner of an asbestos-processing plant, rather than spending 50,000 dollars on ventilation today, could elect to use his capital, pay a worker's compensation claim, send the worker's kids to school, bury him in a gold coffin, and still be ahead financially. That is the way the numbers work out at first blush.

There are, however, four detractors from that generalization, and they are becoming significant. One is that continuing to recognize occupational disease and compensating as many people as possible are symbolic reminders that can feed other systems and create pressures for prevention in a social sense, even if not in an economic sense. Second, it is important to bear in mind that the workers' compensation filing is very often only the first step, which leads ultimately to awarding punitive damages in a tort suit. With punitive damages, which bear no relation to actual financial loss, you are beginning to talk about real money. Then the economics begin to change. A third factor, which is now beginning to appear in tort suits, and which ultimately may appear in compensation, is the issue of exposure-related immune system damage. Such damage can now be detected long before disease becomes manifest. The California system is now awarding damages through the tort system for immune system compromises which are not sufficient to produce clinically evident manifestations of disease, that is, they are providing for subclinical damages. Finally, a very powerful social tool in the current talk of revitalization is the disclosure requirement under the Security and Exchange Laws, whereby a firm must tell its stockholders about the substances to which it is exposing its workers that might lead to workers' compensation claims in the future. The point is that people ought to know about the corporation in which they are investing.

In addition, we ought to have a mechanism to put the tort system and compensation system into a relationship of tension. One way to create such tension would be to require that workers who have a threshold showing of being exposed to toxic substances ought to receive, right up front, compensation for medical monitoring expenses. Such initial compensation would be provided, if necessary, from a fund created from a tax on production. Currently, the pressures to settle or not settle, to file or not file, derive greatly from the fact that workers do not have the means to deal with their health problems, and thus are sick, unemployed, and poor. Those are small actual costs at the beginning of the system, but they would greatly humanize the process. After that point we ought to have a selection system whereby, in the case of wanton negligence, the worker retains his right to use the tort system and is not bound by the compromise that was made years ago to stay in the workers' compensation system.

A further way to create tension between the two systems is to allow a second selection to occur. That second selection is triggered when an employer contests the occupational disease claim. Sixty percent of occupational disease claims are currently contested. However, if the employer who contested a case were to be automatically put in jeopardy of having to return to the tort system, which pays not just for damages, but also for pain and suffering and punitive damages, many fewer cases would be contested.

The great compromise that was made with the workers' compensation system never moved ahead with inflation, never dealt acceptably with the issue of pain and suffering, and certainly did not deal with the issue of punitive damages.

If we recommit and make the so-called compromise between an administrative system, which really compensates workers because we are sorry, and one that prevents the bad actors from operating—and if we recreate a dynamic tradeoff in a system that connects the two systems—we might not have the trouble we are having.

JOHN CHONG (*McMaster University, Hamilton, Ontario, Canada*): I would like to give some examples where education, compensation and the efforts of health professionals have resulted in measurable prevention. For the last five or six years, various groups in Ontario have attempted to bring together various models of worker health clinics. The sequence of events goes somewhat like this: first, worker education is funded; and second, the occupational health professionals and the unions can organize their own health-hazard evaluations and, coupled with publicity and community campaigns, clinics can appear and disappear in various parts of Ontario. Action is taken basically through a rank-and-file organizing approach, where the information is provided to those at risk and various outcomes occur such as cleanup orders from the government and, in certain instances, major shutdowns of industries.

So too, the chain of events can occur in terms of compensation. Physicians who have been trained to recognize specific diseases from those particular high-risk populations do file claims and the events are tallied. In a number of cases, workers, essentially through their own resources, do their own organizing, draw on a number of resources they require, and, on their own, enact the prevention and compensation they desire.

This sequence of events deals ultimately with empowerment. It deals with the role of professionals as strict advocates and moves off the safe ground of neutrality.

DOMINICK TUMINARO (*New York State Assembly, Albany, N.Y.*): Until we do begin to adopt an advocacy role and take seriously the need to fashion coalitions to address these problems, the fundamental problems of existing power relations make these discussions academic. And while some of us might enjoy an academic discussion, these are serious issues that affect people.

I had a letter last week from a worker in New York who explained that he used to earn 650 dollars a week. He is now injured. Initially his maximum compensation was 300 dollars a week. Then, he was sent to the insurance carrier's doctor and he was certified as partially disabled; on the basis of the percentage of disability, he now receives a percentage of the maximum allowable compensation—150 dollars a week. Now that system puts people into poverty. Unless we can implement a variety of solutions to address the problems and deficiencies that presently exist, we are not going to get anywhere. To that end, those of us with expertise and understanding have to begin to participate with community groups, COSH groups, trade unions, and others in bringing visibility to these issues and participating in a political process that is aimed at addressing them. Otherwise, we will come here year after year just talking about the issues, how we might restructure them, and what the legislative agenda should be.

Achieving the agenda that we have discussed is fundamentally a political question. It speaks to the need for those of us who have this concern to actually participate and not simply to avoid public policy discourse by invoking the concept of neutrality.

PETER BARTH (*University of Connecticut, Storrs, Conn.*): I am glad that Peg Seminario, whose remarks were excellent, alerted people to the work that is beginning and is now ongoing at the state levels.

The point has been made that the provinces of Canada, in fact, serve as laboratories for change. We all—Canadians and Americans both—ought to benefit from the experience of these laboratories.

I also think that it is worth noting that some people have spoken forcefully for the need for the federal government to assert its role in the workers' compensation issue. It is well worth remembering, though, that the federal government is not necessarily a savior. Recall the work that has not been done at OSHA and the role that the OMB has played, not simply in the Reagan years, but, in the Carter years, the Ford years, and in the Nixon years as well. Bear that in mind when you speculate that the savior in all of this is going to be that same federal government.

My own speculation is that real improvement in this system will occur at the state level. I despair of the "one fell swoop" or national approach, despite the fact that the national approach has some degree of attractiveness. Clearly, if I represented organized labor, that might be an approach that would have a special attraction in the light of the weakness that organized labor faces in this country. However, I think the action is going to be in the Albanys and the Hartfords and the Sacramentos and not here in Washington. Much more work remains to be done, and while it would be nice to get the brass ring by doing it once here in Washington, I am not sure it is ever going to happen. Furthermore, if it happens in Washington, the difference between the legislative promise and the actual delivery may be vast, given the quality of the interaction between the Executive and the Legislative branches. These considerations lead me to think that there is not a tremendous amount of hope for a single, national solution, or that if there is hope, it may be misplaced.

MALLINO: In reply, I would suggest that if we were to have this conference again in two years, we would be debating whether a national workers' compensation law could, in fact, be implemented. There is no way that we can wait for the collection of fifty states to act correctly. We have been waiting for them for at least fifteen years, and indeed, many states have regressed in dealing with this issue over the past decade. Therefore, I believe that you are going to see an effort at a national solution to reform workers' compensation laws in two years. Our debate then will not be about whether it is going to happen, but about how best it is going to happen.

Three years ago I suggested we could have had a nice discussion about the High-Risk Notification Bill. Today we are having more than a discussion about that bill. We have a live piece of legislation that I believe is going to become law.

BARTH: If you are right, that would be exciting. If that legislation goes through in two years I predict that seventeen years hence we will be meeting to ask how can we get that law to do what we thought it was supposed to do! Remember you were the one who said we have been waiting fifteen years. That reference, of course, is to the report issued in the early 1970s that called for a federal presence in workers' compensation laws. The issue there, though, in terms of the federal legislation, has been for fifteen years the existence of federal minimum standards with the retention of administration and the rest of the compensation system at the state level. I have not heard anyone talking about anything beyond those federal minimum standards. I am not saying that we should forget working in Washington; I am just saying that if we wait for that, it is going to be a very long wait.

Closing Remarks

PHILIP J. LANDRIGAN

Division of Environmental and Occupational Medicine
The Mount Sinai School of Medicine
New York, New York 10029

The operative words of this workshop are contained in the title: "disease prevention," "platform," and, of course, "occupational health." The task of this workshop has been to assemble a group of speakers who would look very fundamentally at approaches to the prevention of occupational disease and who would design a platform for the next decade.

We were concerned that a reasonable, although incomplete, legislative framework exists for the prevention of occupational disease in this country, with the Occupational Safety and Health Act as the cornerstone of that structure. We were also concerned, however, that the Act was not working properly, that gaps and cracks had appeared in the system, and that they needed to be fixed if disease was to be prevented.

Also, we were not ignorant of the fact that the four-year cycle is beginning again. This is an election year. It is a good year to talk about these issues, because it is a year in which candidates who are seeking issues may be persuaded on the merits of the case to look at occupational health and occupational safety as issues that they ought to embrace.

We hope that we have taken at least some steps in that direction. I know that we have had many people here from all three branches of the government—the Executive, the Judicial and the Legislative—people from both parties, and people from north and south of the Canadian border as well as from Europe.

In the course of this process of mutual education, we hope to have opened some eyes, to have expanded some horizons, and to have gotten people thinking about aspects of occupational health and disease prevent that perhaps had not previously occurred to them.

I have learned a great deal, and I hope that you have as well.

I would like to conclude by thanking the folks who made this workshop successful. At the top of the list are the speakers. They have done a superb job and I want to thank all of them for the obvious care and thought that were put into the presentations.

I would also like to thank the many people who generously and energetically participated in the process of commentary and dialogue.

Finally, I would like to thank all of the staff people who made the meeting work. Mrs. Marise Burger from our staff at Mount Sinai participated very vigorously. A dedicated core of persons from the New York Academy of Sciences also must be acknowledged. Mr. Cyril Lichtensteiger operated the slides; his wife, Mrs. Lichtensteiger, was in charge of the audio. Renée Wilkerson and Ellen Marks operated the front desk along with Karen Green and five ladies from the Washington Convention Bureau. Thanks to you all.

Index of Contributors

Ahlers, H. W., 100–106
Ashford, N. A., 76–78
Atherley, G., 200–206

Baker, E. L., 144–150
Barth, P. S., 278–281
Batawi, M. A. El, 207–211
Bell, R. H., 90–92
Berney, B., 67–71
Bingham, E., 61–66
Boden, L. I., 228–234
Brandt-Rauf, P. W., 151–154
Brandt-Rauf, S. I., 151–154
Burger, E. J., Jr., 282–283

Cheek, L., III, 17–22
Connor, M. F., 126–129
Corn, M., 184–188
Cottine, B. R., 89

Elling, R. H., 240–255
Engelberg, A. L., 130–132

Fisher, T. F., 256–260
Fowler, B. A., 46–54
French, J. G., 144–150
Froines, J. R., 177–183

Greenberg, M., 212–215

Hickman, T. A., 216–220

Laird, F. N., 79–83
Landrigan, P. J., 27–45, 295–296
Lee, J. S., 93–99
Lemen, R. A., 100–106

Lilly, S., 110–112

Maguire, A., 166–171
Mallino, D. L., 271–277
Markowitz, S., 27–45
Mazzocchi, A., 155–156
Mazzuckelli, L. F., 100–106
Melius, J. M., 124–125
Millar, J. D., 113–123
Mirer, F. E., 10–16

Nagin, D., 67–71
Nicholson, W. J., 74–75
Niemeier, R. W., 100–106

Ozonoff, D., 23–26

Park, R. M., 10–16
Parkinson, D. K., 157–159

Ringen, K., 133–141
Rothstein, M. A., 160–162

Samuels, S. W., 172–176
Schulte, P. A., 144–150
Selikoff, I. J., 4–9
Seminario, M., 235–236
Silbergeld, E. K., 46–54
Silverstein, M. A., 10–16
Simon, R., 261–270
Steingut, R., 284–285

Tuminaro, D. J., 286–290

Weeks, J. L., 189–199
Wegman, D. H., 224–227